LOCAL FOOD ENVIRONMENTS
FOOD ACCESS IN AMERICA

LOCAL FOOD ENVIRONMENTS
FOOD ACCESS IN AMERICA

EDITED BY KIMBERLY B. MORLAND

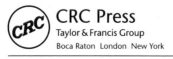

CRC Press
Taylor & Francis Group
Boca Raton London New York

CRC Press is an imprint of the
Taylor & Francis Group, an **informa** business

Cover photos courtesy of Mary Catrow, Rainlake Productions.

CRC Press
Taylor & Francis Group
6000 Broken Sound Parkway NW, Suite 300
Boca Raton, FL 33487-2742

© 2015 by Taylor & Francis Group, LLC
CRC Press is an imprint of Taylor & Francis Group, an Informa business

No claim to original U.S. Government works

Printed on acid-free paper
Version Date: 20150309

International Standard Book Number-13: 978-1-4987-3697-8 (Paperback) 978-1-4665-6778-8 (Hardback)

Library of Congress Cataloging-in-Publication Data

Local food environments : food access in America / editor, Kimberly B. Morland.
        pages cm
    "A CRC title."
    Includes bibliographical references and index.
    ISBN 978-1-4665-6778-8 (alk. paper)
      1. Diet--United States. 2. Diet--Canada. 3. Local foods--Health aspects--United States. 4. Food supply--United States. 5. Nutrition policy--United States. I. Morland, Kimberly B., editor of compilation.

    TX360.U6L63 2014
    363.8'5610973--dc23   2014007000

Visit the Taylor & Francis Web site at
http://www.taylorandfrancis.com

and the CRC Press Web site at
http://www.crcpress.com

Contents

SECTION I Introduction and Contextualizing the Local Food Environment into the American Food System

SECTION II   Local Food Environments: Research, Methods, and Analytical Issues

SECTION III Moving Forward: Local Food Environment Now and in the Future

Foreword

In the summer of 2013, Spencertorry Brown, a 49-year-old African-American woman from Hamtramck, a tiny city within the boundaries of Detroit, did what she often did when her Supplemental Nutrition Assistance Program (SNAP) benefits came in and prompted her monthly grocery-shopping trip. She put on sweats and an Ecko T-shirt, did what she could to remove the patina of pet hair from both, and persuaded her niece to drive her to the grocery store. Today, they aimed for the newest one in town: Whole Foods.

Once there, Spencertorry, who is pretty certain she weighs more than 300 pounds, took her cane and walk-limped to the entryway. Her niece stayed in the car, with her two daughters. Her two sons—Spencertorry's grandnephews—went along with Spencertorry, who procured a green shopping cart, tossed her cane into the basket, and headed in. While she was contemplating the refrigerated bins stacked with trays of wild-caught salmon, farm-raised tilapia, and step-1-animal-welfare-rated chicken breast, one of her grandnephews found the make-your-own peanut butter machine amid the bulk bins of quinoa and barley, pressed a button, and churned a smooth dollop of ground peanuts onto the counter before anyone thought to stop him.

"No, no, honey," called out a nutritionist, hired by the store, to educate customers about healthy eating. She ran over and turned off the machine. "Don't do that." He scurried wordlessly over to Spencertorry and gripped the side of the cart. Spencertorry looked up and seeing the friendly face of the nutritionist, began to ask for some advice. As it turned out, Spencertorry was looking to turn her diet around.

In Spencertorry, I saw a familiar figure. In my ten years as an investigative food reporter, I've gone undercover in farm fields and Walmart produce aisles; I've hung out on bodega corners in Brooklyn; I've helped keep the kitchen moving at an Applebee's. And nearly everywhere I've worked, undercover or as an open journalist, I've seen the same thing. There are always a handful of people who declare allegiance to burgers and fries and who decry salads as rabbit food. But it's been more common for me to meet people like Spencertorry, people who care about their health but are overwhelmed by the logistics of trading the diet they know for the health of another. For folks like this, diet choices are not solely determined by the stores closest to them. And the food in their cabinets reflects more than a hedonistic desire for fat and sugar and salt. What most people eat, I've become convinced, reflects a complicated set of pressures and structures and priorities. And it's not just the personal priorities we set at home that matter; the priorities we set as a nation matter quite a bit, too.

I ended up spending many hours with Spencertorry, who was earnestly trying to improve her diet. She spent more than $60 on that first visit to Whole Foods, a trip she cut short when her niece came into the store, trailing her daughters and asking when they could go. It was an expensive trip for Spencertorry, who put not just chicken breast into her cart but marinated kebabs and turkey–spinach patties, barbecue tofu salad, and a rotisserie chicken, ignoring the suggestion of the nutritionist to include a can of steel-cut oatmeal. She justified the spending, in part, by using her $16 in SNAP benefits.

But more notable than my meeting Spencertorry were the circumstances that led to it. I was working on a journalistic assignment that would have been unheard of a decade ago. I was in Detroit not to cover the declaration of the biggest municipal bankruptcy in history, but the opening of that Whole Foods. In 2013, a national news magazine deemed the opening of a grocery store in a broke, and in some ways broken, city to be worthy of in-depth coverage.

It hasn't always been like this. A decade ago, the fact that low-income neighborhoods frequently had poorly run grocery stores—when they had grocery stores at all—was considered a fact of life. Grimy supermarkets were considered intractable signs of a lower income, the same as well-worn clothes lacking designer labels, cars that have visibly endured dents and repairs, and tall boys of Budweiser. But while most Americans have understood the omnipresence of battered cars as an indication of limited means rather than a preference for unreliable transportation, the traditional explanation for the lack of supermarkets had been, simply, that there was no market for what they were trying to sell. There was, in other words, no consumer demand for their product. And it is only in the last decade or so that the inherent flaw in this logic has been clearly articulated and set forth: a lack of demand for supermarkets can only exist where people do not, in fact, eat.

Advocates, more than researchers, have coined a term for these neighborhoods without enough grocery stores. It is *food desert*, and it has served to focus attention on the fact that a healthy diet is easier to attain in certain places than in others. But for all the good done by naming and grappling with food deserts, the term is best understood as a starting point—the opening shot—for an honest discussion of why Americans, as a whole, are so ensnared by diet-related disease.

Food deserts may only be a beginning, but the conversation they have launched is groundbreaking. For decades, we have approached diet-related disease as if it were one more unfortunate result of a pathogen residing in each patient's bloodstream. The questions we've asked of people eating poor diets have been ground level and specific: What did you order at the restaurant? What do you pluck off the grocery store shelf, and what do you put in your pot? We have tried to change diet by changing each person's choice; by telling the Spencertorrys of the world to choose the steel-cut oatmeal, even though it's unfamiliar and requires 40 minutes of cooking. And today we see the kind of diets we get by relying on personal advice alone: at most, just one-quarter* of Americans eat their recommended five servings of fruits and vegetables each day.

That may be why we've begun—hearteningly—to look beyond each person's plate. The discussion of access to supermarkets is the first step beyond the dinner table, and it's an important one. Most of the food we eat at home is bought in grocery stores, and nearly all of our produce; even with the boom in farmers' markets, just about 2%† of our food shopping happens there. In practice, no community can eat well without ready access to a supermarket.

---

* Twenty-six percent of Americans eat 3–5 servings of vegetables per day and 14% eat 3–5 servings of vegetables per day. http://www.rda.com/news/unhealthy-state-of-the-union-new-study-reveals-roots-of-americans-unhealthy-lifestyles.

† http://www.ers.usda.gov/publications/err-economic-research-report/err97.aspx#.UjcJ_GRgaNw.

Yet, most poor diets begin in grocery stores, too. The discussion of food deserts does not account for this, and that's why any serious discussion of health in the United States needs to go beyond it. Researchers and journalists alike have already begun to dig deep down into the food system, looking at the dramatic disconnect between what we are told we should eat and what our farmers are encouraged to grow. Today, American farmers don't grow anywhere near enough fruits and vegetables for every American to meet their recommended daily allowances.* Meanwhile, 42%† of farm subsidies go to commodity crops like corn destined for animal feed or fuel tanks, and 5% go to fruits and vegetables. Policies like those are what determine whether our food system is full of processed food or fruits and vegetables; they are the things that determine which options will face us on the supermarket shelf.

We can return to home kitchens, of course, and observe that home cooking is on the decline—a practice that typically means a greater use of high-salt and high-sugar processed foods. And we can observe that shoppers do, after all, seek affordable and quick foods. But it would be shortsighted to do that without also observing the steady decline in real wages and the steady increase in the hours of work per week that are considered normal. Yes, modern capitalism has given us food that is cheap and ubiquitous, but it has not given us food that is quick and easy and healthy at that same price. Instead, we have jobs that pay less and demand more, so much so that eating healthy—eating whole grains and fruits and vegetables, cooking without preservatives and chemicals—has come to be understood largely as a hobby for the affluent.

All of this—poor access to food, unhealthy food on the shelves, higher prices for quality produce, the resulting assumption that health requires wealth—comes at a cost that stretches past our dinner and shopping carts. Today, obesity-related disease in the United States rings in at roughly $190 billion a year,‡ more than the annual cost expected for the Affordable Care Act.§

I don't know what Spencertorry thinks about the broad problems of food deserts in the United States or about farm subsidies; I didn't ask her that. I asked her why she came to Whole Foods, and where she usually shopped.

"I don't shop here every week," she said, looking around placidly at the piles of produce, bustling lines, and flower display at the front of the store. She had gone on disability a few years ago, she said, after her epilepsy got too severe; before that, she had cleaned the city's iconic Fisher Theater and some of its offices, a job her mother and grandmother had done before her. Money was scarce, and since she didn't know how to cook very well, she often bought junk food; vanilla Oreos were a particular weakness.

This is America's food dilemma in a nutshell: Why did Spencertorry eat the Oreos? Was it because a supermarket was too far away? Was it because the cookies were cheap and ubiquitous? Was it because she just wanted cookies, health consequences be damned? Was it because of the corn syrup lobby or because of government subsidies?

---

* http://www.farmland.org/news/pressreleases/13-Million-More-Acres.asp.
† https://www.documentcloud.org/documents/292783-ewg-casubsidiesreport.html.
‡ http://www.sciencedirect.com/science/article/pii/S0167629611001366.
§ http://www.cbo.gov/publication/44176.

My hunch is that, for Spencertorry, the answer is "a little bit of everything." But when it comes to broad social trends, the kinds of things we can change through policy, we really don't know. But here's something we *do* know: if we want people to start eating healthy foods, we're going to have to make it as easy for people to eat healthy as it is for Spencertorry to get her hands on the Oreos.

Tracie McMillian
Author of the *New York Times* bestseller,
The American Way of Eating: Undercover at Walmart,
Applebee's, Farm Fields and the Dinner Table

Preface

My awareness of local food environments began in 1994 when I entered a masters program in public health at the University of California, Berkeley. I enrolled in the epidemiology and biostatistics track, but also had an interest in nutrition. For my electives, I became engrossed by facts about diet-related diseases, methods for assessing nutrition, and the role of nutrition in the primary prevention of illness. In terms of primary prevention, access to healthy foods seemed to me to be a logical and accessible solution to many growing diet-related health problems in the United States.

As I thought more about food access, I looked around my own neighborhood in Oakland and wondered about the people living in the adjacent neighborhood of West Oakland. At that time, I resided in an area of Oakland called Rockridge. In terms of my neighborhood food options, there was a supermarket literally across the street and a Whole Foods Market, which opened 10 blocks to the north. Two blocks to the south, located next to the Bay Area Transit Station, were a bakery, fresh fruit and flower market, and a number of established restaurants ranging in cuisines from Chinese, Japanese, Mexican, Mediterranean, and Italian. Some of the restaurants were full-service, whereas others were limited service; however, none of these establishments were franchised fast-food restaurants.

I thought a lot about the difference between my neighborhood and West Oakland. At that time, West Oakland had a demographic of low-income and predominantly African-American residents and was known for higher levels of crime, dilapidated housing, and hardship. As you drove through the heart of West Oakland, it was actually hard to find any supermarkets; rather, retailers were primarily small corner markets, liquor stores, and occasionally a franchised fast-food restaurant. I became curious as to how someone living in West Oakland managed to follow any health education they might receive about what they should or should not eat. During my training at Berkeley, I asked a nutritionist how public health professionals make sure everyone has access to recommended foods. The nutritionist responded that access to food is not a problem in the United States, only for people living in developing nations. I thought about West Oakland as I listened to her reply and wondered where she lived.

I later moved to Chapel Hill, North Carolina, to start a doctoral program in epidemiology. Having decided to focus on nutritional epidemiology during my first year at the University of North Carolina, I became involved with the cardiovascular group and an ongoing multistate cohort, where diet and diet-related health outcomes were being measured. Excited by the possibility to use this cohort to investigate disparities in food store availability and the impact of those disparities on the diets of the participants, I developed a dissertation proposal to link the residential addresses of the cohort participants to the location of local food stores and restaurants. My nutrition advisor reviewed my proposal and, after several days, rejected it with the reasoning that my research questions were not important to public health and the National Institutes of Health would never fund such research.

It seemed very odd to me at that time that accessibility to recommended foods was not an issue that public health and clinical nutritionist were addressing. But given my experiences and continued interest, I decided it was time to start pedaling my ideas to faculty in other disciplines. After failing to convince a social epidemiologist that this was an important public health issue, I had the pleasure of meeting Dr. Steve Wing, an environmental epidemiologist. Over the next 4 years, Steve helped me to develop methods for the investigation. At that time, there were very few studies that discussed local food access in the United States; in fact, the literature and common wisdom were narrowly focused on the use of health education to modify eating behaviors. Therefore, we needed to develop language to talk about the topic of purchasing food from routine sources within people's neighborhoods. Steve suggested *local food environments*.

Over the years, I presented my research and posed these ideas to community groups, public health professionals, medical doctors, and others. What has resonated with me in all of these situations is how people respond very passionately to this area of research. For affected communities, the validation of what is already known is met with a certain hopefulness that things might change. But for professionals, reactions have sometimes been very different. For instance, I have received strong reactions from public health and medical professionals who disagree with the research and firmly believe that we live in a free-market-driven economy. In other words, if certain foods are not available in particular areas, it is because the people who live in those areas would not eat them. As an example, after presenting my research in a postdoctoral seminar several years ago, a distinguished professor became so angry by the results that supermarkets are positively associated with the healthy diets of African-Americans that he walked out of the seminar early after yelling his objections to the findings. Although the reaction was extreme, the response to dismiss the findings has not been uncommon. Taken further, at some level the need to measure the extent to which equitable food access affects the behaviors and health of people could be viewed as misguided. But as this area of research has evolved over the past two decades, there has been a growing fixation with the improvement of methods and statistical models needed to distinguish between the contextual effects of local food environments on residents' health and the selection of residential environments by some groups of people, in other words, a concern for reverse causation. The reasoning that people intentionally sort themselves into areas with restricted access to healthy foods has been used to explain some cross-sectional findings. In many ways, this direction of research inquiry further supports the belief system held by the aforementioned distinguished professor and many others who remain leery of the potential effect of equitable food access on the public's health.

The notion that individuals are entirely responsible for their own behaviors and health outcomes is very pervasive within the medical and public health community. This area of research may strike a chord with some individuals because it provides evidence that health education may not be enough to change food behaviors for some groups of people. Therefore, this blame shifting results in a greater responsibility among those of us in public health, medicine, and/or government service for the poor dietary practices among some American populations. This book is intended to present the current literature regarding disparities among local food environments across the United States, the influence of local availability of healthy foods on the dietary choices of Americans, and how these environments and choices subsequently affect disease occurrence. The aim is to summarize the current literature and to discuss methodological issues related to this area of public health research. Equally important are the chapters that precede and follow the research summary. These chapters describe the decades of U.S. food policies that have influenced the distribution of foods across the nation and the recent novel approaches for decreasing disparities within the United States.

Despite the ongoing challenges, I am inspired by all of the researchers who have questioned the common wisdom and measured local food environment disparities all across the United States and abroad, and documented how these disparities affect people's lives. The findings have added to what was once a very bleak literature. I am equally encouraged by the local, state, and federal policy makers who have acknowledged this body of research, and moved forward by implementing policies and programs to address these disparities, sometimes with conflicting empirical evidence. It is because of this prior work and the effort of everyone involved in this field of research that a book like this is now needed. This text intends to summarize the direction this area of public health has taken since I moved away from Oakland. My hope and intention are that the book will be useful to individuals within a wide range of disciplines who are currently working in this area of public health and for those interested in becoming involved in addressing how local food environments influence the food consumption and health of Americans.

Acknowledgments

As stated earlier, this book is made possible by the work of many people who have conducted research on local food environments and those who have put forth new programs and policies to address disparities in the United States. Without this collective effort, this book would not be possible.

I am also indebted to the contributors of this book who collaborated in an effort to develop a book intended to provide future direction to this area of public health. These contributors have worked with me over the past year to develop and revise chapters to put forth a comprehensive evaluation of the evidence on local food environments and human health in the United States and abroad as well as contextualize this evidence within the American food production/distribution industries and the policies that support those systems. The authors' commitment to the field and the expertise they provided for this book are esteemed.

In addition, I am grateful to Susan Filomena for her tireless work in preparing multiple drafts of each chapter and coordinating communications and changes with contributors, and to Dr. Philip Landrigan for providing the academic support for this book. I also greatly appreciate the review of specific content within the book from the following experts: William B. Morland at SCORE© and Dr. Helena Furberg at Memorial Slone Kettering. Finally, I am forever beholden to my life partner, Corrine Munoz-Plaza, for her overall support and encouragement, as well as her editing of this work.

Editor

Kimberly B. Morland, PhD, M.P.H., is an epidemiologist who has focused her research on the impact of local environments on health. She is a pioneer in the public health arena of local food environments and a leader in advancing evidence-based research. Dr. Morland has developed new epidemiologic methods for geographically based data collection and analysis to investigate associations between neighborhood environments and residents' behaviors that have been replicated by investigators in areas across the United States and other countries, as well as used by community-based organizations to support local changes to commercial environments. She has served on a number of national and local review panels, worked with community-based organizations, and implemented one of the first interventions to address food access by developing a community-owned and community-operated food store in Brooklyn. She is currently an associate professor at Mount Sinai School of Medicine in New York City.

Contributors

Jennifer Black
Food, Nutrition and Health
University of British Columbia
Vancouver, British Columbia, Canada

Carol M. Devine
Division of Nutritional Sciences
Cornell University
Ithaca, New York

Ana V. Diez-Roux
Drexel University School of Public
  Health
Philadelphia, Pennsylvania

Bethany Hendrickson
Public Health Nutrition
School of Public Health
University of California
Berkeley, California

Allison Karpyn
The Food Trust
Philadelphia, Pennsylvania

Barbara A. Laraia
Public Health Nutrition
School of Public Health
University of California
Berkeley, California

Yael Lehmann
The Food Trust
Philadelphia, Pennsylvania

Latetia V. Moore
Division of Nutrition, Physical Activity,
  and Obesity
Centers for Disease Control and
  Prevention
Atlanta, Georgia

Kimberly B. Morland
Department of Preventive
  Medicine
Mount Sinai School of Medicine
New York, New York

Angela Odoms-Young
Department of Kinesiology and
  Nutrition
School of Applied
  Health Sciences
University of Illinois
Chicago, Illinois

Margarita Reina
Department of Biostatistics and
  Epidemiology
School of Public Health
University of Illinois
Chicago, Illinois

Arlene Spark
Hunter College and the CUNY
  Graduate Center
City University of New York School of
  Public Health
New York, New York

Esther Thatcher
School of Nursing
University of Virginia
Charlottesville, Virginia

Jordan Tucker
The Food Trust
Philadelphia, Pennsylvania

April White
The Food Trust
Philadelphia, Pennsylvania

Jennifer L. Wilkins
Division of Nutritional
   Sciences
Cornell University
Ithaca, New York

Steve Wing
Department of Epidemiology
School of Public Health
University of North Carolina
Chapel Hill, North Carolina

Shannon N. Zenk
Department of Health Systems Science
College of Nursing
University of Illinois
Chicago, Illinois

Yun T. Zhang
Public Health Nutrition
School of Public Health
University of California
Berkeley, California

Section I

Introduction and Contextualizing the Local Food Environment into the American Food System

1 Introduction

Kimberly B. Morland

> Environmental disparities between white communities and communities of color reflect larger societal inequalities. Over the years, disparities have been created, tolerated and institutionalized by local, state and federal action.
>
> **Robert D. Bullard (1994)**

The fundamental purpose of this book is to engage readers to appreciate the empirical evidence demonstrating disparities in access to healthy affordable foods across the United States, and that these disparities may explain food consumption patterns for some Americans as well as potential risk for diet-related illness. Furthermore, the book describes the current body of research that has investigated these associations and presents the methodological issues pertinent to this area of public health specifically. Evidence from these studies is put into the context of current and historical American food policies that have supported the existing food retail market, including the production and retailing of foods within the United States and the ways in which the consolidation of the U.S. food system has affected Americans. Although the focus of this book pertains to local food environments within the United States, similar issues regarding access to food are concurrently taking place outside the United States. For instance, research on this subject has been conducted in Europe, Australia, and Canada. Therefore, research conducted regarding local food environments in Canada has been included as a point of comparison. In Chapters 4 through 8, methods and the current state of knowledge regarding the factors associated with disparities between local food environments, the effect of these disparities on the diets of residents within those communities, and finally the impact local food environments have on diet-related health outcomes, such as obesity, are discussed. In the final chapters, we describe solutions garnered to minimize local food environment inequalities that are currently being conducted by federal, state, and local government agencies in the United States to reduce imbalances between local food environments. Within all chapters, readers are encouraged to critically consider the current research methods as well as recent programs and policies that aim to address local food environments. This is an emerging area of public health that requires a range of multidisciplinary experts from fields such as nutrition, business, city planning, policy, epidemiology, health behavior, and geography to conceive, implement, and evaluate environmental changes that will promote health for all Americans.

DEFINING LOCAL FOOD ENVIRONMENTS

Simply put, local food environments are areas where people conveniently shop for food. These areas consist of retail food stores such as supermarkets, convenience stores, and other stores where people can purchase food to prepare at home. But, local food environments also contain restaurants where people might eat away from home or *take-out* food. The word *local* refers to the immediate availability of these types of retailers. This local provision of food may be thought of as food availability within a neighborhood, a small walkable urban area, or short driving distance within suburban and rural areas. These geographic regions vary depending on residential urban/rural geography (as discussed in Chapter 4), but conceptually, local food environments are places that are conveniently located for residents to buy food. Notably, food stores are just one type of retail business in the United States, and the federal government surveys retailing by categorizing businesses by the type of goods they sell and how these sales are procured. Food retailers are composed of food stores and food service places according to the North American Industry Classification System (NAICS), previously known as Standard Industry Classifications. These categories and definitions for food retail businesses are a good reference for the types of food retailing in the United States and are summarized in Table 1.1 (U.S. Census Bureau 2012).

The terminology *local food environments* is used in this book. As stated earlier, this is an emerging area of public health research, and hence the language developed to describe concepts must be clear and meaningful. In fact, other language has developed over time that may cause confusion for the reader; therefore, this section defines the term in greater detail, with a justification as to why this definition is preferable for research over others.

First, local food environments are not to be confused with the local production of food, referred to as *local food*. There has been an increased interest in the demand by some consumers to support regional and small farmers, sometimes through farmers markets and, to a smaller extent, through regular supply chains (King et al. 2010). Rather, local food environments pertain solely to the retailing of foods (that may or may not be *locally* grown) within convenient distances to residential establishments.

Another expression used to describe disparities in food access is *food desert*. The word desert is synonymous with *wasteland, abandonment,* or *desolation*, and initially the terminology meant to identify areas with no food retailers, areas that have literally been *abandoned*. However, over time, research has revealed that few of these types of areas actually exist in the United States, and as a result, the terminology has since been used to refer to local areas with *few healthy food options*. This definition is ultimately problematic for research and evaluation purposes because it is difficult to quantify with any consistency across studies.

First, there is a value judgment of the word *healthy*, which is difficult to measure. In reality, a single food item is neither healthy nor unhealthy because any food item can be incorporated into a healthy diet within moderation. Likewise, any food retailer sells a variety of foods, containing varying levels of calories, saturated fat, sugar, and other nutrients. Therefore, quantifying food retailers as either healthy or unhealthy becomes difficult when aiming for precision of quantifiable measurements for research purposes. Taking this to the extreme, investigators have

TABLE 1.1

**2012 North American Industry Classification System (NAICS)
Definitions and Codes of Food Stores and Service Places**

NAICS Industry Classification	NAICS Index	Examples
Supermarkets and other groceries	445110 Supermarkets	A&P
	445110 Grocery stores	
	445110 Food stores	
Convenience stores	445120 Convenience	7-Eleven
Gasoline stations with convenience	447110 Gasoline station with convenience	Chevron
Specialty food stores	445210 Meat markets	
	445220 Fish markets	Fulton fish market
	445230 Fruit/Vegetable markets	
	445291 Baked goods	Magnolia bakery
	445292 Confectionery/nut stores	Godiva Chocolatier
	445299 All other	
Delicatessens, retailing groceries	445110 Delicatessens	Carnegie Deli
Commissaries, primarily groceries	445110 Commissaries	
Full-service restaurants	722511 Steak houses, full service	Peter Lugar Steak House
	722511 Pizzerias, full service	Grimaldi's
	722511 Fine dining, full service	The River Café
	722511 Family restaurants, full service	Applebee's
	722511 Diners, full service	
	722511 Bagel shop, full service	Ess-A-Bagel
	722511 Doughnut shop, full service	
Limited-service restaurants	722513 Fast-food restaurants	McDonald's
	722513 Pizza parlor, limited service	Famous Famiglia
	722513 Pizza delivery shops	Dominos
Cafeterias, grill buffets, and buffets	722514 Cafeteria	
	722514 Buffet	
Snack and nonalcoholic	722515 Beverage bar (nonalcoholic)	Starbucks
	722515 Doughnut shops, carry-out	Dunkin' Donuts
	722515 Ice cream parlor	Baskin Robbins
	722515 Pretzel shops, carry out	Aunt Annie's
	722515 Cookie shops, carry out	Mrs. Field's Cookies
	722515 Bagel shops, carry out	Bruegger's Bagels
Drinking places	722410 Bars	
	722410 Cocktail lounges	
	722410 Taverns	
	722410 Nightclubs	

(*Continued*)

TABLE 1.1 (*Continued*)
2012 North American Industry Classification System (NAICS)
Definitions and Codes of Food Stores and Service Places

NAICS Industry Classification	NAICS Index	Examples
Mobile food services	722330 Mobile food concession stands	
	722330 Mobile food carts	NYC Green Carts
	722330 Mobile canteens	
	722330 Mobile refreshment stands	
	722330 Mobile snack stands	
Caterers	722320 Banquet halls with catering staff	
	722320 Caterer	

Source: United States Census Bureau, North American Industry Classification System (http://www .census.gov/eos/www/naics).

targeted franchised fast-food restaurants as *unhealthy food retailers* and supermarkets as *healthy food retailers*. But, using these heuristics for healthy retailers, even supermarkets contain foods that are considered undesirable in large quantities for American diets.

The second issue with the terminology of food desert for research purposes is that the definition suggests a binary categorization of food and nonfood deserts. In reality, food retail landscapes are complicated by the number and types of food retailers within a given geographic area, and the interaction between those retailers. This becomes problematic when one aims to quantify *few healthy food stores*. Questions arise, such as, *How many fast-food restaurants does it take to make a food desert? What if there are supermarkets in the area as well? How many supermarkets are needed in the area to offset the fast-food restaurants—5, 10, 15, or more? What if the only supermarket is a Whole Foods Market where the foods are relatively expensive?* Because there are no specific answers to the questions, the need to quantify few healthy food options may actually lead to nonspecific main effects that weaken the ability to detect any true effect between local food environments and diet or disease.

Nevertheless, the U.S. Department of Agriculture (USDA), as part of the Healthy Food Financing Initiative, has recently defined food deserts as "a low-income census tract where a substantial number or share of residents has *low access* to a supermarket or large grocery store." However, this definition has been newly defined and used primarily for descriptive purposes. To quantify *low-access communities*, the USDA has made a definition that "at least 500 people and/or at least 33% of the census tract's population must reside more than 1 mile from a supermarket or a large grocery store (for rural census tracts, the distance is more than 10 miles)." These definitions have been used by the USDA to characterize local food environments as food deserts across the United States. The USDA focuses on low-income communities and on a single type of food retailer (USDA Food Desert Locator 2013). Investigators have used other definitions to define food deserts.

It is preferable for research purposes that all food retailers within a targeted geographic region are considered in multivariate models* as predictors of diet and/or diet-related health outcomes. The rationale is that the effect of each type of food store or food service place can be evaluated individually and can also be adjusted† for the effect of the number and types of other food purveyors. This is particularly important during the early stages of investigations because we rely on the ability to reproduce results within different human populations as evidence of causation‡ in observational studies. Within these models, the independent variables§ are value neutral and allow for the effects of each type of food store and restaurant to be observed without assumptions built into composite definitions of variables such as the one created by the USDA regarding food deserts. Modeling the count or density of each type of retailer also allows for continuous distributions of retailers to be measured, increasing statistical power for these models. The terminology *local food environments* then represents the evaluation of all of the food retailers within a geographic area where an individual can purchase food. Some of those places will produce positive effects on diet and some will produce negative effects. Ultimately, the concept and terminology of local food environments reflects the Gestalt¶ of all types of food retailers and the connections between those places.

The other issue surrounding the definition of local food environment pertains to the need for these counts or density of food stores/restaurants to be measured within a certain geographic area (e.g., census tract, 1 mile from home, within a 400-m buffer zone). The size of the geographic unit needs to be specific to the target population being studied, and different geographic units may be necessary for different populations. For instance, defining *local* may have a larger geographic boundary in a rural area of Montana, whereas an intensely urban area of New York City may require a smaller geographic unit. Such variability is inherent to this area of research and, although it may present issues when comparing findings across studies that are discussed in more detail in Chapters 4 through 7, the specificity of the main effect requires determination of the best boundary for the population being studied.

Moreover, the concept of local food environments pertains to places where people *routinely* buy food. Therefore, this definition is restricted to food retailers and excludes service organizations such as food banks, soup kitchens, community centers, and other places where food may be provided for free or at a nominal cost. Food environments are intended to represent establishments in areas where anyone could purchase food regardless of socioeconomic circumstances or other issues. These retail environments also exclude schools or workplaces where foods may be

---

* A multivariate statistical model is a regression equation where the relationship of the dependent variables is measured with more than one independent variable (Rosner 1995).

† Within multivariate regression, the effect of a given variable has taken into account or held constant the effect of other variables in the statistical model (Rosner 1995).

‡ Causation can be defined as "an event, condition, or characteristic that plays an essential role in producing an occurrence of a disease" (Rothman and Greenland 1998).

§ A variable is an individual's environmental or behavioral factor that is measured and hypothesized to influence disease occurrence.

¶ Gestalt is a theory that posits the whole is greater than the sum of its parts. Related to local food environments, it can be interpreted that the entirety of local food access, as a concept, is greater than the measurement of its single components (e.g., supermarkets, fast-food restaurants).

offered and eaten, but not available to any person at any time. Although there has been research conducted to evaluate these types of food environments, they are not included in the definition of local food environments for this book. Finally, farmer markets and other seasonal retailers have typically been excluded from the local food environment research because foods cannot be purchased year round and farmers markets were not as prevalent when local food environment research began (USDA Directory Records 2013). However, with the burgeoning of local farmers markets and the movement to increasingly rely on locally produced food, these types of food purveyors may become important targets for addressing disparities in food access. These issues are discussed in greater detail in Chapter 10.

In summary, the terminology *local food environment* is value neutral and ideally represents a noncomposite definition of food retailers or foods sold by a retailer. It is descriptive of the environmental exposure being assessed, such that the term *local* refers to the availability of foods that can be procured within convenient distances from residential homes. Furthermore, the term *food environment* refers to the collective space where the food retailers conduct business to sell food to consumers and is distinguished from food producers and manufacturers further up the food chain.

The definition of local food environments relies heavily on the placement of food retailers because Americans obtain most of their food from the food retail market, specifically food stores (USDA ERS Food at Home 2013). From a public health perspective, it is important to acknowledge right from the start that this U.S. food retail market is a for-profit industry. Moreover, this retail market is embedded into a larger for-profit food industry, which is discussed in detail in Chapters 2 and 3. The result is that food retailers make profit-driven decisions about the placement of their store(s), including what they will sell, the volume of items sold, and the prices of those products. Therefore, as health promoters are interested in changing the availability, cost and/or quality of food items sold to Americans, solutions must be conceived in conjunction with for-profit food retailers. Although sometime in the future the United States may adopt new food policies outside a free market domain, it is unlikely that free enterprise will not continue to influence the food industry at any level, given that the United States is a capitalistic society. Understanding the U.S. food industry, and how the U.S. government interacts and influences the industry, is paramount for discerning sustainable changes to food retailing for Americans (Chapter 2). It is also important to understand how food retailers conduct business in the United States.

FOOD RETAILING IN THE UNITED STATES

There are several ways to set up a retail business in the United States (Dunne et al. 2011). Most U.S. retailers are in the business of making money, and food retailers are no exception. Therefore, the success of a food retailer is based on the ability to make a profit on the foods they sell. Profits are measured in several ways (Pinson 2004; Beesley 2013; Food Marketing Institute 2008; Inc. 2013). For instance, a *profit margin* is the ratio of the amount of money gained and the cost of selling a given item. The gross profit margin does not account for the operational costs that are needed to sell the food items, such as rent, salaries for employees, insurance, and so forth. Thus, when operational costs are subtracted from the gross dollar margin, the result is the *net profit margin*. Food retailers price individual items for a gross profit margin but often discuss total profit in terms of net profit margins. An example of how the profit margins are calculated is described in Table 1.2.

Profit margins are calculated within certain periods, sometimes thought of as production cycles (e.g., quarterly or annually). Although profit margins are often expressed for a given store or industry, they are actually an average of the profit margins of every item sold in the store; in other words, every food item within a given store has a unique gross profit margin. A *profit rate* is another measure of profitability. A profit rate uses the profit margin, but also takes the amount of inventory turnover into consideration. For instance, a profit margin for item A could remain stable, but if the food store was able to turn over item A multiple times during a production cycle, then the amount of money earned from item A would increase without an increase in the profit margin. This rate is sometimes known as the *rate of return*. Thus, the rate of return can be increased by increasing the profit margin or increasing the rate of inventory turnover (this is referred to as *shortening the production cycle*). The concept of stimulating a high volume of sales with small net profit margins is the fundamental principal behind *mass merchandising.*

These concepts are very important for understanding how food stores operate. It is well known in the food industry that supermarkets operate with a low net profit margin, roughly 2% (Pinson 2004). One might conclude that supermarket owners do not have much wiggle room to lower prices without risking going out of business. However, there are two things to remember with the low net profit margins for food retailers. First, the industry has very high turnover rates of their products. For example, consider a food retailer versus a car dealer. All people need food to live, eat every day, and typically make food purchases for families multiple times a month. Conversely, not everyone owns a car and for those that do, a new car may be purchased every 5 years or longer. The car dealers have slow production cycles, and subsequently they need their profit margins to remain high to remain profitable. In contrast, for food store retailers, profits within a given period can be quite high because of the high turnover of food products sold, even though the profit margins are low. Second, it is important to remember that the gross profit margin of every

---

TABLE 1.2
Dollar Profits and Profit Margins (Example)

Annual Report for Store A

Total gross sales	$10,000.00	
Cost to purchase inventory	−$4,000.00	
Gross profit	**$6,000.00**	
Operational costs	−$3,500.00	
Net profit	**$2,500.00**	
Gross profit margin	6,000/10,000	**60%**
Net profit margin	2,500/10,000	**25%**

food item within a store is not low. For instance, a supermarket may run a sale on a commonly used food item to draw customers into the store. The owner may accept a very low profit margin (or even a loss) on that item because it is expected that shoppers will purchase more than that one item. Thus, the low profit margin of a particular item might be offset by a high margin on another product. This concept is known to food retailers as *loss leading* (McMillian 2012).

These economic principles have been behind the development of larger chain grocers in the early part of the last century. Prior to the development of large food stores, such as Kroger and A & P, Americans would shop for food from what we would now call smaller specialty food stores, such as meat markets and produce stands. Large markets that drew different vendors into public spaces, such as La Marqueta in the neighborhood of East Harlem in New York City, were not uncommon and sold both food and nonfood items (East Harlem Online 2012). The development of larger stores, such as A&P, allowed retailers to offset the lower profit margin of one type of product with the higher margins of many other products. A typical supermarket sells roughly 38,000 items, which allows for greater turnover and flexibility of profit margins. However, it was in the early part of the twentieth century that an additional cost-saving innovation made its way into the American food system—and truly revolutionized the way food is retailed in the United States (Food Marketing Institute 2010). That innovation was processed nonperishable foods, which became available after World War II. The development of this class of food products allowed grocers to increase their stock without being concerned about perishable waste, such as fresh produce, milk, eggs, meat, and cheese, all of which have limited shelf lives and result in a loss to the business owner if not sold. Stocking nonperishables allowed retailer Michael Kullen to open the first American supermarket on August 4, 1930 (Kullen 2013). By selling nonperishables, Kullen was able to increase the volume of goods sold and accept a smaller profit margin, which translated to lower prices for customers and increased turnover of his products. This business model of mass merchandising, often referred to as *economy of scale*, has proven to be very successful and has been used by other food retailers including Walmart. The increase in the proportion of food retailer's profits garnered by supermarkets in the early part of the last century can be seen in Figure 1.1 where the proportion of total sales by type of food vendor is presented. This graph also depicts how other smaller grocery stores lost a significant market share of food dollars as supermarkets increased profits over time. Other types of food retailers have shared a small portion of profits (under 10%), with the profit share from warehouse and supercenters rising in the most recent years.

Consequently, there remains stiff competition for consumers' food dollars, even after taking into account the very low net profit margins within the industry. U.S. supermarkets sell more than $556 billion worth of products each year and sales are nearly five times greater than other types of food retailers (Figure 1.2).

The success of mass merchandising within this industry has brought non-food retailers and wholesalers into this marketplace, thereby altering the American food retail landscape over the past several decades. Retailers such as Walmart have replaced food retailers such as Kroger and Safeway as leaders in the field (Food Marketing Institute 2008; Food & Water Watch 2010). Food retailers have also boosted margins with private label sales and stronger control over producers.

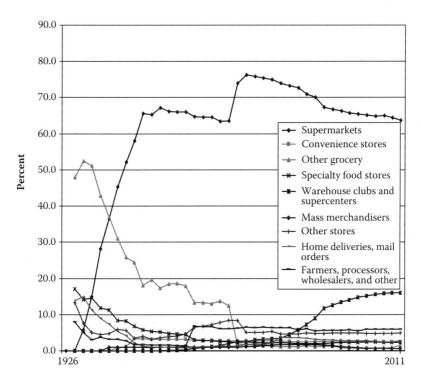

FIGURE 1.1 Proportion of food sales by type of food retailer in the United States: 1926–2011. (Calculated by the Economic Research Service from various dataset from the U.S. Census Bureau and the Bureau of Labor Statistics—USDA ERS AER-575.)

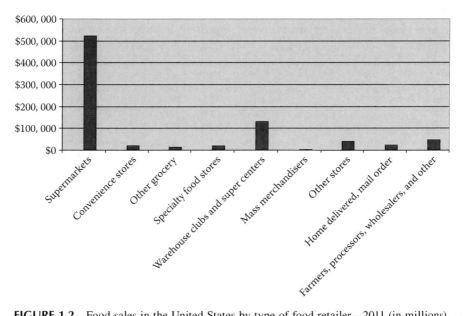

FIGURE 1.2 Food sales in the United States by type of food retailer—2011 (in millions). (Modified from USDA ERS Food Expenditures, AER-575 Table 14 [dollar amounts].)

The bottom line for Americans is that these business practices have translated into greater availability of inexpensive food items. In fact, over the years, Americans are spending less of their income on food, even with an increase in the expenditures from foods eaten away from home (Figure 1.3). In 2005, Americans spent under 6% of their income on food (Food Marketing Institute 2007). This is three times less than people living in Western European countries and more than five times less than people living in China during the same time period (USDA 2004). It is estimated by the USDA that, in 2009, American families spent an average of $6,389 a year on food, roughly $500 per month. This estimate includes purchases of foods prepared at home as well as those purchased away from home (at limited- and full-service restaurants). This annual food expenditure is 40% higher than in 1984 ($4,552, annual household expenditure) (USDA 2012). Interestingly, the proportion of the American annual household food budget earmarked for foods eaten away from home has increased substantially in recent years (1984: 29% vs. 2009: 41%).

The food service industry has also grown, particularly during the past decade. Although there were an equal number of supermarkets and restaurants per American in 2000, there has been an increase in the number of full- and limited-service restaurants in the last decade, with a decreasing trend in the availability of supermarkets (Figure 1.4). It is estimated that over 75% of Americans eat outside of their homes at least once a week and the proportion of caloric intake from foods purchased away from home has nearly doubled since the 1970s (Stewart et al. 2006). This trend has let to some concern about changes in the nutritional quality of Americans' diets with the understanding that, in general, meals eaten away from home have higher caloric content and are nutritionally poorer than foods prepared at home (Lin et al. 1999). Restaurant owners have business goals similar to those of food stores owners, which is to make a profit. Therefore, it is not surprising that moderate reactions were received from chain restaurant executives regarding the suggestion of more *healthy meal options*; with officials being skeptical that these types of changes in menus would increase patronage (Technomic 2006).

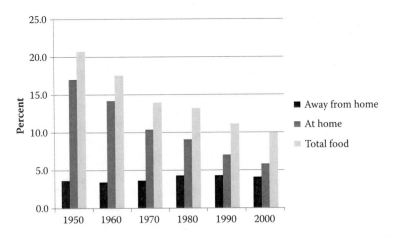

FIGURE 1.3 Percent of U.S. family incomes spent on food to be eaten at home and away from home between 1950 and 2000.

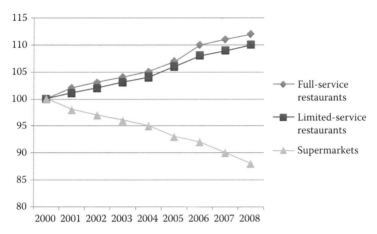

FIGURE 1.4 Number of supermarkets and restaurants per capita, 2002–2008. (From USDA, A Revised and Expanded Food Dollar Series: A Better Understanding of Our Food Costs, Economic Research Report No. (ERR-114), Figure 6, p. 30, 2011.)

FOOD CONSUMPTION TRENDS IN THE UNITED STATES

Americans are consuming more food, which in turn supports the growing food retail markets. It is estimated that Americans eat several hundred more calories per day compared to 50–60 years ago. The food supply in 2000 provided 3,800 calories per American per day—500 calories more than that produced in the 1970s (USDA 2003). Some of the 3,800 calories per person are estimated to be lost to spoilage, plate waste, or cooking; nevertheless, it has been documented that caloric intake by Americans has increased by 24.5% between 1970 and 2000 (Technomic 2006). The types of foods that have contributed the greatest to the increase in calories have been refined grain products, added fats and oils, and added sugars. However, there has been an increased consumption in nearly every food category. Estimates in Table 1.3 are based on USDA food disappearance data as an approximation of human consumption. The data are unadjusted for spoilage and overestimate consumption to some extent. Nevertheless, this overestimation is constant over time; therefore, differences across the decades can be discerned with these data.

Looking at specific categories of foods, there is an increase in the consumption of almost every food item between 1950 and 2000 with the exception of veal and lamb, eggs, dairy products (such as cottage cheese, ice cream, sherbet, nonfat dry milk, condensed and evaporated milks, and whole milk), butter and margarine, cane and beet sugars, and other non-corn caloric sweeteners. For fruits and vegetables, comparisons are available from 1970 to 2000. During that time, there was also an increase in almost all fresh and processed fruits and vegetables except fresh citrus fruit, canned non-citrus fruit, and fresh potatoes and canned vegetables, other than tomatoes.

The greatest difference observed over time is in the consumption of high-fructose corn syrup. This corn sweetener entered the market in the 1970s, when cane and beet sugars still outranked corn sweeteners by 3:1. By 2000, the

TABLE 1.3

Average Annual American Food Consumption by Food Category: 1950–2000

Food Item	Decade					
	1950	1960	1970	1980	1990	2000*
Animal products (*pound per capita, boneless-trimmed weight+; number per capita**)						
Total meats+	138.2	161.7	177.2	182.2	189.0	195.2
Red meats	106.7	122.3	129.5	121.8	112.4	113.5
Beef	52.8	69.2	80.9	71.7	63.2	64.4
Pork	45.4	46.9	45.0	47.7	47.6	47.7
Veal and lamb	8.5	6.2	3.5	2.4	1.7	1.4
Poultry	20.5	28.7	35.2	46.2	61.9	66.5
Chicken	16.4	22.7	28.4	36.3	47.9	52.9
Turkey	4.1	6.0	6.8	9.9	13.9	13.6
Fish and shellfish	10.9	10.7	12.5	14.2	14.7	15.2
Eggs*	374.0	320.0	285.0	257.0	236.0	250.0
Dairy products (*per pound+; 1/2 pint*; and gallon^*)						
Total dairy products+	703.0	619.0	548.0	573.0	571.0	593.0
Cheese	7.7	9.5	14.4	21.5	26.7	29.8
Cottage cheese	3.9	4.6	4.9	4.1	2.9	2.6
Frozen dairy products	23.0	27.5	27.8	27.4	28.8	27.8
Ice cream	18.1	18.3	17.7	17.7	16.0	16.5
Low-fat ice cream	2.7	6.2	7.6	7.2	7.5	7.3
Sherbet	1.3	1.5	1.5	1.3	1.3	1.2
Other (e.g., frozen yogurt)	1.0	1.5	1.0	1.2	4.0	3.1
Nonfat dry milk	4.9	5.9	4.1	2.4	3.1	3.4
Dry whey	0.2	0.6	2.1	3.2	3.5	3.4
Condensed and evaporated milks	21.6	15.7	9.4	7.5	7.3	5.8
Cream products*	18.1	13.3	10.1	12.8	15.7	18.6
Yogurt	0.2	0.7	3.2	6.5	8.5	9.9
Beverage milk^	36.4	32.6	29.8	26.5	24.3	22.6
Whole	33.5	28.8	21.7	14.3	9.1	8.1
Lower fat	2.9	3.7	8.1	12.2	15.3	14.5
Grains (*pound per capita*)						
Total grain products	155.4	142.5	138.2	157.4	190.6	199.9
Wheat flour	125.7	114.4	113.6	122.8	141.8	146.3
Corn products	15.4	13.8	11.0	17.3	24.5	28.4
Rice	5.3	7.1	7.3	11.3	17.5	19.7
Sweeteners (*per capita, dry weight basis*)						
Total caloric sweeteners	109.6	114.4	123.7	126.5	145.9	152.4
Cane and beet sugar	96.7	98.0	96.0	68.4	64.7	65.6
Corn sweeteners	11.0	14.9	26.3	56.8	79.9	85.3
High-fructose corn syrup	0.0	0.0	5.5	37.3	56.8	63.8
Glucose	7.4	10.9	16.6	16.0	19.3	18.1

TABLE 1.3

Average Annual American Food Consumption by Food Category: 1950–2000

Food Item	Decade					
	1950	1960	1970	1980	1990	2000*
Dextrose	3.5	4.1	4.3	3.5	3.8	3.4
Other caloric sweeteners	2.0	1.5	1.4	1.3	1.3	1.5
Added fats and oils (*product weight basis*)						
Total added fats and oils	44.5	47.8	53.4	60.8	65.5	74.5
Salad and cooking oils	9.8	13.9	20.2	25.0	28.2	35.2
Baking and frying fats	21.4	20.7	20.5	23.6	26.2	29.0
Shortening	10.9	14.6	17.4	20.5	22.7	23.1
Lard and beef fallow	10.5	6.1	3.5	3.1	4.0	6.0
Table spreads	17.0	16.5	15.9	15.3	14.0	12.8
Butter	9.0	6.6	4.7	4.6	4.4	4.6
Margarine	8.0	9.9	11.2	10.7	9.6	8.2
Fruits and vegetables (*pound per capita, fresh weight equivalent*)						
Total fruits and vegetables	N/A	N/A	587.5	622.1	688.3	707.7
Total fruit	N/A	N/A	248.7	269.0	280.1	279.4
Fresh fruit	N/A	N/A	99.4	113.1	123.7	126.8
Citrus	N/A	N/A	27.2	24.2	23.7	23.4
Non-citrus	N/A	N/A	72.2	88.9	100.0	103.0
Processed fruit	N/A	N/A	149.3	155.9	156.5	152.7
Frozen fruit non-citrus	N/A	N/A	3.4	3.4	3.8	3.7
Dried fruit, non-citrus	N/A	N/A	9.9	12.2	11.7	10.5
Canned fruit, non-citrus	N/A	N/A	24.7	21.3	19.7	17.4
Fruit juices	N/A	N/A	110.7	118.6	120.8	120.6
Total vegetable	N/A	N/A	338.8	353.1	408.2	428.3
Fresh vegetables	N/A	N/A	147.9	157.2	181.9	201.7
Potatoes	N/A	N/A	52.5	48.5	48.8	47.2
Other	N/A	N/A	95.4	108.7	133.1	154.5
Processed (canned)	N/A	N/A	101.1	98.9	109.4	104.7
Tomatoes	N/A	N/A	62.9	63.5	74.4	69.9
Other	N/A	N/A	38.2	35.4	35.0	34.8
Processed (frozen)	N/A	N/A	52.1	61.0	76.8	79.7
Potatoes	N/A	N/A	36.1	42.8	54.9	57.8
Other	N/A	N/A	16.0	18.2	21.9	21.9
Dehydrated vegetables/ chips	N/A	N/A	30.8	29.4	32.0	33.7
Pulses	N/A	N/A	7.0	6.5	8.1	8.6

*Estimates based on single year.

Source: U.S. Department of Agriculture, Chapter 2: Profiling Food Consumption in America, In
          Agricultural Fact Book 2001–2002, U.S. Government Printing Office, Washington DC, 2003.
          http:www.usda.gov/factbook/chapter2.htm.

Note: N/A = not available.

consumption of corn sweeteners was higher than cane and beet sugars with the category of corn sweeteners, high-fructose corn syrup, being consumed at the same rate as cane and beet sugars. Overall, the use of sweeteners in the American diet has increased dramatically, where levels in 2000 were comparable to 32 teaspoons of added sugar per day, adjusted for waste. This amount is in reference to the recommendation of 10 teaspoons per day for a 2000 caloric diet at that time. For clarity, added sugar does not refer solely to the addition of cane sugar to meals by Americans, but is also inclusive of sugars added to the food supply by producers and is ubiquitous in foods ranging from beverages such as soda to other staples such as breads.

Corn also appeared in larger consumption over this time period through grain products (84.4% increase). This increase, coupled with a similar increase in rice consumption (77.5%), has resulted in a greater intake of grains, usually refined grains, for Americans. It is estimated with these data that Americans are eating approximately 10 servings of grains per day, although the distinction between whole and refined grains is not apparent with these data. Americans are continuing to increase consumption of added fat as well. Although, there seems to be a shift away from fats such as butter to heart-healthy monounsaturated fats found in salads and cooking oils (e.g., olive and canola oils).

In terms of other food groups, there has been a change in food production during this time that may also be influencing consumption. Producers have responded to consumers' need for convenient ready-made foods as the demographics of working families have changed over this time period. Producers have packaged food differently to allow for single servings, time-saving preparations such as prewashed vegetables or prepackaged shredded cheeses. These changes in the manufacturing of foods have also allowed producers and retailers to charge more for these items. These types of items are referred to as value-added items. The value to the retailer is the increased profit, whereas the value to the consumer is the increased convenience. Interestingly, there has been a dramatic increase in cheese consumption (287%) over the past decades, translating to a change of 7.7 lb per person in the 1950s to 29.8 lb per person in 2000. During this same time period, Americans are drinking less milk, with a trend toward lower fat milks for those that do consume milk. One hypothesis is that the increased consumption of soft drinks has replaced milk consumption and that Americans' increasing dependency on fast-food restaurants has likely played a role in this shift. The value-added offerings of prewashed and precut vegetables in particular are thought to have contributed to the increase in fresh vegetable consumption between the 1950s and 2000, which increased at a greater rate than processed vegetables. Regarding fruit consumption, non-citrus fresh fruit and fruit juice intake increased the greatest. American diets are also reliant on meat products and intake has increased from years earlier. For instance, in 2000, each American ate 195 pounds of meat on average or roughly 16 pounds per month, which is a 40% increase since the 1950s. The greatest proportion of meat consumed is red meat (58%) followed by poultry (34%). American diets consist of relatively little fish. Within the category of red meats, consumption of pork has remained relatively stable over time; however, there was an increase in beef consumption between 1950 and 1970. After that time, beef consumption has decreased moderately, but still remains higher in 2000 compared to 50 years ago. Although Americans continue to consume red meat in large quantities, it is the consumption of poultry that has really made significant changes to the American diet. In the 1950s, poultry was only 15% of the meat consumed by Americans. But over time, there has been an incremental increase in both chicken and turkey in the diets of Americans. The increase in meat consumption over the 50-year period is also thought to be attributed, in part, to value-added foods provided by the meat industry and the low cost of meat.

HUNGER AND OBESITY IN THE UNITED STATES

Although the local food environment literature has mainly focused on outcomes such as healthy food intake and obesity, hunger is an outcome that may also be a result of disparities between local food environments in the United States. Quite remarkably, it was not until 1966 that the federal government began to measure hunger in the United States (Brown 2006). It was at this time that a group of physicians conducted a study to measure the nutritional status in areas of poverty across the United States and found an extensive amount of hunger within the communities studied. The physicians reported to the U.S. Congress that households were without food for several days a month and babies were without milk. Furthermore, within inner cities, the investigators found cases of severe malnutrition. Fortunately, this study led to an expansion of the Food Stamp Program, as well as the initiation of: (1) the School Breakfast Program, (2) the Special Supplement Food Program for Women, Infants, and Children, and (3) elderly feeding programs under President Nixon's administration (U.S. Senate 1973; Citizens' Board of Inquiry 1977). Further investigations of hunger in the United States and the communities specifically impacted by poverty were conducted in 1983 by the USDA. These studies determined that hunger was continuing to grow and estimated to affect 20 million Americans (Physicians Task Force on Hunger 1985; Brown and Allen 1988). The issue quickly became a political one given that the United States produces more than enough food to feed its population. The USDA began to evaluate hunger in the United States by measuring the food security of households, which is quantified with responses to a number of questions related to one's ability to obtain food, and is presented in Figure 1.5 by food security status of adults in 2011. Figure 1.5 shows that Americans who are food secure do not worry about food and do not experience hunger, whereas as food security decreases, there is a greater proportion of Americans reporting experiences of hunger and hardship managing regular food intake.

The direct measurement of hunger, used by the federal government, as "painful sensations" associated with inadequate food intake or "chronically inadequate nutritional intake due to low income status" defined by others has been abandoned, which makes the comparison of hunger rates over time problematic (Brown 2006; Hunger Notes 2012). Nevertheless, as recently as 2010, it was estimated that 14.5% of American households were food insecure and that proportion is the highest recorded by the USDA (Coleman-Jensen et al. 2011). Hunger presents itself in the United States as what the World Health Organization has called *silent undernutrition*

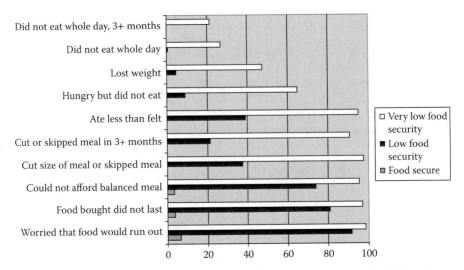

FIGURE 1.5 Percentage of American households reporting indicators of adult food insecurity, by food security status, 2011. (Calculated by the Economic Research Services of the USDA using data from the December 2011 current Population Survey Food Security Supplement.)

(World Health Organization 1980). Unlike protein–calorie malnutrition experienced by children in developing nations, U.S. children with inadequate nutrition appear thin and experience growth failure. Because growth is monitored for American children and standardized to pediatric growth charts, this is the easiest group of Americans to study and detect the effects of nutrition deficiencies. Conversely, the effect of hunger on American adults is not as well characterized.

It is argued that for some people hunger may be a component cause* of obesity (Townsend et al. 2001; Darmon et al. 2002). The rationale is that to avoid the experience of hunger when resources are limited, individual's choices are limited to cheaper foods that are more filling. Individuals are forced to make decisions related to food choices weighing quantity versus quality and in this regard, obesity is thought to be "an adaptive response when food availability is unreliable" (Brown 2006). At this stage, the U.S. Public Health Service has identified obesity as a leading health concern in our society, and the prevalence of obesity had been increasing in the United States through 2009 (Flegal et al. 2012; U.S. Department of Health and Human Services 2012). Although there has been no change in the prevalence of obesity among adults between 2007–2008 and 2009–2010, the prevalence of obesity among adults in the United States was 35.5% for individuals 20 years and older and 39.7% for those 60 years and older during this time period (Flegal et al. 2012). Disparities in obesity prevalence exist by race/ethnicity and socioeconomic status (Flegal et al. 2002). Obesity has both health and economic consequences, as individuals who are obese are at greater risk of developing comorbidities (Allison et al. 1999; Must et al. 1999;

_____

* A component cause is an individual's environmental or behavioral factor that often works in conjunction with other factors sufficient for disease occurrence (Rothman and Greenland 1998).

Finkelstein et al. 2003). The cause of obesity is likely to be multifactorial, resulting from the interaction of environmental and behavioral factors. Although genetic traits may be important for determining an individual's susceptibility to becoming obese, given the short time period during which the sharp increase has occurred, individual exposure to environmental factors, such as the contextual effect of residential areas, is likely to have a more proximal role as component causes of the obesity epidemic. Environmental factors affect obesity through their influence on individual's behavior—specifically, dietary intake and physical activity. Local food availability at the neighborhood level has recently received attention as a possible environmental determinant of dietary intake (Sooman et al. 1993; Fitzgibbon and Stolley 2004). For instance, in Figure 1.6, the association between the prevalence of obesity for people living in varied types of local food environments compared to people living in areas with only supermarkets are presented. People living in areas with only supermarkets and small grocery stores have a very small increased risk of obesity. But, as other types of food stores are included into environments, such as convenience stores, the prevalence of obesity increases. In addition, as supermarkets are excluded from environments, even when small grocers remain, risk also increases (Morland et al. 2006). It should be noted that the direction of these findings cannot be determined with the data provided. In other words, the associations described may be a function of neighborhood characteristics that do not attract supermarket retailers, or obese people may sort themselves into these types of areas. Nevertheless, these data do demonstrate that there is a geographic distribution of supermarkets and that distribution is associated with the geographic pattern of obesity.

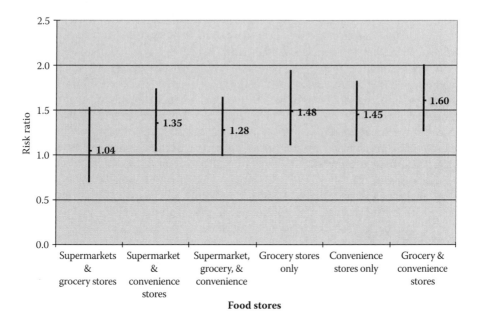

FIGURE 1.6 Associations between components of local food environments and obesity. (From Morland, K. et al., *Am J Prev Med*, 30, 333–9, 2006.)

CONCEPTUAL MODELS AND LOCAL FOOD ENVIRONMENTS

Baranowski et al. (1997, 2003) have provided a useful discussion of the selection of specific health behavior models that may be helpful for furthering our understanding of the causal mechanisms between local food environments and dietary intake. The investigators compared several health behavior models in terms of their applicability for understanding dietary and physical activity behaviors: (1) knowledge–attitude–behavior model, (2) behavioral learning theory, (3) health belief model, (4) social cognitive theory, (5) theory of reasoned action or theory of planned behavior, (6) transtheoretical model and stages of change, (7) ecological and social ecological models, and (8) social marketing. The authors show that these theories/models only moderately predict behavior ($r^2 < 0.3$) (Baranowski et al. 1999) and there is little evidence to suggest that one model has a better ability to predict dietary or physical activity behavior over another. That being said, an additional problem arises in the applicability of these health behavior models for understanding the influence of individuals' built environments on behaviors and health, as most of these models fail to acknowledge the influence of the environment, particularly the physical environment.

Factors Involved in Obtaining Food, Physical Activity, and Disease Development

Investigators have described factors that influence diets. For instance, dietary choices have been shown to be influenced by a number of factors described previously, such as food preferences, as well as self-efficacy and home availability (Neumark-Sztainer et al. 2003; Steptoe et al. 2003; Bere and Klepp 2004; Blanchette and Brug 2005). More recently, investigators have been describing environmental influences in the context of mediating variables that directly impact behavior (Baranowski et al. 1998; Cullen et al. 2000; McNeal et al. 2004; Ball et al. 2006; Kremers et al. 2006; Jago et al. 2007; Stafford et al. 2007). Home availability has been shown to be a strong and proximal predictor of healthy food intake. In addition, investigators have described food intake as a result of a series of hierarchical processes that begin with a wider environment, whereby household resources (i.e., money), food acquisition, food management (i.e., storage), and food preparation techniques are used to understand food consumption (Campbell and Desjardins 1989). Building on these concepts, Figure 1.7 describes the proposed causal relationships between observable behaviors and nonobservable decision-making processes that influence these behaviors and subsequent health outcomes. It is through these behavioral pathways that the relationship between local food environment, dietary intake, and disease can be conceptualized.

For instance, the process by which a single food or meal is eaten is described on the left-hand side of Figure 1.7. Beginning with a decision to eat, and then followed by a decision about what to eat, an individual moves in one of two directions. However, the simple decision of what to eat is influenced by several factors, including the time of day (foods for breakfast, lunch, or dinner), how much time there is to prepare food, food preferences, and so forth. If the decision is to eat and the type

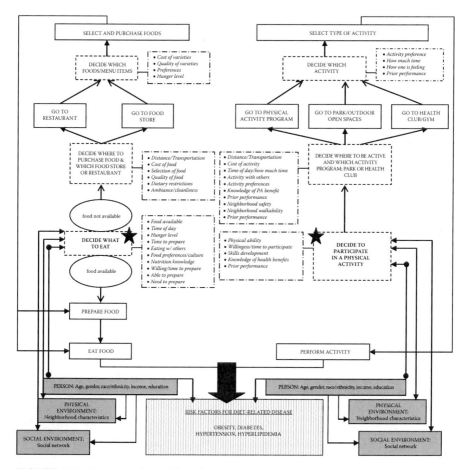

FIGURE 1.7 Proposed observable behaviors and nonobservable decision making based on environmental influences that effect behaviors and diet-related disease risk.

of food desired is readily available at home, then the person moves to the behavior of preparing the food to be eaten and subsequently eating. However, if the chosen food is not readily available, then the person must make a different decision that will ultimately lead to eating a food or meal. Specifically, after determining that foods are not readily available (i.e., at home), an individual then must decide where to buy the food (food store or restaurant). Once this decision is made, the individual must choose a specific restaurant or food store to patron. Similar to the preceding decision, several factors influence this decision-making process: (1) the distance to a food store or restaurant, (2) access to transportation, (3) the cost of foods, (4) the quality of food, (5) the desire to eat with other individuals or alone, and (6) ambience preferences. These decisions are followed by the observable behavior of going to the store/restaurant. Additional decisions are made at the food store/restaurant when selecting food/menu items, which may be influenced by particular sale items, specials, the overall quality of the food, and so forth. Nevertheless, the decision-making process ends with either (1) the food(s) being purchased at the food store and subsequently prepared and eaten or (2) direct food intake at a restaurant. This complex web of behaviors and decision making repeats itself several times per day (as foods are eaten or avoided), which then results in various types of food that are consumed, as well as where and when they are purchased and/or consumed, if they are eaten alone or with others, and the number of calories per day and different macro- and micronutrients that are ultimately consumed.

An individual's environment (social and physical) and personal attributes are expected to modify this decision-making process and affect behavior. Moreover, the modifying effects can be bidirectional. Using the physical environment as an example (food environment in this case), the decision of what to buy may be influenced by the selection, cost, and quality of foods at nearby restaurants or food stores, accessibility of transportation, and/or willingness to travel to purchase foods. A reciprocal effect between the physical environment and the decision of what to eat may be observed if a preferred food was carried by a local store because a resident recommended it to the store manager. The reciprocal effects are more difficult to describe with individual factors such as age, gender, race/ethnicity, income, and education. Whereas these factors may influence decisions on what to eat through pathways of food preferences or social environments, for instance, what an individual chooses to eat will not influence his/her gender, race, education, or income. However, individual attributes are expected to influence the physical environment (i.e., determining the racial makeup of an area) and social environment (i.e., gender-specific social networks).

Because outcomes such as obesity are a result of energy balance, the causal pathway describing the behaviors and decision to participate in a physical activity are described on the right-hand side of Figure 1.7. The behavior—to perform an activity—is preceded by a similar number of factors influencing the decision-making process for dietary intake. Although these decisions and behaviors may not happen repeatedly each day, in the way they are likely to with regard to diet, the influence of both the social environment (other people to be active with or other people supportive of a person's physical activity level) and the physical environment (availability of a place to be active, safety of outdoor spaces, etc.) are likely to have similar reciprocal effects regarding an individual's decision to partake in a given physical activity. It is through this complex web of decision making that individuals decide to perform and follow through with certain physical activities. The bottom of Figure 1.7 describes how these series of decisions and behaviors (diet and physical activity) can lead to the presence of diet-related disease outcomes.

CAUSATION IN LOCAL FOOD ENVIRONMENT STUDIES

As we develop specific methods to quantify hypothesized relationships between the local availability of food for Americans and the impact on diets and diet-related diseases, it is important to be clear about how causation is inferred from the studies. The aim of epidemiologic studies is to identify causes of disease. In other scientific disciplines, the causal effect of an exposure can be controlled within lab experiments, thereby isolating the causal effect between the exposure and the out-come. Randomized control trials simulate laboratory studies by randomizing expo-sures to people and are used in settings such as the investigation of the effects of pharmaceuticals on disease or health education on behavioral changes. Also, with regard to environmental exposures, some small controlled chamber studies have been conducted where humans are exposed to particulate matter or other environ-mental compounds; however, studies that investigate the effects of environmental exposures on large human populations rarely use randomized controlled trials for ethical and practical reasons. Certainly in the case of investigating the effects of local food environments, it would be impractical to randomly *expose* humans to different types of local food environments and wait to observe a behavior or health outcome. Thus, one of the first challenges in determining causation between local food environments and behaviors or health is *isolating the exposure and directly observing the effect*. This issue is compounded by the fact that most diseases (and behaviors) develop because of *multiple component causes* (Rothman and Greenland 1998). In epidemiology, component causes are often referred to as *risk factors*. It often takes the presence of more than one risk factor to develop a disease. For instance, using the Framingham Risk Score, an individual's 10-year risk of having a heart attack can be calculated using an algorithm that includes values for several component causes of heart disease such as total cholesterol, smoking status, and blood pressure (http://cvdrisk.nhlbi.nih.gov/calculator.asp). The greater number of risk factors is associated with a higher risk of heart attack. These component causes are biological and behavioral, but environmental factors could also be included in such models. For instance, the number of supermarkets, fast-food restaurants, conve-nience stores, and so forth, may be considered potential component determinants of eating the recommended servings of fruits and vegetables per day or risk factors for diet-related health outcomes such as obesity. There is a third issue that makes mea-suring the causal effects of environmental exposures from randomized controlled trials challenging, which is the *length of time it takes for environmental exposures to produce an observable outcome*. The development of any disease often occurs over years, with much of the disease development happening without any diagnos-able symptoms, and therefore unmeasurable. Again, in the example of measuring the effect of exposure to local food environments, the duration of exposure required to cause a distal effect, such as obesity, may be lengthy, thereby making the use of randomized controlled trials impractical for these types of investigations.

For these reasons, the studies, which aim to measure causal relationships between local food environments and diet or disease, are typically observational studies. With these types of studies, investigators aim to simulate a randomized controlled trial by measuring the exposures and disease occurrence of a study population, using a comparison group to function as the *counterfactual* experience of the targeted study population (Rothman and Greenland 1998). The comparison group is intended to represent the matched experience of each person in the target study population such that only the exposure levels vary. This is of course in theory as it is not feasible to find comparison groups that match participants to this degree; however, it is the intended meaning of the comparison groups when reporting results from observa-tional studies.

Other criteria for inferring causation from observational studies of humans have been used in epidemiology. For instance, evidence of causation within a single study is evaluated with: (1) the magnitude and precision of the effect estimates, (2) dose–response of effects, (3) control for confounding factors, (4) consideration of effect modification, and (5) determination that the exposure precedes the outcome. These concepts are discussed in detail in Chapter 8. Overall, however, statistical inference is based on the concept that each study is aiming to measure the true relationship between local food environments and the behavior or health outcome. Hence, causation is inferred though statistical inference with a body of research where findings have been replicated in several study populations.

There are several causal questions within this area of public health that include, but are not limited to the following:

- Does the racial makeup of a geographic area cause food retailers to locate in an area?
- Does the income of the residents cause food retailers to locate in an area?
- Does the income or racial makeup of an area cause food retailers to sell different food products at different prices?
- Do the types of food retailers (and foods sold) in a given area cause local residents to purchase and consume the foods from those retailers?
- Do the types of food retailers (and food sold) in a given area cause local residents to gain weight, develop diabetes, have poor management of diet-related diseases, and so forth?

Although Figure 1.7 is helpful in terms of describing the minutiae involved in health decisions, statistical models would be oversaturated and require very large sample sizes to include this level of detail into models aimed to predict behaviors and health. Therefore, in the most basic terms, these questions require a more simplistic model that would lend itself to the development of statistical models and research protocols (Figure 1.8). Statistical models and research design can benefit from the development of simple visual descriptions such as these that describe the hypothesized pathways of associations between variables. The pathways for how factors such as racial segregation affect health can be quite complicated. The aim here is to develop very specific descriptions of the hypothesized relationships between the environment and individual level factors, and the directions of the hypothesized relationships. Again, these depictions can be used to develop protocols for measuring factors within the studies and also in building statistical models. Causes for human behavior and disease development are admittedly complicated multifactorial processes and other influences may play roles as modifiers of the main effects of interest, such as the effect of physical activity on the relationship between local food environments and obesity.

A very simple diagram describing the direction of the proposed relationships aims to describe the hypothesis that local food environments influence dietary intake through the local purchasing of food (Figure 1.8). The direction between local food environments and diet is hypothesized here to be unidirectional, from the environment to behavior. This may in fact be an oversimplified representation, as it is possible that people with better diets locate in areas where local food environments

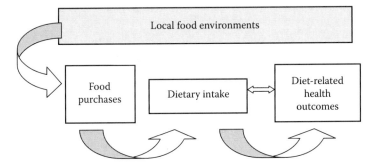

FIGURE 1.8 Simplified model of the relationship between local food environments, diet, and diet-related health outcomes.

are less restricted. In order for the direction of the relationship between local food environments and diet to be explored, specific types of study designs are needed, which are generally rather expensive. Therefore, early studies aimed to measure any association between local food environments and dietary intake with the rationale that if there are no associations, then the direction of those associations becomes a moot point.

Furthermore, local food environments influence diet-related health outcomes, such as obesity, through a pathway of difference in dietary intake. Here, the schematic hypothesizes a bidirectional relationship from diet to obesity whereby dietary choices influence weight gain and individuals' personal weight status influences their dietary choices. Note the relationship between diet-related health outcomes and the local food environment is not independent, rather dietary intake and food purchasing are intermediates of that relationship.

Whether the outcome of interest is fresh produce consumption, meeting federal guidelines for healthy eating, or more distal outcomes such as obesity or hunger, the ability of an investigator to detect any true effect is dependent on the specificity of the measurements of the independent and dependent variables included in statistical models. The ability to recognize, measure, and include in statistical modeling other factors that modify these effects also becomes important in interpreting the complicated relationships between environmental exposures and proximal and distal outcomes. The simplified causal model (Figure 1.8) is used in Chapters 4 through 6 to include other important factors that may be influencing the associations between local food environments and the health so that targeted interventions can be proposed and evaluated to improve the public health. In the final chapters (Chapters 9 and 10), we aim to describe solutions garnered for minimizing local food environment inequalities that are currently being conducted by federal, state, and local government agencies in the United States to reduce existing imbalances between local food environments that may stem from the American Food System described in Chapters 2 and 3. This is an emerging area of public health that requires the cooperation of a range of multidisciplinary experts from within and outside traditional public health, including members of affected communities, to conceive, implement, and evaluate environmental changes that will promote health for all Americans.

REFERENCES

Allison D. B., Fontaine K. R., Manson J. E., Stevens J., Vanitallie T. B. 1999. Annual deaths attributable to obesity in the United States. *JAMA* 282:1530–8.

Ball K., Timperio A. F., Crawford D. A. 2006. Understanding environmental influences on nutrition and physical activity behaviors: Where should we look and what should we count? *Int J Behav Nutr Phys Act* 3:33.

Baranowski T., Anderson C., Carmack C. 1998. Mediating variable framework in physical activity interventions: How are we doing? How might we do better? *Am J Prev Med* 15:266–97.

Baranowski T., Cullen K., Baranowski J. 1999. Psychosocial correlates of dietary intake: Advancing dietary intervention. *Ann Rev Nutr* 19:17–40.

Baranowski T., Cullen K. W., Nicklas T., Thompson D., Baranowski J. 2003. Are current health behavioral models helpful in guiding prevention of weight gain efforts? *Obes Res* 11:23S–43S.

Baranowski T., Perry C. L., Parcel G. S. 1997. How individuals, environments, and health behavior interact: Social cognitive theory. In *Health Behavior and Health Education* 2nd Edition, edited by K. Glanz, F. M. Lewis, and B. K. Rimer. San Francisco: Jossey-Bass.

Beesley C. Understanding gross margin and how it can make or break your startup. U.S. Small Business Administration. http://www.sba.gov/community/blogs/community-blogs/small-business-cents/understanding-gross-margin-and-how-it-can-make- (Accessed February 1, 2013).

Bere E. and Klepp K. I. 2004. Correlates of fruit and vegetable intake among Norwegian schoolchildren: Parental and self-reports. *Public Health Nutr* 7:991–8.

Blanchette L. and Brug J. 2005. Determinants of fruit and vegetable consumption among 6–12-year-old children and effective interventions to increase consumption. *J Hum Nutr Diet* 18:431–43.

Brown J. L. 2006. Nutrition. In *Social Injustice and Public Health*, edited by B. S. Levy and V. W. Sidel. New York: Oxford University Press.

Brown J. L. and D. Allen. 1988. Hunger in America. *Ann Rev Public Health* 9:503–26.

Bullard R. D. 1994. Introduction. In *Unequal Protection: Environmental Justice & Communities of Color*, edited by R. D. Bullard. San Francisco, CA: Sierra Club Books.

Campbell C. C. and Desjardins E. 1989. A model and research approach for studying the management of limited food resources by low-income families. *J Nutr Educ* 21:162–71.

Citizens' Board of Inquiry into Hunger and Malnutrition in America. 1977. *Hunger U.S.A. Revisited*. New York: NY Field Foundation.

Coleman-Jensen A., Nord M., Andrews M., Carlson S. 2011. Household Food Security in the United States in 2010. ERR-125, U.S. Department of Agriculture Economic Research Service.http://www.ers.usda.gov/publications/err-economic-research-report/err125.aspx (Accessed February 25, 2013).

Cullen K. W., Baranowski T., Rittenberry L., Olvera N. 2000. Social-environmental influences on children's diets: Results from focus groups with African-, Euro- and Mexican-American children and their parents. *Health Educ Res* 15:581–90.

Darmon N., Ferguson E. L., Briend A. 2002. A cost constraint alone has adverse effects on food selection and nutrient density: An analysis of human diets by linear programming. *J Nutr* 132:3764–71.

Dunne P. M., Lusch R. F., Carver J. R. 2011. *Retailing*. Mason, OH: South-Western.

East Harlem Online. 2012. East Harlem's History. http://www.east-harlem.com/cb11_197A_history.htm. (Accessed February 25, 2013).

Finkelstein E. A., Fiebelkorn I. C., Wang G. 2003. National medical spending attributable to overweight and obesity: How much and who's paying? *Health Aff* W3:219–26.

Fitzgibbon M. L. and Stolley M. R. 2004. Environmental changes may be needed for prevention of overweight in minority children. *Pediatr Ann* 33:45–9.

Flegal K. M., Carroll M. D., Kit B. K., Ogden C. L. 2012. Prevalence of obesity and trends in the distribution of body mass index among US adults, 1999–2010. *JAMA* 307:491–7.

Flegal K. M., Carroll M. D., Ogden C. L., Johnson C. L. 2002. Prevalence and trends in obesity among US adults, 1999–2000. *JAMA* 288:1723–7.

Food Marketing Institute. 2007. 2005 to Mark 75th Anniversary of the Supermarket—The Epitome of Consumer-Driven Innovation, Free Choice, Free Enterprise. http://www.fmi.org/news-room/news-archive/view/2004/11/29/2005-to-mark-75th-anniversary-of-the-supermarket-the-epitome-of-consumer-driven-innovation-free-choice-free-enterprise (Accessed July 7, 2013).

Food Marketing Institute. 2008. Competition and profit. http://www.fmi.org/docs/facts-figures/competitionandprofit.pdf?sfvrsn=2 (Accessed February 1, 2013).

Food Marketing Institute. 2010. http://www.fmi.org (Accessed February 1, 2013).

Food & Water Watch. 2010. Consolidation and Buyer Power in the Grocery Industry. http://documents.foodandwaterwatch.org/doc/RetailConcentration-web.pdf (Accessed October 30, 2013).

Hunger Notes. 2012. Hunger in America: 2012 United States Hunger and Poverty Facts. http://www.worldhunger.org/articles/12/us.htm (Accessed July 7, 2013).

Inc., Profit Margin. http://www.inc.com//encyclopedia/profit-margin.html (Accessed February 1, 2013).

Jago R., Baranowski T., Baranowski J. C. 2007. Fruit and vegetable availability: A micro environmental mediating variable? *Public Health Nutr* 10:681–9.

King R. P., Hand M. S., DiGiacomo G. et al. 2010. Comparing the Structure, Size, and Performance of Local and Mainstream Supply Chains. ERS Report Summary June 1, 2010. http://www.ers.usda.gov/publications/err-economic-research-report/err99.aspx#.UdomBBbPl8s (Accessed July 7, 2013).

Kremers S., de Bruijn G., Visscher T., van Mechelen W., de Vries N. K., Brug J. 2006. Environmental influences on energy balance-related behaviors: A dual-process view. *Int J Behav Nutr Phys Act* 3:9.

Kullen K. About King Kullen Supermarkets. http://www.kingkullen.com/about-us/ (Accessed July 7, 2013).

Lin B. H., Frazao E., Guthrie J. 1999. Away-From-Home Foods Increasingly Important to Quality of American Diet. AIB-749, United States Department of Agriculture (USDA), Economic Research Service. http://www.ers.usda.gov/publications/aib-agricultural-information-bulletin/aib749.aspx.

McMillian T. 2012. *The American Way of Eating: Undercover at Walmart, Applebee's, Farm Fields and the Dinner Table*. New York: Scribner.

McNeal R. B., Hansen W. B., Harrington N. G., Giles S. M. 2004. How all stars works: An examination of program effects on mediating variables. *Health Educ Behav* 31:165–78.

Morland K. B., Diez Roux A. V., Wing S. 2006. Supermarkets, other food stores and obesity: The atherosclerosis risk in communities study. *Am J Prev Med* 30:333–9.

Must A., Spadano J., Coakley E. H., Field A. E., Colditz G., Dietz W. H. 1999. The disease burden associated with overweight and obesity. *JAMA* 282:1523–9.

Neumark-Sztainer D., Wall M., Perry C., Story M. 2003. Correlates of fruit and vegetable intake among adolescents. Findings from Project EAT. *Prev Med* 37:198–208.

Physicians Task Force on Hunger in America. 1985. *Hunger in America: The Growing Epidemic*. Middletown, CT: Wesleyan University Press.

Pinson L. 2004. *Keeping the books: Basic Record Keeping and Accounting for the Successful Small Business*. Chicago. IL: Dearborn Trade Publishing.

Rosner B. 1995. *Fundamentals of Biostatistics*, 4th Ed. Boston, MA: Duxbury Press.

Rothman K. and S. Greenland. 1998. Causation and causal inference. In *Modern Epidemiology*, edited by K. J. Rothman and S. Greenland, pp. 7–28. Philadelphia: Lippincott-Raven.

Sooman A., Macintyre S., Anderson A. 1993. Scotland's health—a more difficult challenge for some? The price and availability of healthy foods in socially contrasting localities in the west of Scotland. *Health Bull* 51:276–84.

Stafford M., Cummins S., Ellaway A., Sacker A., Wiggins R. D., Macintyre S. 2007. Pathways to obesity: Identifying local, modifiable determinants of physical activity and diet. *Soc Sci Med* 65:1882–97.

Steptoe A., Perkins-Porras L., McKay C., Rink E., Hilton S., Cappuccio F. P. 2003. Psychological factors associated with fruit and vegetable intake and the biomarkers in adults from a low-income neighborhood. *Health Psychol* 22:148–55.

Stewart H., Blisard N., Joliffe D. 2006. Let's Eat Out: Americans Weigh Taste, Convenience, and Nutrition. EIB-19, United States Department of Agriculture (USDA), Economic Research Service.

Technomic.2006. *Trends in Healthier Eating and Fruit and Vegetable Usage in Chain Restaurants*. Wilmington, DE: Produce for Better Health Foundation.

Townsend M. S., Peerson J., Love B., Achterberg C., Murphy S. P. 2001. Food insecurity is positively related to overweight in women. *J Nutr* 131:1738–45.

U.S. Census Bureau. 2012. North American Industry Classification System: 2012 NAICS Definitions. http://www.census.gov/eos/www/naics (Accessed February 1, 2013).

U.S. Department of Agriculture. 2003. Profiling food consumption in America. In *Agriculture Fact Book 2001–2002*. Washington DC: U.S. Government Printing Office. http://www.usda.gov/factbook/chapter2.pdf (Accessed July 7, 2013).

U.S. Department of Agriculture (USDA). USDA Directory Records More Than 7,800 Farmers Markets. http://www.usda.gov/wps/portal/usda/usdamediafb?contentid=2012/08/0262.xml&printable=true&contentidonly=true (Accessed July 7, 2013).

U.S. Department of Agriculture (USDA), Economic Research Service. 2004. Food CPI, Prices and Expenditures: Expenditures on Food by selected Countries. http://www.ers.usda.gov/topics/food-markets-prices/food-prices,-expenditures-costs.aspx#.Udoy_hbPl8s (Accessed July 7, 2013).

U.S. Department of Agriculture (USDA), Economic Research Service. 2012. The Demand for Disaggregated Food-Away-From-Home and Food-at-Home Products in the United States. http://www.ers.usda.gov/publications/err-economic-research-report/err139.aspx (Accessed February 5, 2013).

U.S. Department of Agriculture (USDA) Economic Research Services. Food Desert Locator. http://www.ers.usda.gov/data-products/food-desert-locator.aspx.

U.S. Department of Agriculture (USDA), Economic Research Service. Food at Home: Total Expenditure (Table 2). http://www.ers.usda.gov/data-products/food-expenditures.aspx#26634 (Accessed February 1, 2013).

U.S. Department of Health and Human Services. 2012. Healthy People 2020. Nutrition and Weight Status. http://www.healthypeople.gov/2020/topicsobjectives2020/overview.aspx?topicid=29 (Accessed July 7, 2012).

U.S. Senate. Select Committee on Nutrition and Human Needs. 1973. "Hunger 1973" and press reaction: November 1973, pp. 1–74. Washington, DC: Government Printing Office.

World Health Organization. 1980. *Towards a Better Future: Maternal and Child Health*. Geneva, Switzerland: WHO.

2 U.S. Agricultural Policies and the U.S. Food Industry
Production to Retail

Arlene Spark

When there is a single power as large as Walmart connecting food processors and food consumers, individual consumers are no longer the food manufacturing industry's most important customer.

Wenonah Hauter (2012)

U.S. GOVERNMENT OVERSIGHT OF AGRICULTURE

For 150 years, food producers have worked intensely, if not intimately, with the House of Representatives and Senate Agricultural Committees and the United States Department of Agriculture (USDA) to develop what is informally known as the *agriculture establishment*. This establishment has united in a way to secure federal policies and legislation related to land use and food distribution that support the food industry. This has been done in several ways. First, many members of the Congressional Agricultural Committees are from the Great Plains farm states (see Figure 2.1). Second, committee members serve long terms, sometimes decades. Third, committee members are sometimes replaced with former food industry lobbyists and, conversely, some committee members become lobbyists themselves. As Marion Nestle says, "Today's public servant is tomorrow's lobbyist." The Congressional Agricultural Committees are important targets for the food industry lobby because it is legal to lobby for committee members, whereas it is not permitted for USDA members to interact with lobbyists (Nestle 2007).

FOOD INDUSTRY LOBBY

The food industry consists of four primary players: (1) producers, (2) processors, (3) distributors, and (4) retailers. Lobbying is a practice whereby companies hire people to influence political action (i.e., policies and legislation). In general, lobbyists offer expertise, make campaign contributions, provide perquisite (perks) such as lavish meals, and use other methods of persuasion to influence politicians to pass laws that support the companies that hire them. Note that lobbying is not technically

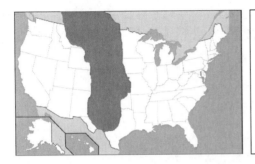

The Great Plains reaches from Mexico north into Canada and spreads west to the Rocky Mountains, encompassing parts of Colorado, Kansas, Montana, Nebraska, New Mexico, North Dakota, Oklahoma, South Dakota, Texas, and Wyoming, and the Canadian provinces of Alberta, Manitoba, and Saskatchewan.

FIGURE 2.1   Map of the Great Plains States. (From Wikipedia Commons, Map of the Great Plains,   http://upload.wikimedia.org/wikipedia/commons/4/49/Map_of_Great_Plains2.jpg, accessed July 28, 2013.)

TABLE 2.1
Lobbying Expenditures for Selected Agribusiness Companies: 1998–2010

Company	Type of Business	Amount
Wal-Mart	Retailer	$33,245,000
Kraft Foods	Food company	$13,155,000
Smithfield Foods	Food producer and processor	$9,635,000
Archer Daniels Midland	Food processor	$6,270,000
Tyson Foods	Food producer	$13,876,285
Dole Food Company	Food producer and distributor	$3,375,000
Monsanto	Seed producer	$46,522,720

Source: Food & Water Watch, *Farm Bill 101*, January 2012, http://www.foodandwaterwatch.org/tools -and-resources/farm-bill-101, accessed May 4, 2014.

or legally considered a form of bribery, although at times, there seems to be a fine line between the two practices. Lobbying refers to the act of trying to influence members of a legislative body to vote in favor of the lobbyist, whereas acts of bribery are defined as cases where cash or property is offered in exchange for a specific influence that tips in the briber's favor. Almost every major U.S. company has some sort of active lobby, and the corporations within the food industry are no exception. Food producers dominate the agricultural lobby, although it is estimated that there are hundreds of businesses within the food industry, ranging from producers to retailers that currently lobby to promote specific policies that favor their ability to profit within the industry. The agribusiness lobby spent about $65 million in 2011–2012; hence the interests of agricultural corporations remain highly represented (OpenSecrets 2012). Examples of monetary amounts paid to lobby by different types of companies within the food industry are presented in Table 2.1.

The reason agricultural policy has favored farmers over the course of U.S. history is also attributed, in part, to the fact that farmers tend to have favorable proportional political representation in Congress. Since there are two senators per state, regardless of how small the population of that state may be, people living in rural states are effectively granted more power per person than people in populated states. Also, because the 435-member House of Representatives is reapportioned only once every 10 years (following the constitutionally mandated decennial census), and because the population tends to shift from rural to urban areas,[*] farmers are often left with greater proportional power until the reapportionment is complete.

U.S. Department of Agriculture

The United States Department of Agriculture (informally, the Agriculture Department or USDA) is the U.S. federal executive department responsible for developing and executing national policy on farming, agriculture, and food. The department was formed in 1862 by President Abraham Lincoln and received cabinet status in 1889 under President Grover Cleveland. The department's aims are both bold and daunting. They include meeting the needs of farmers and ranchers, promoting agricultural trade and production, working to assure food safety, protecting natural resources, fostering rural communities, and ending hunger in the United States and abroad.

The USDA is headed by a secretary, whose nomination by the president must be approved by Congress. The secretary has historically represented agribusiness in some form. For instance, during the Reagan administration, USDA Secretary John Block was a hog farmer from Illinois. Other high-ranking positions at the USDA have been filled with a former director of the American Meat Institute and a lobbyist from the National Cattlemen's Association (Nestle 2007). Currently, the Senate unanimously confirmed Democratic President Barack Obama's choice of Thomas J. Vilsack, a Democrat and 1999–2007 governor of Iowa (home of the largest number of pork producers) as the 30th USDA Secretary. From 2008 to 2012, Secretary Vilsack oversaw a budget of almost $300 billion and more than 100,000 employees (USDA 2012a).

U.S. FARM BILL

The United States supports the agricultural sector through a variety of programs, and the primary legal framework for agricultural policy is set through a legislative process that occurs periodically through the development of a Farm Bill. *The Farm Bill* is a phrase that refers to omnibus legislation—a giant piece of multiyear legislation that deals with many subjects and programs. Congress drafts, debates, and passes a Farm Bill every 5–7 years. In legal terms, functions of the bill include amending some provisions of laws enacted through earlier farm bills and suspending many; reauthorizing, amending, or repealing provisions of preceding temporary agricultural acts; and establishing new policy provisions for a limited time into the

---

[*] The U.S. Census reports a decrease in rural population and increase in urban population decennially from 1790 to 2010. The urban population increased from 5.1% of the total population in 1790 to 80.7% in 2010. The migration of labor geographically, out of rural areas, and occupationally, out of farm jobs, is one of the most pervasive features of agricultural transformations and economic growth. This is true for developed and less developed countries.

future (USDA 2012b). Actually, the term *farm bill* is a misnomer (USDA 2011). In addition to farming, the legislation involves ecology, economics, employment, energy, nutrition, research, and trade. Thus, food activists and many others feel the legislation should be called the *Food and Farm Bill* as most of the money involved is earmarked for domestic antihunger nutrition programs (Johnson 2008a,b).

NAMING AND TITLES OF THE U.S. FARM BILLS

Since 1965, each farm bill has been given a new name; the name is a significant marketing tool, because it reflects both what is important in the bill and what the authors want the public to think is important about the bill. In the 2008 Farm Bill titled the Food, Conservation, and Energy Act, the word *food* signals that the bill contains provisions that are important to consumers; *conservation* calls attention to the importance of the environment; and *energy* points to concerns about high fuel prices and its effect on food prices. Beginning in 1973, farm bills have included titles for major issue areas. New titles are added as new scopes of work become crucial to the food and farm economy. The 2008 Farm Bill had 15 titles, up from 10 in 2002. Organic agriculture appeared for the first time in 2008. Table 2.2 presents the current Farm Bill's titles, major issues, and functions.

As indicated in Table 2.3, the 5-year price tag of the 2008 Farm Bill was estimated at about $290 billion (and $604 billion over 10 years). The bulk of the multibillion dollar cost was borne by two titles: Nutrition, primarily Supplemental

---

TABLE 2.2

2014 Farm Bill (P.L. 113-79): Functions and Major Issues, by Title

  I.   **Commodity Programs:** Provides farm payments when crop prices or revenues decline for major commodity crops, including wheat, corn, soybeans, peanuts, and rice. Includes disaster programs to help livestock and tree fruit producers manage production losses due to natural disasters. Other support includes margin insurance for dairy and marketing quotas, minimum price guarantees, and import barriers for sugar.

 II.   **Conservation:** Encourages environmental stewardship and improved management practices. Working lands programs include Environmental Quality Incentives Program (EQIP) and Conservation Stewardship Program (CSP). Land retirement programs include the Conservation Reserve Program (CRP). Other aid is in the Agricultural Conservation Easement Program (ACEP) and Regional Conservation Partnership Program (RCPP).

III.   **Trade:** Provides support for U.S. agricultural export programs and international food assistance programs. Major programs included Market Access Program (MAP) and the primary U.S. food aid program, Food for Peace, which provides emergency and nonemergency food aid, among other programs. Other provisions address program changes related to World Trade Organization (WTO) obligations.

 IV.   **Nutrition:** Provides nutrition assistance for low-income households through programs including the Supplemental Nutrition Assistance Program (SNAP, formerly known as food stamps) and The Emergency Food Assistance Program (TEFAP). Also supports the distribution of foods in schools.

  V.   **Credit:** Provides support for federal direct and guaranteed loans to farmers and ranchers, and loan eligibility rules and policies.

TABLE 2.2
2014 Farm Bill (P.L. 113-79): Functions and Major Issues, by Title

VI.   Rural Development: Supports business and community programs for planning, feasibility assessments, and coordination with other local, state, and federal programs. Programs include grants and loans for infrastructure, economic development, broadband and telecommunications, among other programs.

VII.   Research, Extension, and Related Matters: Supports a wide range of agricultural research and extension programs that help farmers and ranchers become more efficient, innovative, and productive. Other types of research programs include biosecurity and response, biotechnology, and organic production.

VIII.   Forestry: Supports forestry management programs run by USDA's Forest Service.

IX.   Energy: Supports the development of farm and community renewable energy systems through grants, loan guarantees, and procurement assistance initiatives. Provisions cover the production, marketing, and processing of biofuels and biofuel feedstocks, and research, education, and demonstration programs.

X.   Horticulture: Supports specialty crops—fruits, vegetables, tree nuts, and floriculture and ornamental products—through a range of initiatives, including market promotion; plant pest and disease prevention; and public research; among other initiatives. Also provides assistance to support certified organic agricultural production.

XI.   Crop Insurance: Enhances the permanently authorized federal crop insurance program. New plans include Stacked Income Protection (STAX) for cotton and Supplemental Coverage Option (SCO) for other crops.

XII.   Miscellaneous: Programs not covered in other titles, including provisions affecting livestock and poultry production and limited-resource and socially disadvantaged farmers, among other provisions.

TABLE 2.3
Budget for the 2014 Farm Bill: Ranked by Projected Outlays

Rank	Title Number	Title	Projected Outlay
1	IV	Nutrition	756,432
2	XI	Crop insurance	89,827
3	II	Conservation	57,600
4	I	Commodities	44,458
5	III	Trade	3,574
6	XII	Miscellaneous	2,634
7	X	Horticulture	1,755
8	VII	Research	1,256
9	IX	Energy	1,122
10	VI	Rural development	241
11	VIII	Forestry	13
12	V	Credit	−2.240

Source: R. M. Chite, Congressional Research Service, 2014, The 2014 Farm Bill (P.L. 113-79): Summary and Side-by-Side, CRS 7-5700 R43076, February 12, 2014. http://www.farmland.org/programs/federal/documents/2014_0213_CRS_FarmBillSummary.pdf, accessed May 5, 2014.

Note: 10 year total, FY2014-FY2023. Outlays in millions of dollars.

Nutrition Assistance Program (SNAP) ($188.9 billion), and Commodity Programs ($41.6 billion). The next two most costly titles were Conservation ($24.1 billion) and Crop Insurance and Disaster Assistance Programs ($21.9 billion). The 5-year cost of the 2008 Farm Bill was estimated to be slightly less than that of its predecessor, the 2002 Farm Security and Rural Development Act ($241 billion). Despite the overall lower cost of the 2008 Bill, several titles within the 2008 Bill actually increased in cost (Conservation, Trade, Nutrition, Rural Development, Research, and Energy). Although a full 5-year Farm Bill was not passed in 2012, the then current policies contained in the 2008 Bill were extended through September 30, 2013.

Traditionally, farm bills have not provided livestock and poultry producers with price- and income-support programs such as those established for the commodity crops (e.g., grains and oilseeds). Instead, the livestock and poultry industries have looked to government for leadership to bolster buyers' confidence that their products are safe, of high quality, and free from pests and diseases, and the 2008 Farm Bill was the first to include a title (XI) that specifically covered livestock and poultry issues. Some groups favor more government oversight of the industry to address competition issues. Other groups, such as the National Cattleman's Beef Association, oppose a separate livestock title in future farm bills to minimize government's oversight of their industry (Chite 2012).

There are other areas of the farm bill that concern livestock and poultry producers. For example, the government authorizes conservation programs that take croplands out of production, and also provides incentives that might shift corn to fuel use, both of which increase the price of corn as a feed ingredient. Other farm bill *conservation* programs, such as the Environmental Quality Incentives Program (EQIP) (USDA 2012c), have supported building the actual infrastructure for large animal feeding operations to process their waste (Imhoff 2010); so in this regard the legislation may actually damage natural resources. Not surprisingly, the livestock industry lobbied for EQIP, whereas the progressive farm groups, such as the National Sustainable Agriculture Coalition and the National Family Farm Coalition, supported the large conservation program, the Conservation Stewardship Program (CSP) (USDA 2012d).

New Farm Bill Signed into Law in 2014

The 2008 farm law, the *Food, Conservation, and Energy Act*, remained in effect through 2012. Many provisions of the 2008 Farm Bill expired in 2012, but were extended through the American Taxpayer Relief Act of 2012 (P. L. 112-240, also known as *the fiscal cliff bill*). The 2014 bill is the latest chapter in the legislation's history, which dates back to its origin during the Great Depression. Almost a trillion dollars in mandatory outlays will be available for programs for the 10-year period 2014–2023. Within this total, about three-quarters will be available for nutrition programs such as Food Stamps (now known as the SNAP) within the Nutrition title, about one-quarter for farm commodity support, crop insurance, and conservation). The remaining roughly less than one-half of 1% of mandatory funding would cover the other farm bill titles. All of these programs have mandatory funding, meaning that their continuation is virtually guaranteed. On the other hand, programs with discretionary funding survive, or fall, at the hands of the Appropriations Committee. They are authorized in the farm bill but paid for separately in annual appropriations bills (Johnson and Monke 2013).

OVERVIEW AND HISTORY OF THE FARM BILL

To fully understand how U.S. federal agriculture policies are driven almost entirely by one bill, it is important to understand how the Farm Bill was created. For instance, the first Farm Bill was created during the Great Depression at the height of a severe worldwide economic depression in the decade preceding World War II. It was the longest, most widespread, and deepest depression of the twentieth century. In the 1920s, production surpluses aggravated unemployment and lack of consumer buying power. The depression originated in the United States, after the fall in stock prices that began in September 1929, and became worldwide news with the stock market crash of October 29, 1929 (known as Black Tuesday). The timing of the Great Depression varied across nations, but in most countries it started in 1930 and lasted until the late 1930s or middle 1940s. The Great Depression had devastating effects in countries both rich and poor. Personal income, tax revenue, profits, and prices dropped, whereas international trade plunged by more than 50%. Unemployment in the United States rose to 25%, and in some countries rose as high as 33%. People nationally and internationally could not afford to buy the crops and animals that the U.S. farms produced, and the drought made it increasingly difficult for farmers to plant and harvest their crops. As a result, many farmers lost their farms, and many moved out of the agricultural Great Plains states (Figure 2.1) in search of any kind of work they could find. Many relocated to the West Coast where they became migrant farm laborers.

Thus, the Farm Bill was originally developed as an emergency measure for farmers during the Great Depression. When Franklin D. Roosevelt (FDR) became president, U.S. farmers were producing extraordinary amounts of corn. According to the law of supply and demand, the glut on the market led to an increased supply, which caused a decrease in demand per unit of crop, resulting in decreased profits for the farmers. Thus, farmers who produced large amounts of crops suffered financially. To remedy the situation, one of FDR's first acts of his *New Deal** was authorizing the Agricultural Adjustment Act of 1933, regarded as the first farm bill. The legislation restricted agricultural production so commodity prices would increase. Farmers were paid a subsidy to restrict their output, which was paid to farmers through a tax levied exclusively on companies that processed farm products.

The Act established the USDA's Agricultural Adjustment Administration (AAA) to implement a *domestic allotment* plan that subsidized producers of basic commodities for cutting their output. Its goal was the restoration of prices paid to farmers for their goods to a level equal in purchasing power to that of 1909–1914, a period of relatively comparative prosperity.

---

* The New Deal was a series of economic programs enacted between 1933 and 1936, during FDR's first term as president. In response to the Great Depression, the programs focused on what historians call the three R's: Relief (for the unemployed and poor), Recovery (of the economy to pre-Depression levels), and Reform (of the financial system to prevent another depression).

The Food Surplus Commodities Corporation, previously known as the Federal Surplus Relief Corporation, was established in 1935 with funding through the Agricultural Adjustment Act to reestablish farmers' purchasing power by supporting agricultural exports and encouraging domestic consumption of surpluses, called commodity crops. In 1936, the U.S. Supreme Court ruled the act was unconstitutional because the tax structure used to fund the program was deemed an overreach of the powers of the federal government. Congress promptly replaced it with the Soil Conservation and Domestic Allotment Act, which encouraged conservation by paying benefits for planting soil-building crops that would not be sold on the market, such as alfalfa, instead of staple crops such as corn and wheat. On signing the Soil Conservation and Domestic Allotment Act in 1936, FDR said,

> The new law has three major objectives which are inseparably and of necessity linked with the national welfare. The first of these aims is conservation of the soil itself through wise and proper land use. The second purpose is the reestablishment and maintenance of farm income at fair levels so that the great gains made by agriculture in the past 3 years can be preserved and national recovery can continue. The third major objective is the protection of consumers by assuring adequate supplies of food and fiber now and in the future.

Peters and Woolley 1936

Another piece of New Deal legislation, the Agricultural Adjustment Act of 1938, empowered the AAA in years of good crops to make loans to farmers on staple crop yields and to store the surplus produce, which could then be released in years of low yield. The Agriculture Adjustment Act instituted the recurring farm bill every 5 years, and created price supports for corn, cotton, and wheat. This was later expanded to include soybeans, barley, oats, rice, other grains, and dairy. Fruits and vegetables, as well as livestock, were largely excluded. Farmers' cash income doubled between 1932 and 1936, but it took the enormous demands of World War II to reduce the accumulated farm surpluses and to increase farm income. The following subsections contain a further discussion of commodity crops.

U.S. COMMODITY CROPS AND SUBSIDIES

Commodity food crops include wheat, feed grains (grain used as fodder, such as maize or corn, sorghum, barley, and oats), milk, rice, peanuts, sugar, and oilseeds, such as soybeans. An agricultural subsidy is governmental assistance paid to farmers and agribusinesses to supplement their income, manage the supply of agricultural commodities, and influence the cost and supply of such commodities.

COMMODITY CROPS AND SUBSIDIES RESULT IN "CHEAP FOOD"

Artificially low prices may result from commodities that are subsidized. Since the 1970s, when Earl Butz was Secretary of Agriculture (1971–1976), U.S. agriculture has operated under a *cheap food* policy that was spurred by the production of a few commodity crops, and thus American's consumption of the calories from these commodity crops. In an interview from the movie *King Corn*, Earl Butz said that beforeprior to his term as the 18th Secretary of Agriculture (1971–1976), farmers were paid not to produce, which he then described as, "...one of the stupidest things we ever did, I think" (*King Corn* 2007). The policy shifts enacted under Butz came about when oil shortages and inflation pushed up food prices—provoking widespread hunger abroad, as well as the rise of major agribusiness corporations and the declining financial stability of small family farms in the United States. He has been associated with starting the rise of corn production, large commercial farms, and the abundance of corn consumed in American diets. In the *King Corn* interview, Butz claims that the current system of increased agricultural production in the United States has driven food prices down, such that now we only pay about 17% of our incomes on food (whereas earlier generations paid twice that amount). Consequently, we now live in an *age of plenty*. He acknowledged that his policies led to large-scale farming created by farmers who took out huge bank loans in response to his repeated exhortation to *get big or get out*. Ultimately, this practice was responsible for thousands of smaller farms foreclosing during the farm financial crisis of the 1980s.

Because government subsidizes the production of corn, soybeans, and other commodity crops, farmers are incentivized to grow prodigious quantities of these commodities. In and of themselves, commodity crops are not unhealthy; rather, the problem lies in the fact that we do not directly consume some of these crops, such as corn and soybeans. For example, only about 1% of U.S.-produced corn is consumed directly by humans with the majority instead turned into biofuels, fed to livestock, or processed into additives such as high-fructose corn syrup (HFCS),* or hydrogenated vegetable oils (Russo 2011).

Subsidies have resulted in market distortions, leading to the following current situations:

- Corn processed into HFCS has become a ubiquitous ingredient in American food processing since the 1970s because of its low cost, ease of production, and widespread availability.
  - Health consequences: This, in turn, has led the average American who consumes processed foods to ingest large amounts of HFCS. Although increased fructose consumption in many developed nations coincides with the increased prevalence of obesity, this association does not prove causation. However, fructose metabolism in the liver does favor lipogenesis (fat production), and a number of studies have shown that fructose consumption induces hyperlipidemia (elevated blood levels of fat) and particularly increases the kind of fat known as triglycerides after meals. These effects may be pronounced in people with the metabolic syndrome (existing hyperlipidemia and insulin resistance) (Havel 2005).

---

* Table sugar (that is, sucrose) is disaccharide (two-sugar unit) made up of a molecule of glucose bonded to a molecule of fructose—a 50–50 mixture of the two. The fructose, which is almost twice as sweet as glucose, is what distinguishes sugar from other carbohydrate-rich foods such as bread or potatoes that break down upon digestion to glucose alone. The more fructose in a substance, the sweeter it will be. In comparison, HFCS is about 55% fructose, and the remaining 45% is nearly all glucose. After digestion, each of these sugars ends up as glucose and fructose in our small intestines.

- Soybeans ground up into a meal, with the meal going to feed cows, and the liquid skimmed off and turned into fat-based additives such as trans-fatty-acid-rich, partially hydrogenated vegetable oils.
  - Health consequences: Trans fatty acids have been shown to be athero-genic—they increase the risk of coronary heart disease by raising levels of low-density lipoproteins and lowering levels of high-density lipopro-teins. Starting in 2007, New York City banned trans fats in restaurants, bakeries, and other food-service establishments, the first major city to institute such legislation. Within 5 years, the average trans fat content of fast-food restaurant meals dropped from about 3 to 0.5 g (Lichtenstein 2012).
- Corn fed to cattle in corporate animal feed operations known as concen-trated animal feeding operations (CAFOs). This is an industrial farming practice that pushes down the price of meat, poultry, and eggs with the ability to raise huge numbers of animals at once in a small space. In the industrial system of meat production, meat animals are raised where their mobility is restricted. They are fed a high-calorie, grain-based diet, often supplemented with antibiotics and hormones. Feed is brought to the ani-mals rather than the animals grazing or otherwise seeking feed in pastures, fields, or on rangeland. Their waste is concentrated and becomes an envi-ronmental problem (UCS 2012b).
  - Health consequences: A lower overall fat content of grass-fed cattle may reduce the risk of some types of cancer. Steak from grass-fed animals tends to have higher levels of the omega-3 fatty acid alpha-linolenic acid (ALA) and sometimes has higher levels of the omega-3 fatty acids eicos-apentaenoic acid (EPA) and docosahexaenoic acid (DHA). Ground beef from grass-fed cattle usually has higher levels of conjugated linoleic acid (CLA). Milk from pasture-raised cattle tends to have higher levels of ALA and consistently higher levels of CLA. The evidence supporting the health benefits of omega-3 fatty acids and CLA is mixed; the data are stronger for some fatty acids than for others. The strongest evidence, encompassing animal studies as well as experimental and observational studies of humans, supports the effects of EPA/DHA on reducing the risk of heart disease. ALA also appears to reduce the risk of fatal and acute heart attacks. Finally, animal research on CLA has shown many positive effects on heart disease, cancer, and the immune system, but these results have yet to be duplicated in human studies (Clancy 2006).

COMMODITY FOODS AND USDA NUTRITION PROGRAMS

Because of the overproduction of dairy products, eggs, flour, and seasonal fruits and vegetables, some of these commodity foods are purchased by the USDA for distribu-tion to nutrition assistance programs. Thus, the USDA's commodity foods programs serve a dual purpose, maintaining the price of certain food products and ensuring that at-risk populations receive calories. This arrangement is believed to benefit both farmer and consumer alike (Table 2.4).

TABLE 2.4
USDA's Commodity Domestic Nutrition Assistance Programs

Food Distribution Programs

1. Commodity Supplemental Food Program (CSFP) provides nutritious USDA commodity foods to supplement the diet of the same population served by WIC but who are not WIC participants.
2. Food Distribution Program on Indian Reservations provides commodity foods to low-income households, including the elderly, living on Indian reservations, and to Native American families residing in designated areas near reservations.
3. The Emergency Food Assistance Program (TEFAP) makes USDA commodity foods available to States, which provide the food to local agencies that they have selected, usually food banks, which in turn, distribute the food to soup kitchens and food pantries that directly serve the public.

Child Nutrition Programs

1. Child and Adult Care Food Program (CACFP) provides nutritious foods to day care centers, to adults who receive care in nonresidential adult day care centers, and to children residing in homeless shelters, and youths participating in eligible after-school care programs.
2. Fresh Fruit and Vegetable Program provides free fresh fruits and vegetables in selected low-income elementary schools nationwide.
3. National School Lunch Program (NSLP) provides cash subsidies and donated USDA commodities to school districts and independent schools that choose to take part in the lunch program. In return, the organizations must serve lunches that meet federal requirements, and they must offer free or reduced-price lunches to eligible children. School food authorities can also be reimbursed for snacks served to children through age 18 in after-school educational or enrichment programs.
4. School Breakfast Program, like the NSLP, provides cash subsidies to participating schools that serve breakfast.
5. Special Milk Program provides milk to participating schools and institutions, which receive reimbursement from the USDA for each half pint of milk served. They must operate their milk programs on a nonprofit basis. They agree to use the Federal reimbursement to reduce the selling price of milk to all children.
6. Summer Food Service Program (SFSP) helps fill the hunger gap during summer when the NSLP and SPP are not available.

Women, Infants, and Children (WIC) provides nutritious foods to supplement diets, information on healthy eating, and referrals to health care to low-income women, infants, and children up to age five who are at nutritional risk.

1. Farmers' Market Nutrition Program provides fresh, unprepared, locally grown fruits and vegetables from local farmers' markets to WIC recipients.
2. Senior Farmers' Market Nutrition Program awards grants to States to provide low-income seniors with coupons that can be exchanged for eligible foods at farmers' markets, roadside stands, and community-supported agriculture programs.

Source: R. A. Aussenberg and K. J. Colello, Domestic food assistance: summary of programs, Congressional Research Service, January 27, 2014, http://www.fas.org/sgp/crs/misc/R42353.pdf, accessed May 4, 2014.

Historically, the government subsidized food purchased through the Food Stamp Program for those in need, as long as those purchases were viewed as helping to reduce the nation's agricultural surplus. From the inception of the Food Stamp Program (now called SNAP), the government had a say in what could be purchased, and because surpluses change with the natural cycle of the seasons, the list was updated monthly.

Emergency Food Assistance Program

The Emergency Food Assistance Program (TEFAP) helps supplement the diets of low-income Americans, including elderly people, by providing them with emergency food and nutrition assistance at no cost. Under TEFAP, the USDA makes commodity foods available to state distributing agencies. The amount of food that each state receives out of the total amount of food that is provided is based on the number of unemployed persons and the number of people with incomes below the poverty level in the state. States provide the food to local agencies that they have selected, usually food banks, which in turn, distribute the food to local organizations such as soup kitchens and food pantries that directly serve the public. States also provide the food to other types of local organizations, such as community action agencies that distribute the foods directly to needy households. These local organizations distribute the donated commodities to eligible recipients for household consumption, or use them to prepare and serve meals in a congregate setting. Recipients of food for home use must meet income eligibility criteria set by the states. Under TEFAP, the states also receive administrative funds to support the storage and distribution of the donated commodities. These funds must, in part, be passed down to local agencies.

First authorized in 1981 to distribute surplus commodities to households, the program was designed to help reduce federal food inventories and storage costs, while assisting the needy. Stocks of some foods held in surplus had been depleted by 1988. Therefore, the Hunger Prevention Act of 1988 authorized funds to be appropriated for the purchase of commodities specifically for TEFAP. Foods acquired with appropriated funds are in addition to any surplus commodities donated to TEFAP by the USDA.

Congress appropriated almost $300 million for TEFAP for FY 2009—$250 million to purchase food, and the remainder for administrative support for state and local agencies. With enactment of the American Recovery and Reinvestment Act of 2009,* Congress provided an additional $100 million for FY 2009 TEFAP food purchases and $25 million for administrative support. In addition to commodities purchased with appropriated funds, TEFAP receives surplus commodities. In FY 2008, almost $180 million worth of commodities were made available to TEFAP.

---

* The American Recovery and Reinvestment Act of 2009, commonly referred to as the Stimulus or The Recovery Act, is an economic stimulus package enacted in 2009 in response to the 2008 recession. The primary objective for the Act was to save and create jobs and, secondarily, to provide temporary relief programs for those most impacted by the recession.

Commodity Supplemental Food Program

Commodity Supplemental Food Program (CSFP) works to improve the health of low-income pregnant and breast-feeding women, other new mothers up to 1 year post-partum, infants, children up to age 6, and elderly people at least 60 years of age by supplementing their diets with USDA commodity foods. CSFP food packages do not provide a complete diet, but rather are good sources of some nutrients typically lacking in the diets of the target population. Among the foods provided are canned fruits and vegetables, canned meats, bottled unsweetened fruit, and dried beans. The population served by CSFP is similar to that served by Women, Infants, and Children (WIC), but CSFP also serves the elderly, and provides actual food rather than the food vouchers that WIC participants receive. The income limit for the elderly is 130% or below the Federal Poverty Income Guidelines,* and for others it is 185% or below the guidelines, but not below 100% of the guidelines. CSFP recipients are provided with referrals to other welfare, nutrition, and health-care programs such as SNAP, Medicaid, and Medicare. Eligible people cannot participate in CSFP and WIC at the same time. For FY 2012, Congress appropriated $176.8 million for CSFP (USDA 2012e).

National School Lunch Program Profit Programs

The National School Lunch Program Profit Program (NSLP) provides after-school snacks to children, using the same income eligibility basis as school meals. However, programs that operate in areas where at least 50% of students are eligible for free or reduced-price meals may serve all their snacks for free. Most of the support USDA provides to schools comes in the form of a cash reimbursement for each meal served. The most recent basic cash reimbursement rates, if school food authorities served less than 60% free and reduced-price lunches during the second preceding school year, are as follows:

- Free lunches (and snacks): $2.86 ($0.78)
- Reduced-price lunches (and snacks): $2.46 ($0.39)
- Paid lunches (and snacks): $0.27 ($0.07)

School food authorities that are certified to be in compliance with the most recent meal requirements receive an additional 6 cents of reimbursement for each meal served. Higher reimbursement rates are also in effect for Alaska and Hawaii, as well as for schools with high percentages of low-income students. The latest reimbursement rates can be viewed from USDA (USDA 2013a).

Summer Food Service Program

The Summer Food Service Program (SFSP) helps assure that eligible populations have access to nutritious meals during the summer months. When school is not in session, SFSP provides reimbursement to community agencies offering the required

---

* The poverty guidelines are designated by the year in which they are issued. The 2012 Federal Income Guidelines are available at http://aspe.hhs.gov/poverty/12poverty.shtml#guidelines. To put the government's definition of *poverty* in perspective, for the period July 1, 2012, through June 30, 2013, 130% of the poverty level is $29,965 and 185% is $42,643 for a family of four living in one of the 48 contiguous states or the District of Columbia.

continuum of meals. Eligible participants include children 0–18 years of age whose family incomes are less than or equal to 185% of the Federal Poverty Guidelines, and income-eligible adults over 18 years of age who have been determined by a state educational agency to have a disability and who participate in a school-based program for the disabled during the school year. SFSP contracts with schools and other community-based organizations to sponsor the local programs and provide meals that meet established guidelines (USDA 2013b).

Child and Adult Care Food Program

The Child and Adult Care Food Program (CACFP) plays a vital role in improving the quality of day care and making it more affordable for many low-income families. Each day, 3.3 million children receive nutritious meals and snacks through CACFP. The program also provides meals and snacks to 120,000 adults who receive care in nonresidential adult day care centers. CACFP reaches even further to provide meals to children residing in emergency shelters, and snacks and suppers to youths participating in eligible after-school care programs.

Eligible public or private nonprofit child care centers, outside-school-hours care centers, Head Start programs, and other institutions that are licensed or approved to provide day care services may participate in CACFP, either independently or as sponsored centers. *At-Risk* after-school care programs that offer enrichment activities for at-risk children and youth after the regular school day ends can provide free meals and snacks for those aged 18 and under through CACFP. Programs must be offered in areas where at least 50% of the children are eligible for free and reduced-price meals based on school data. Emergency shelters that provide residential food services offer up to three meals a day to homeless children and youth. Adult day care centers that provide structured, comprehensive services to nonresidential adults who are functionally impaired, or aged 60 and above, may participate in CACFP either as independent or as sponsored centers (USDA 2013c).

IMPORTS AND EXPORTS

In addition to use in domestic programs, the overproduction of commodity crops are leveraged within international markets, a tradition that dates back to World War II. As the war began, what had been a small but steady flow of agricultural exports suddenly dropped as shipping became dangerous. Then the U.S. Navy began protecting convoys, and demand from the Allies grew. The quantity of agricultural exports increased and remained high for the next 40 years. As demand for exports increased, the American farmers came to rely on exports to prop up prices and farm incomes. As the United States grew and farmers moved west, the domestic market grew faster than the world market. Exports were still important, but it was cheaper to ship produce across the country than across the seas. All of that changed during and after World War II.

By 1943, the government bought most of all the lower grades of beef produced in the United States, and up to one-half of all other beef cuts, butter, veal, lamb, and canned fruits and vegetables. The war made the government the de facto controller of the export market, and the export market proved to be the foundation for farm incomes.

When World War II ended, the United States provided monetary support to help rebuild European economies by removing trade barriers, modernizing industry, and making Europe prosperous again through the Marshall Plan (1948–1952, officially, the European Recovery Program). Thus, the Marshall Plan continued the U.S. government's involvement in exports.

International trade is a two-way street and the United States simultaneously imports many agricultural products and exports others. Before World War II, imports into the United States were dominated by rubber, coffee, and sugar. By the end of the twentieth century, fruits and vegetables were the largest agricultural imports, followed by coffee, grains, and meat. In some cases, these commodities compete directly with U.S. production. But in other ways, they provide U.S. consumers with new choices, such as the ability to eat fruits and vegetables that are not in season. For instance, produce grown during the summer months in Central and South America supplies U.S. citizens with fresh produce during the country's winter months (Genzel 2012).

As indicated in Figure 2.2, from 1998 to 2011, U.S. agricultural exports almost tripled, from about $51.8 billion to about $141.3 billion. During the same period, U.S. agricultural imports more than tripled from about $36.9 billion to $102.9 billion. In general, agricultural trade increases have paralleled gross farm income (Schnepf 2012).

Over the years, continued and ever-expanding subsidies for corn, soy, and other *commodity crops* have helped to fuel increased supplies of these crops, which gave rise to a number of phenomena. First, there are increased exports, which disadvantage farmers in countries such as Mexico that cannot produce their crops at competitive prices. Second, corn is fermented into ethanol (the residual grains are fed to

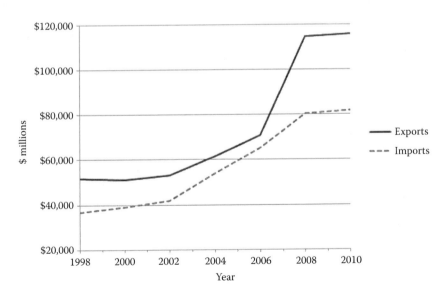

FIGURE 2.2 U.S. Agricultural trade since 1998. (From USDA, Economic Research Service, Foreign Agricultural Trade of the United States [FATUS], http://www.ers.usda.gov/data-products/foreign-agricultural-trade-of-the-united-states-(fatus)/calendar-year.aspx, accessed July 24, 2013.)

animals). Third, most corn grown by American farmers is not eaten by people, but rather is fed to animals in feedlots and livestock warehouses, thus effectively lowering the cost of animal protein in the United States. Fourth, corn is used to produce sweeteners, such as HFCS,* which has primarily replaced sucrose (table sugar) in U.S. food production. In addition to corn subsidies, other factors that have resulted in the proliferation and ubiquity of HFCS include governmental production quotas on domestic sugar and a tariff on imported sugar, which combine to raise the price of sucrose to levels above those of the rest of the world, thus making HFCS cheaper for many sweetener applications (Groombridge 2001). In short, we have become a nation with a preference for meats and items containing HFCS because these foods are comparatively cheap. Corn subsidies have driven the popularity of food such as hamburgers and soft drinks in the United States, and as cheap food agricultural policies were enacted, obesity has replaced hunger as the more prevalent nutritional problem in the United States.

Specialty Crops

Since 1996, farm bills traditionally treated fruits and vegetables as specialty crops separately from program crops, such as wheat and cotton, which have subsidies tied to their acres. However, many public health advocates and agricultural economists are now calling for a change in Farm Bill legislation that currently rewards the production of commodity crops over fruits and vegetables. All recent credible food guidance systems stress the importance of vegetables, fruits, dry beans, and nuts in the diet. Choose My Plate, USDA's food guidance graphic (Figure 2.3), recommends that (excluding dairy) at least one-half of our food intake and calories should come from fruits and vegetables.

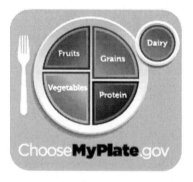

FIGURE 2.3 ChooseMyPlate.gov. (From U.S. Department of Agriculture, Food and Nutrition Service, Center for Nutrition Policy and Promotion, 2011a, MyPlate, June 2011, http://www.cnpp.usda.gov/MyPlate.htm, accessed May 4, 2014.)

---

* In 2010, the Corn Refiners Association petitioned to allow it to use the term *corn sugar* instead of HFCS, arguing that consumers have a bad impression of HFCS, in part, because of its complicated name. The petition was denied in 2012. See: http://www.fda.gov/aboutFDA/CentersOffices/OfficeofFoods/CFSAN/CFSANFOIAElectronicReadingRoom/ucm305226.htm; accessed December 8, 2012.

Yet, only a small amount of funding authorized by recent farm bills goes toward programs supporting fruits and vegetables. Since 1995, the USDA paid just $262 million to subsidize apples, which is the only significant federal subsidy of fresh produce (Russo 2011). The production of fruits and vegetables, tree nuts, and dried fruits are referred to by the government as *specialty crops*,* and the sales of fruits, vegetables, and tree nuts account for nearly one-third of U.S. crop cash receipts and one-fifth of U.S. agricultural exports. However, despite their relatively large share of crop receipts, these specialty crops occupy only about 3% of the U.S. harvested cropland. Despite the call for increased consumption of fruits and vegetables, they are planted on only 3% of U.S. farmland.

Sadly, U.S. farm policy presents obstacles for farmers who want to plant healthy food. Farmers who plant fruits and vegetables are eligible for federal crop insurance, but they are not eligible for direct support under USDA's farm commodity price- and income-support programs. Farmers that grow commodity crops are largely restricted from planting fruits and vegetables on land that receives government subsidies. The 2008 Farm Bill extends this planting restriction through FY 2012. Growers of fresh fruits and vegetables (especially vegetables) support this statute, arguing that because specialty crop growers do not get subsidies, it would be unfair if other farmers who do get subsidies started to compete with them by growing specialty crops. In other words, growers of produce would like to limit the competition of the market, which allows the market prices to be controlled by fewer farmers, where prices will remain high. Advocates for the expanded production of healthy foods, such as the Union of Concerned Scientists, recommend that the federal government eliminate restrictions that provide disincentives for farmers to plant fruits and vegetables and argue that Americans would eat better if more of our agricultural land supported the production of fruits and vegetables rather than the commodity crops.

The USDA offers support to fruit and vegetable farmers by direct purchases and then donates a variety of fruit, vegetables, and tree nut products for consumption through domestic nutrition and food assistance programs. These purchases and donations help groups of nutritionally vulnerable recipients (such as low-income school children, participants at family child care homes, and others) to eat a healthy diet and avoid hunger. In addition, purchasing produce for domestic food-assistance programs and crop insurance, the USDA promotes opportunities for specialty crop producers through other initiatives, such as the Specialty Crop Block Grant Program and the Specialty Crop Research Initiative (SCRI). In FY 2012, block grants were awarded to all the states, which in turn funded more than 700 initiatives across the country to strengthen markets and expand economic opportunities for local and regional producers. At the same time, the SCRI awarded $46 million to support new and continuing research and extension activities to address challenges and opportunities for growers and businesses that rely on a sustainable, profitable specialty crops industry.

---

* When discussed in this book, specialty crops refer to fruits, vegetables, and nuts. Technically, USDA defines specialty crops as fruits and vegetables, tree nuts, and dried fruits, as well as horticulture, and nursery crops. A detailed definition of specialty crops is available at http://www.ams.usda.gov /AMSv1.0/getfile?dDocName= STELPRDC5082113.

STRATEGIC INITIATIVES

In addition to domestic nutrition assistance programs that are funded primarily by the mandatory authorization of funds, earlier food bills have encouraged small-scale strategic initiatives that support the production at local levels and/or consumption of fresh produce, such as the People's Garden and Know Your Farmer–Know Your Food (KYF2) (USDA 2012f,g). These programs are described in detail in the following sections.

People's Garden

Since 2009, this initiative has grown into a collaborative effort of over 700 local and national organizations that work together to establish community and school gardens across the country. The simple act of planting a garden can help unite neighborhoods in a common effort and inspire locally led solutions to challenges facing our country—from hunger to the environment. For example, Washington State University (WSU) was selected to implement the People's Garden School Pilot Program. WSU develops school gardens in 70 high-poverty schools located in various urban, suburban, and rural areas to provide youth-led garden projects during the school year as well as throughout the summer. The program also works with school food purveyors to incorporate fresh garden produce into the school snack and meals programs.

Know Your Farmer, Know Your Food

This program has no budget. It is an internal initiative launched by the USDA in 2009 that aims to lead a national conversation about food and agriculture to strengthen the connection between consumers and farmers. The USDA Deputy Secretary chairs a task force of USDA employees representing every agency within the Department to break down bureaucratic silos, develop commonsense solutions for communities and farmers, foster new partnerships inside USDA and across the country, and otherwise humanize the huge bureaucracy that the USDA has become over the past decades. The KYF2 website lists programs inside the USDA as well as those not related to the USDA that can help build local and regional food systems. One of KYF2's innovations is a digital guide and map, the KYF Compass, which highlights USDA-supported local food projects around the country. The 2.0 version features thousands of local food projects in all 50 states and includes keyword and zip code search features.

CROP INSURANCE

In addition to crop subsidies, crop insurance is another farm safety net program originally designed to protect farmers and agriculture. Crop insurance is purchased by agricultural producers, including farmers and ranchers to protect themselves against the loss of their crops due to natural disasters (e.g., hail, drought, floods) or the loss of revenue due to declines in the prices of agricultural commodities.

Crop insurance was authorized in 1938 as part of the first farm bill to help agriculture recover from the combined effects of the Great Depression and the Dust Bowl. Four crops—corn, cotton, soybeans, and wheat—now account for three-quarters of the total acres enrolled in crop insurance. But the program is not limited to crops and relatively new or pilot programs protect livestock and dairy producers from loss of gross margin or price declines. The government pays, on average, 60% of the premium for coverage and the farmer pays the rest. Over the past decade, crop insurance has become the most important crop subsidy program in the United States. In 2013, crop insurance is expected to account for 63% of all budgeted outlays for farm subsidies (Shields 2010; USDA 2012h). In total, policies are available for more than 100 crops (including coverage on a variety of fruit trees, nursery crops, pasture, rangeland, and forage) (Chite 2012). Many specialty crop producers depend on crop insurance as the only *safety net* for their operation, unlike field crop producers, who are also eligible for farm commodity program payments. Crop insurance covers about 75% of the total area for selected specialty crops.

Although farmers who are insured may be more inclined to embrace some sustainable forms of agriculture, such as using fewer chemicals against pests, government-subsidized insurance has also encouraged corn farmers to take risks that were not foreseen when the program was developed. Because crop insurance reduces financial risk, insured farmers may engage in risky practices, such as failing to rotate the kinds of crops planted, and expanding and planting on marginally productive land that could be conserved or used for grazing. Indeed, heavily subsidized agricultural operations are associated with plowing up environmentally sensitive wetlands and grasslands. For example, of the more than 23 million acres of grass and wetlands that were plowed under for cash crops such as corn and soybean from 2008 through 2011, the land losses were greatest where crop insurance subsidies were largest (Sumner and Zulauf 2012).

In addition to threatening wildlife and the environment, these subsidies also take a heavy toll on American taxpayers. A decade ago, USDA paid 30%, on average, of the cost of crop insurance premiums. To encourage more farmers to buy the insurance, Congress in 2000 dramatically increased the subsidies for farmers, from less than $2 billion in 2001 to $7.4 billion in 2011. Today, USDA pays, on average, 62% of farmers' premium subsidies and $1.3 billion to insurance companies and agents that sell the policies. Soon, the annual cost of this program is expected to be $9 billion (Sumner and Zulauf 2012).

The existing farm safety net programs should be reformed, according to many groups that champion sustainable agriculture, such as the American Farmland Trust* and the Environmental Working Group (EWG).[†] The Trust argues that a modern farm safety net needs crop insurance and crop subsidies that are complementary rather than duplicative, which would save taxpayers significant amounts of money. In addition, farmers should only receive assistance if they suffer unavoidable losses, which would do away with subsidies for not planting (American Farmland Trust 2012). The EWG advocates making conservation compliance a condition of

---

* American Farmland Trust is a lobbying group, the only national conservation organization dedicated to protecting farmland, promoting sound farming practices, and keeping farmers on the land.
[†] EWG is a nonprofit 501(3)(c) organization that publishes a database of agricultural subsidies and their recipients. Their lobbying arm, the EWG Action Fund, advocates for farm bill reform in the form of decreased disaster payments and subsidies for commodity crops, and increased funding for nutrition programs, conservation, specialty crops (i.e., fruits and vegetables), and organic agriculture.

receiving crop insurance subsidies, placing limits on who can receive subsidies and how much they can receive, and rejecting cuts to voluntary conservation programs (Faber and Cox 2012).

HEALTHY FOOD FINANCING INITIATIVE

Currently, there is no integrated approach among government departments and agencies to address healthy food access. As illustrated throughout this chapter, the USDA is in the forefront of supporting food-related programs. Programs are also supported by other federal departments and agencies. First, we examine the joint efforts of three departments: the U.S. Department of Agriculture, the U.S. Department of the Treasury, and the Department of Health and Human Services (HHS). Then we list programs supported by cabinet-level departments and several federal agencies.

The Departments of Agriculture, Treasury, and HHS are partnering to support the development of sustainable projects and strategies to increase access to healthy, affordable foods and eliminate food deserts. The program created by these departments is the Healthy Food Financing Initiative (HFFI). Table 2.5 contains a summary of the 19 programs from these three departments that are involved. The FY 2013 budget requested for HFFI includes $10 million from HHS and $25 million from the Treasury Department. In addition, the budget calls for the USDA to target additional resources toward the overall goals of combating food deserts and increasing access to healthy food.

Priority consideration for HFFI support is given to organizations located in communities identified as food deserts and whose projects seek to eliminate food deserts in these designated areas, but projects that demonstrate the need for improved healthy food access in communities that are not officially designated as food deserts are also eligible for funding (USDA 2012i). The aim is to reduce the number of low-income Americans living in areas with inadequate access to healthy food—all the while helping combat the childhood obesity crisis nationwide and potentially creating or preserving thousands of permanent and construction jobs. The addition of HFFI will significantly strengthen nationwide efforts to increase access to healthy foods—particularly in low-income communities and communities of color. It will also help to revitalize low-income communities by bringing in new, vibrant, healthy food retail and by creating and preserving quality jobs for local residents. The incorporation of HFFI into the Farm Bill is a powerful step toward creating equitable and sustainable access to fresh and healthy foods across America.

The proposed HFFI budget for FY 2013 also called for a $250 million set-aside request within the broader New Markets Tax Credit (NMTC). The NMTC permits taxpayers to receive a credit against Federal income taxes for making qualified equity investments in designated Community Development Entities (CDEs). In this regard, the HFFI is intended to be an economically sustainable solution to the problem of limited access to healthy foods and to reduce health disparities by improving the health of families and children, creating jobs, and stimulating local economic development in low-income communities. HFFI would attract investment in underserved communities by providing critical loan and grant financing. This one-time resource would help fresh food retailers overcome the higher initial barriers to

TABLE 2.5
Programs That Support the Development of Sustainable Strategies to Increase Access to Healthy, Affordable Foods

Agency and Grant Program	Purpose
U.S. Department of the Treasury	
Community Development Financial Institutions (CDFI) Fund	To expand the capacity of CDFIs to provide credit, capital, and financial services to underserved populations and communities in the United States
The New Markets Tax Credit (NMTC) Program	Permits taxpayers to receive a credit against federal income taxes for making qualified equity investments in designated CDEs. Substantially all of the qualified equity investment must in turn be used by the CDE to provide investments in low-income communities
U.S. Department of Health and Human Services	
Community Economic Development Program	To award competitive grants to Community Development Corporations whose primary purpose is planning, developing, or managing low-income housing or community development activities to support projects that finance grocery stores, farmers markets, and other sources of fresh nutritious food. These projects will serve the dual purposes of facilitating access to healthy, affordable food options while creating job and business development opportunities in low-income communities, particularly as grocery stores often serve as anchor institutions in commercial centers
U.S. Department of Agriculture	
Community Facilities Program	To develop essential community facilities and services for public use in rural areas, to improve the quality of life of rural residents. Projects that may qualify include farmers markets, school and community kitchens/equipment, community food banks, refrigerated trucks, meals-on-wheels delivery vehicles, and community gardens. These projects will support local and regional food systems and increase access to healthy, locally grown foods
Rural Business Opportunity Grant Program	To promote sustainable economic development in rural communities with exceptional needs through provision of training and technical assistance for business development, entrepreneurs, and economic development officials and to assist with economic development planning. Funds may be provided for development of export markets, feasibility studies, development of long-term trade strategies, community economic development planning, business training and business-based technical assistance for rural entrepreneurs and business managers, establishment of rural business incubators, and assistance with technology-based economic development
Business and Industry Loan Guarantee Program	To help new and existing businesses based in rural areas gain access to affordable capital. Loans can be used for a wide variety of business-related activities, including business development, repair, or modernization; purchase and development of land; and purchase of equipment, machinery, supplies, and/or inventory

(Continued)

TABLE 2.5 (Continued)

Programs That Support the Development of Sustainable Strategies to Increase Access to Healthy, Affordable Foods

Agency and Grant Program	Purpose
Rural Microentrepreneur Assistance Program	To support the development and ongoing success of rural microentrepreneurs and microenterprises
Intermediary Relending Program	To provide loans to local organizations (intermediaries) for the establishment of revolving loan funds. These revolving loan funds are used to assist with financing business and economic development activity to create or retain jobs in disadvantaged and remote communities
Rural Business Enterprise Grant Program	To provide grants for rural projects that finance and facilitate the development of small and emerging rural businesses and help fund employment-related adult education programs
Farmers Market Promotion Program	To support the development, promotion, and expansion of direct, producer-to-consumer marketing and consumption of domestic agricultural commodities
Specialty Crop Block Grants	To enhance the competitiveness of specialty crops—fruits, vegetables, and tree nuts
Federal-State Marketing Improvement Program	To provide matching funds to state departments of agriculture, state agricultural experiment stations, and other appropriate state agencies to assist in exploring new market opportunities for U.S. food and agricultural products, and to encourage research and innovation aimed at improving the efficiency and performance of the marketing system
Farmers Market Nutrition Program	Associated with the WIC, to provide fresh, unprepared, locally grown fruits and vegetables to WIC participants, and to expand the awareness, use of, and sales at farmers markets
Senior Farmer's Market Nutrition Program	1. To provide resources in the form of fresh, nutritious, unprepared, locally grown fruits, vegetables, honey, and herbs from farmers markets, roadside stands and community-supported agriculture programs to low-income seniors 2. To increase the domestic consumption of agricultural commodities by expanding or aiding in the expansion of domestic farmers markets, roadside stands, and community-supported agriculture programs 3. To develop or aid in the development of new and additional farmers markets, roadside stands, and community-supported agriculture programs
Special Supplemental Nutrition Program for Women, Infants, and Children (WIC)	To provide federal grants to states for supplemental foods, health care referrals, and nutrition education for low-income pregnant, breast-feeding, and non–breast-feeding postpartum women, and to infants and children up to age five who are found to be at nutritional risk
Supplemental Nutrition Assistance Program (SNAP)	The federal nutrition assistance program that provides food to low- and no-income people and families

TABLE 2.5

Programs That Support the Development of Sustainable Strategies to Increase Access to Healthy, Affordable Foods

Agency and Grant Program	Purpose
The Emergency Food Assistance Program	To help supplement the diets of low-income people, including the elderly, by providing them with emergency food and nutrition assistance through public or private nonprofit organizations that provide food and nutrition assistance to the needy through the distribution of food for home use or the preparation of meals
The Healthy Urban Food Enterprise Development Center	A grant program that establishes and supports a Healthy Urban Food Enterprise Development Center to increase access to healthy, affordable foods, including locally produced agricultural products, to underserved communities

Source: USDA, Agricultural Marketing Service, Grant Opportunities, n.d., http://apps.ams.usda.gov /fooddeserts/Default.aspx, accessed May 4, 2014.

enter into underserved, low-income communities, and would also support renovation and expansion of existing stores so that they can continue providing healthy foods. The program would be flexible and comprehensive enough to support innovations in healthy food retailing and to assist retailers with different aspects of the store development and renovation process. HFFI is modeled on the successful Pennsylvania Fresh Food Financing Initiative, in which a $30 million investment by the state has led to over $190 million in total project costs. The result has been in the placement of 88 markets in underserved communities across the state, improved access to healthy food for more than 400,000 people, and creation or retention of more than 5,000 jobs (USDA 2012i).

OTHER FEDERAL AGENCIES WITH AUTHORITY ON THE U.S. FOOD SYSTEM

In addition to the USDA and the HFFI partnership, there are other federal agencies with authority over activities that impact the U.S. food system. Those agencies are described in the following section (Gosselin 2010).

The Department of Health and Human Services (HHS) is charged with protecting the health of Americans. The Food and Drug Administration (FDA) carries out the most prominent of HHS's food-related activities, including primary oversight of food safety, food labeling, and veterinary drugs. HHS's Centers for Disease Control and Prevention (CDC) conducts research and educates the public about food- and diet-related topics, and provides information about health-related issues that inform policy and rulemaking. With the USDA, HHS publishes the Dietary Guidelines for Americans every 5 years. HHS funds the Community Service Block Grant Programs, CDC oversees Action Communities for Health, Innovation, and Environmental Change. Some advocates have argued that HHS should support more food system reforms that improve the diets of Americans; the FDA should ban subtherapeutic use of antibiotics in livestock; HHS should consider the ecological impacts of food consumption (Clonan and Holdsworth 2012).

The Department of Commerce (DoC), whose primary purpose is to promote economic development, impacts and informs the food system in many ways. DoC's National Oceanic and Atmospheric Administration manages fishing in all federal ocean waters, conducts research on climate change, and runs the National Weather Service. The department also issues patents and trademarks for all products, including foods and seeds, and plays a role in domestic economic development and international trade. The department plans to develop strict and comprehensive regulations for aquaculture in federal waters to ensure that farming of fish is done without antibiotics and does not threaten wild fish populations or any other marine life.

The Department of Defense (DOD) purchases more than $4.5 billion worth of domestic food annually to feed nearly 1.5 million active service people and to supply food to several other federal programs, including the NSLP. The program will allow school food authorities to (1) purchase fresh fruits and vegetables from purveyors other than DOD, (2) purchase agricultural products from USDA-qualified participants in beginning and minority farmer programs when possible, and (3) include in contracts the requirement to offer organic produce if it is requested and available.

The Department of the Interior (DOI) manages more than 10% of all land in the United States and routes much water in the Western United States through several massive delivery projects. DOI also houses the Fish and Wildlife Service, which is in charge of managing freshwater fisheries and hatcheries, and is the primary administrator of the Endangered Species Act. DOI's Bureau of Land Management allows livestock grazing on about 160 million acres of public land, which functions as a subsidy program to ranchers (many of whom sell their young animals to CAFOs). The DOI plans to create new rules for livestock grazing on public lands that rewards environmental stewardship, prevents environmental degradation, and charges a fair market price for grazing permits.

The Department of Transportation's (DOT) investments in transportation infrastructure affect how food travels, where agricultural industries develop, and how easily Americans can access healthy foods. Although food is among the DOT's most vital interests, no transportation-related laws or regulations address the issues of food access or agricultural transport. The DOT and the Department of Housing and Urban Development (HUD) are in partnership to create livable communities that should include consideration of food environments (Gosselin 2009).

The Department of Homeland Security (DHS) has some oversight of food safety, enforces certain country-of-origin labeling laws at U.S. borders, and affects the supply of labor for farming and food processing industries through immigration enforcement. DHS can contribute to a more sustainable food system by (1) recognizing that food system decentralization is a viable strategy to improve food security and safety and (2) ensuring that imported foods meet food safety requirements before being sold in the United States.

HUD plays an important role in some economically depressed communities in which access to food and the ability to pay for healthy foods is limited. Given this role, HUD's potential to make an impact is significant. Economic revitalization projects, such as those funded through the Community Development Block Grant Program, should consider food access and encourage the inclusion of community gardens and farmers markets in local planning efforts.

The Environmental Protection Agency (EPA) is an independent government body, in charge of regulating environmental pollutants. The agency regulates the application of pesticides and fertilizers, soil tillage, and animal confinement, which are major sources of water and air pollution. The EPA also does research related to climate change and implements the Renewable Fuels Standard. There are plans to improve oversight of water and air pollution generated by CAFOs by properly enforcing existing laws and forming a task force with USDA to develop a plan for on-farm mitigation of greenhouse gas emissions.

U.S. FOOD INDUSTRY

Currently, American agriculture is experiencing one of its most productive periods in history. Both agricultural exports and net farm income are at record levels, whereas farm debt has been cut in half since the 1980s. In addition, American agriculture supports 1 in 12 jobs in the United States.

CONSOLIDATION OF THE U.S. FOOD INDUSTRY

Agribusiness Producers

According to *Food Fight: The Citizen's Guide to the Next Food and Farm Bill*, the farms comprising 50 to 2000 acres are not the problem in today's agricultural landscape (Imhoff 2012). These farms earned an average net income of $30,000 a year from farming, more than half of which came from subsidy payments. In addition to farm income and subsidies, most of these farm households supplemented their income from off-farm employment. Thus, without subsidies these would perish. Rather, it is the large commercial farms that earn over $250,000 per year that turn a profit from subsidies, and it is these mega farms that are flourishing.

Alarmingly, the concentration of production in agriculture has increased significantly in the last 5 years (USDA 2007). In 2002, 75% of the value of U.S. agricultural production was produced by 144,000 farms, but only by 125,000 farms in 2007. Farms with more than $1 million in sales produced 59% of U.S. agricultural products in 2007, up from 47% in 2002 (Figure 2.4).

These facts raise the following questions: How did some farms become so large? Why are these farms able to profit from a subsidy system that was originally designed as a safety net for farmers and not intended to be a cash cow?

Consolidation of Farms. Conducted every 5 years by USDA's National Agricultural Statistics Service (NASS), the Census of Agriculture is a complete count of the U.S. farms and ranches and the people who operate them. The census looks at land use

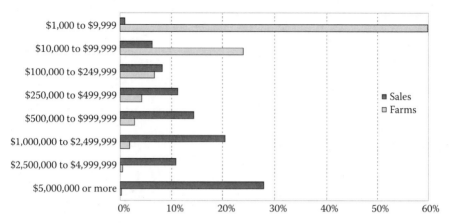

FIGURE 2.4 Number of farms and sales 2007 percent of total. (From U.S. Department of Agriculture, National Agricultural Statistics Services, 2007 Census of Agriculture: Farm Numbers, http://www.agcensus.usda.gov/Publications/2007/Online_Highlights/Fact _Sheets/Farm_Numbers/farm_numbers.pdf, accessed July 24, 2013.)

and ownership, operator characteristics, production practices, income and expenditures, and other topics. It provides the only source of uniform, comprehensive agricultural data for every county in the nation.

NASS defines a farm as any place from which $1,000 or more of agricultural products were, or normally would be, produced and sold during the census year. The 2007 Census tells a story about the increasing concentration of wealth in U.S. agriculture (USDA 2007). In 1935, there were 6.8 million farms in the United States with an average size of 155 acres. In 2008 there were a third as many farms (2.2 million), which were on average almost three times larger (418 acres). However, most (more than 63%) of the value of all agricultural products sold comes from only 9% of all farms—the large family farms (sales between $250,000 and $500,000) and very large family farms (sales over $500,000).

The percentage of Americans who live on a farm diminished from nearly 25% during the Great Depression to about 2% now. Of that population, less than 1% claim farming as an occupation (US EPA 2012a) and even less work full time on a farm. As the agribusiness lobby grew to $65 million in 2011–2012, the interests of agricultural corporations remain highly represented. In recent years, farm subsidies have remained high even in times of record farm profits (OpenSecrets 2012).

The farm sector has been converted to a manufacturing model predicated on providing its consumers with the lowest cost product. That low cost can only be guaranteed by economies of scale—the cost advantages that an enterprise obtains because of expansion. There are factors that cause a producer's average cost per unit to fall as the scale of output is increased. In terms of large-scale farms, wherever possible, labor is replaced with machinery and chemicals. These expensive costs are amortized when spread over a maximum number of acres or animals. Thus, big farms reap more profits per acre than small ones. In addition, these factory farms are structured as complex family corporations configured to circumvent subsidy laws that limit how much a single farming operation can receive.

Animal feed is the livestock and poultry producer's single largest input—and corn, the basis for most feed, is heavily subsidized by the government, which keeps meat and chicken prices down, and is in part responsible for our current low meat costs. As we have seen earlier, cheap corn-fed beef cattle and poultry is the basis for our ubiquitous hamburger and chicken fast-food chains. Typically, the corn is raised via a system of farming known as *monoculture*, an unsustainable agricultural practice that maximizes yield by concentrating on a single crop. Intensive monoculture depletes soil and leaves it vulnerable to erosion. Herbicides and insecticides harm wildlife and can pose human health risks as well. Biodiversity in and near monoculture fields is negatively impacted, as populations of birds and beneficial insects decline (UCS 2012a).

(CAFOs). Essentially, CAFOs are "factory-like buildings into which animals—industrially bred for rapid growth and high output of meat, milk, or eggs" (Imhoff 2010). As an example, ownership and control of the swine industry has become particularly concentrated. Fifty years ago, nearly 3 million farms in the United States raised hogs. By 2003, only about 3% of that number, or 85,000 farms, raised the same number of hogs. The number of hogs per farm has increased dramatically. In addition, the ownership and control is concentrated to specific regions in the United States, with Iowa and North Carolina containing the greatest proportion of confined animal feed operation for hog production. Although hog confinement operations began as early as the 1970s in Iowa, the greatest growth was in the mid-1990s. Iowa produced an average of 250 hogs per farm on 80,000 farms in 1980, with an average of 1,500 hogs per farm on only 10,000 farms in 2002. The number of hogs per farm increased more rapidly in Iowa than in the nation as a whole and by 2002 was nearly double the national average (Flora et al. 2007).

Recently, consumer consciousness about the treatment of food animals, particularly those in CAFOs, has been raised by the films *Fast Food Nation: Do You Want Lies with That?* (2006) and *Food, Inc.* (2008), which contain graphic depictions of animal abuse on farms and in slaughterhouses, and the book *The CAFO Reader* (2010) and its accompanying website (Imhoff 2010). In addition to the inhumane treatment of animals and reliance on monoculture to produce animal feed, there are other consequences of CAFOs—antibiotic resistance in humans and the impact of CAFOs on the environment. Antibiotic resistance in humans results from the ingestion of meat from animals that were administered drugs to keep them from becoming ill, or cure those that are ill, or promote *feed efficiency* (increase the animal's weight gain per unit of feed) (Food & Water Watch 2010b; UCS 2013). In addition, failures to properly manage manure and wastewater at CAFOs can negatively impact the environment. Mismanaged manure and wastewater contribute pollutants (nitrogen and phosphorus, organic matter, sediments, pathogens, heavy metals, hormones, and ammonia) to the environment. The environmental impacts resulting from mismanagement of wastes include excess nutrients in water (nitrogen and phosphorus), which contributes to low levels of dissolved oxygen (fish kills), and decomposing organic matter that contributes to toxic algae blooms. Contamination from runoff or lagoon leakage degrades water resources, and contributes to illness by exposing people to wastes and pathogens in their drinking water. Dust and odors can contribute to respiratory problems in workers and nearby residents (US EPA 2012b). More details about the human and environmental impact of confined animal feed operations can be found in Chapter 3.

Agribusiness Processors

There has been a concentration of food processors since 1990 where megamergers have resulted in the consolidation of food processors. For instance, the top four pork processors (Smithfield, Tyson Foods, Swift [JBS–Swift], and Excel [Cargill Meat Solutions]) slaughter 64% of the pork in the United States. Similarly, Cargill, Tyson Food, JBS, and National Beef slaughter 81% of the beef, and over half of the broiler chicken is slaughtered by Tyson Foods, Pilgrim's Pride Corporation, Perdue Farms, and Sanderson Farms. (Anon 2011a,b; National Pork Board 2011). Smithfield, for instance, is the world's largest pork producer and controls all stages from growing to slaughtering of its swine. Smithfield sales in 2009 reached $11.2 billion, with exports to more than 40 countries (Smithfield Foods 2010). Archer Daniels Midland is the largest corn producer and processor in the world and the leader in manufacturing HFCS with sales in 2009 reaching $61.7 billion. These examples demonstrate the big business involved in processing foods and the global reach of the corporations.

Agribusiness Food Companies

Although it may seem that the variety of food products offered to consumers continues to increase, the reality is that most food is manufactured by a small number of companies. The companies use a number of brand names to sell their products. For instance, Kraft Foods (which is owned by Phillip Morris) is the world's second largest food company, with annual sales of $54.4 billion. Kraft owns Oreo, Cadbury, Nabisco, Oscar Mayer, and Maxwell House, in addition to the products sold under their own name (Kraft Foods 2011).

Agribusiness Food Retailers

Along with consolidation of farms and ranches that produce the foods that enter the U.S. food chain, there is also consolidation of retail food stores that serve as the middlemen between producers (farmers and ranchers), manufacturers, and the consumer. The same law applies to retailers as to producers and manufacturers—economy of scale.

The U.S. Census Bureau tracks annual sales of U.S. retail and food service. In 2010, annual sales from the food and beverage stores and food service and drinking places amounted to almost one-quarter (24%) of the annual retail sales for the country, more than 1 trillion dollars. This is a 40% increase in sales from 10 years earlier. Food and beverage stores are tracked separately from food service and drinking places and consistently produce higher annual sales. Make no mistake, the U.S. food retail sector is big business and therefore similar business practices that have developed in other parts of the food industry are not surprisingly taking place in the food retail sector, such as the concentration of retailers.

In addition, stores such as Walmart and Costco have become increasingly significant nontraditional sources of retail food sales during the past three decades. Grocery mergers that were common in the 1990s resulted in the emergence of national supercenters and discounters as grocery powerhouses, and by the end of the twentieth century, the four largest food retailers controlled 72% of sales in the largest metropolitan areas. The share of sales going to traditional food retailers (supermarkets, super-stores, and food–drug combination stores) fell from 82% in 1998 to 69% in 2003. Walmart became the largest U.S. food retailer in 1988, just 12 years after opening its first supercenter that sold food products, a phenomenon known as "Walmarting the food chain." By 2009, more than half of all grocery sales were controlled by the top four food retailers—Walmart, Kroger, Costco, and Supervalu (Leibtag 2006; Food & Water Watch 2010a).

The proliferation of these stores appears oligopolistic.* The consumer may see the mergers as opportunities for cheap food as these consolidated food retailers may have the wherewithal to sell products at lower prices. But the trade-off in allowing a small number of corporations to control a large proportion of the food retail market is that it creates an environment where a small number of large stores now control prices, selection, quality, and the location of where food can be purchased. If this portion of the food industry's main mission was to provide healthy affordable foods that are recommended for health promotion, this conglomeration of businesses may have a positive effect on the public's health. Unfortunately that is not the case. Food retailers, like other corporations, are in the business of making a monetary profit and those profits are derived from selling a large volume of goods—regardless of the nutritional values of those goods.

Simply put, all humans have to eat. Unlike other retail markets such as electronics or furniture, people cannot modify their need for calories to survive. The question is *where is the government regulation within the food retail sector?* Although the farm bill does address the production of food, where is the title to address the delivery of food to Americans in nonemergency, noncommodity styles of everyday living? The consolidation of food retailers allows them to become so large and so few that they can exert their influence over food producers, processors, shippers, and other suppliers to control the food market and food messaging. For instance, the USDA documented that in 2011, farmers only received 13.9% of the total food retail sales (Canning 2011).

Food retailers such as Walmart and Whole Foods take the processing of foods one step further by branding their own food product, giving customers limited brand variability for purchases. Increasingly, small businesses that are not able to compete with the glut of the consolidated food retailers will go out of business. This affects the lower income Americans disproportionately:

- In 2009, 23.5 million people lacked access to a supermarket within a mile of their home.
- One-fifth (20%) of the rural counties in the United States were *food deserts*, where all residents live more than 10 miles from a supermarket or supercenter.
- Low-income census tracts have half as many supermarkets as wealthy tracts.
- Only 8% of African-Americans live in a tract with a supermarket, compared to 31% of whites (Treuhaft and Karpyn 2010).

---

* When there are only a few sellers, we call the structure an oligopoly and the sellers are oligopolists, from the Greek root *oligo* meaning a few. If there were only one seller, the structure would be a monopoly, from the root *mono*.

REFERENCES

American Farmland Trust. 2012. A New Farm Bill: Farm Policy for the 21st Century. http://www.farmbillfacts.org/farm-safety-net (accessed May 5, 2014).

Anon. 2011a. Feed Marketing & Distribution. http://fdsmagissues.feedstuffs.com/fds/Reference_issue_2012/02_Feed%20Marketing%20&%20Distribution.pdf (accessed May 5, 2014).

Anon. Feed Marketing & Distribution. 2011b. *Feedstuffs*, September 14, 2011. http://fdsmagissues.feedstuffs.com/fds/Reference_issue_2012/02_Feed%20Marketing%20&%20Distribution.pdf (accessed May 5, 2014).

Aussenberg R. A. and K. J. Colello. 2014. Domestic food assistance: summary of programs. Congressional Research Service. January 27, 2014. http://www.fas.org/sgp/crs/misc/R42353.pdf (accessed May 4, 2014).

Brown J. L. 2013. Nutrition. In *Social Injustice and Public Health*, edited by B. S. Levy and V. W. Sidel. New York: Oxford University Press.

Canning, P. 2011. USDA Agriculture Fact Book 1996. A Revised and Expanded Food Dollar Series: A Better Understanding of our Food Costs. Economic Research Report Number 114. http://www.ers.usda.gov/publications/err-economic-research-report/err114.aspx (accessed July 29, 2013).

Chite, R. M. 2012. Previewing the Next Farm Bill. Congressional Research Service. http://www.fas.org/sgp/crs/misc/R42357.pdf (accessed December 18, 2012).

Clancy, K. 2006. Greener Pastures: How Grass-Fed Beef and Milk Contribute to Healthy Eating. Union of Concerned Scientists. http://www.ucsusa.org/food_and_agriculture/solutions/advance-sustainable-agriculture/greener-pastures.html (accessed July 29, 2013).

Clonan, A. and M. Holdsworth. 2012. The challenges of eating a healthy and sustainable diet. *Am J Clin Nutr* 96: 459–60.

Faber, S. and C. Cox. 2012. The Case for Crop Insurance Reform. Environmental Working Group. http://www.ewg.org/farmbill2013/the-case-for-crop-insurance-reform (accessed December 13, 2012).

Flora, J. L., Q. (L.) Chen, S. Bastian, and R. Hartmann. 2007. Hog CAFOS and Sustainability: The Impact on Local Development and Water Quality. The Iowa Policy Project. http://www.iowapolicyproject.org/2007docs/071018-cafos.pdf (accessed July 26, 2013).

Food & Water Watch. 2010a. Fact Sheet: Consolidation and Buyer Power in the Grocery Industry. http://documents.foodandwaterwatch.org/doc/RetailConcentration-web.pdf (accessed December 17, 2012).

Food & Water Watch. 2010b. Factory Farm Nation: How America Turned Its Livestock Farms into Factories. http://www.factoryfarmmap.org/wp-content/uploads/2010/11/FactoryFarmNation-web.pdf (accessed July 29, 2013).

Food & Water Watch. 2012. Farm Bill 101. http://documents.foodandwaterwatch.org/doc/FarmBill101Report.pdf (accessed May 5, 2014).

Genzel, B. 2012. Farming in the 1940s: Exports & Imports. http://www.livinghistoryfarm.org/farminginthe40s/money_09.html (accessed December 3, 2012).

Gosselin, M. 2009. Transportation and sustainable food systems: An open policy window? Think Forward. http://iatp.typepad.com/thinkforward/2009/08/transportation-and-sustainable-food-systems-an-open-policy-window.html (accessed July 26, 2013).

Gosselin, M. 2010. Beyond the USDA: How other government agencies can support a healthier, more sustainable food system. Institute for Agriculture and Trade Policy. http://www.ams.usda.gov/AMSv1.0/getfile?dDocName=STELPRDC5097199 (accessed May 4, 2014).

Groombridge, M. A. 2001. America's Bittersweet Sugar Policy. Executive Summary. CATO Institute. Center for Trade Policy Studies. http://www.cato.org/pubs/tbp/tbp-013.pdf (accessed December 8, 2012).

Hauter, W. 2012. Walmarting the food chain, In *Foodopoly: The Battle over the Future of Food and Farming in America*. New York: The New Press.

Havel, P. J. 2005. Dietary fructose: Implications for dysregulation of energy homeostasis and lipid/carbohydrate metabolism. *Nutr Rev* 63: 133–57.

Imhoff, D. 2010. *The CAFO Reader: The Tragedy of Industrial Farm Animals*. Berkeley, CA: University of California Press.

Imhoff, D. 2012. *Food Fight: The Citizens Guide to the Next Food and Farm Bill*. Healdsburg, CA: Watershed Media.

Johnson, R. 2008a. The 2008 Farm Bill: Major Provisions and Legislative Action. Congressional Research Service 7-5700 RL34696. http://www.leahy.senate.gov/imo /media/doc/CRS%20Report%20Farm%20Bill%20Major%20Provisions.pdf (accessed July 31, 2013).

Johnson, R. 2008b. What Is the "Farm Bill"? Congressional Research Service RS22131. http://fpc.state.gov/documents/organization/107241.pdf. (accessed July 28, 2013).

Johnson, R. and J. Monke. 2013. What is the Farm Bill? Congressional Research Service 7-5700 RS22131. http://fpc.state.gov/documents/organization/211400.pdf (accessed May 4, 2014).

King Corn. DVD. Directed by Aaron Woolf. Amherst, MA: Balcony Releasing, 2007.

Kraft Foods. 2011. 2011 Fact Sheet. http://www.kraftfoodscompany.com/SiteCollection Documents/pdf/kraft_foods_fact_sheet.pdf (accessed July 26, 2013).

Leibtag, E. 2006. The Impact of Big-Box Stores on Retail Food Prices and the Consumer Price Index. USDA. Economic Research Service. Economic Research Report Number 33. http://ageconsearch.umn.edu/bitstream/7238/2/er070033.pdf (accessed December 17, 2012).

Lichtenstein, A. H. 2012. New York City trans fat ban: Improving the default option when purchasing foods prepared outside of the home. *Ann Intern Med* 157:144–5.

Monke, J. and R. Johnson. 2010. Actual Farm Bill Spending and Cost Estimates. CRS Report to Congress. Congressional Research Service 7-5700. http://www.farmpolicy.com /wp-content/uploads/2010/10/CRSFrmBillSpending10Oct7.pdf (accessed May 5, 2014).

National Pork Board. 2011. Quick Facts: The Pork Industry at a Glance. Pork Checkoff. http:// viewer.zmags.com/publication/5bb6aa6d#/5bb6aa6d/4 (accessed July 31, 2013).

Nestle, M. 2007. *Food Politics: How the Food Industry Influences Nutrition and Health, Revised and Expanded Edition*. Edited by Goldstein D. Berkeley, CA: University of California Press.

OpenSecrets.org. Agribusiness. http://www.opensecrets.org/industries/indus.php?Ind=A (accessed December 10, 2012).

Peters, G. and J. T. Woolley. 1936. The American Presidency Project. Roosevelt F. D. Statement on Signing the Soil Conservation and Domestic Allotment Act. http://www.presidency .ucsb.edu/ws/?pid=15254 (accessed December 2, 2012).

Russo, M. 2011. Apples to Twinkies: Comparing Federal Subsidies of Fresh Produce and Junk Food. U.S. PIRG Education Fund. http://uspirg.org/reports/xxp/apples-twinkies (accessed December 10, 2012).

Schnepf, R. 2014. U.S. Farm Income. Congressional Research Service. 7-5700 R40152. http:// www.fas.org/sgp/crs/misc/R40152.pdf (accessed May 4, 2014).

Shields, D. A. 2010. Federal Crop Insurance: Background and Issues. Congressional Research Service. 7-5700 R40532. http://adriansmith.house.gov/sites/adriansmith.house.gov /files/CRS%20-%20Crop%20Insurance.pdf (accessed May 4, 2014).

Smithfield Foods. 2010. Securities and Exchange Commission, 10K Filing. http://www .faqs.org/sec-filings/100618/SMITHFIELD-FOODS-INC_10-K/ex32-2.htm (accessed July 31, 2013).

Sumner, D. A. and C. Zulauf. 2012. Economic & Environmental Effects of Agricultural Insurance Programs. The Council on Food, Agricultural, and Resource Economics (C-FARE). http://ageconsearch.umn.edu/bitstream/156622/2/Sumner-Zulauf_Final.pdf (accessed May 4, 2014).

Treuhaft, S. and A. Karpyn. 2010. The Grocery Gap: Who Has Access to Healthy Food and Why It Matters. PolicyLink and The Food Trust. http://www.policylink.org/atf/cf /%7B97C6D565-BB43-406D-A6D5-ECA3BBF35AF0%7D/FINALGroceryGap.pdf (accessed February 23, 2013).

Union of Concerned Scientists (UCS). 2012a. Eight Ways Monsanto Fails at Sustainable Agriculture: #4—Expanding Monoculture. http://www.ucsusa.org/food_and_agriculture /our-failing-food-system/genetic-engineering/expanding-monoculture.html (accessed December 18, 2012).

Union of Concerned Scientists (UCS). 2012b. Our Failing Food System: Industrial Agriculture. http://www.ucsusa.org/food_and_agriculture/our-failing-food-system/industrial -agriculture (accessed December 18, 2012).

Union of Concerned Scientists (UCS). 2013. Prescription for Trouble: Using Antibiotics to Fatten Livestock. http://www.ucsusa.org/food_and_agriculture/our-failing-food -system/industrial-agriculture/prescription-for-trouble.html (accessed July 31, 2013).

U.S. Department of Agriculture (USDA). 2007. National Agricultural Statistics Service .2007 Census of Agriculture. Farm Numbers. http://www.agcensus.usda.gov /Publications/2007/Online_Highlights/Fact_Sheets/Farm_Numbers/farm_numbers.pdf (accessed December 10, 2012).

U.S. Department of Agriculture, Food and Nutrition Service, Center for Nutrition Policy and Promotion. 2011a. MyPlate. June 2011. http://www.cnpp.usda.gov/MyPlate.htm (accessed May 4, 2014).

U.S. Department of Agriculture (USDA). 2011b. News Transcript. Release No. 0458.11. Agriculture Secretary Vilsack on Priorities for the 2012 Farm Bill: Remarks As Delivered. http://www.usda.gov/wps/portal/usda/usdahome?contentid=2011/10/0458.xml&navid =TRANSCRIPT&navtype=RT&parentnav=TRANSCRIPTS_SPEECHES&edeploymen t_action=retrievecontent (accessed November 25, 2011).

U.S. Department of Agriculture (USDA). 2012a. Homepage. http://www.usda.gov (accessed December 5, 2012).

U.S. Department of Agriculture (USDA). 2012b. Food Safety and Inspection Service. Glossary. http://www.fsis.usda.gov/wps/portal/searchhelp/sitemap/!ut/p/a1/04_Sj9C Pykssy0xPLMnMz0vMAfGjzOINAg3MDC2dDbz8LQ3dDDz9wgL9vZ2dDdx9jY AKIkEKcABHA0L6vSAKcOsHWmBU5Ovsm64fVZBYkqGbmZeWrx-RkZpToB- RnpNfXJxYVIlg6aahsMP1o_A6wMIEpgC3AwpyI6p8HNOCPR0VFQFfJWLk/?1dm y&current=true&urile=wcm%3apath%3a%2FFSIS-Content%2Finternet%2Fsearch- and-help%2Fhelp%2Fglossary (accessed August 1, 2013).

U.S. Department of Agriculture (USDA). 2012c. Natural Resources Conservation Service. Environmental Quality Incentives Program (EQIP). http://www.nrcs.usda.gov/wps/ portal /nrcs/detail/national/programs/financial/eqip/?&cid=stelprdb1044009 (accessed August 1, 2013).

U.S. Department of Agriculture (USDA). 2012d. Natural Resources Conservation Service. Conservation Stewardship Program (CSP). http://www.nrcs.usda.gov/wps/portal /nrcs/detailfull/national/programs/alphabetical/csp/?cid = nrcs143_008316 (accessed August 1, 2013).

U.S. Department of Agriculture (USDA). 2012e. Food and Nutrition Service. Commodity Supplemental Food Program (CSFP). http://www.fns.usda.gov/fdd/programs/csfp/ (accessed August, 2013).

U.S. Department of Agriculture (USDA). 2012f. Food and Nutrition Service. The People's Garden Homepage. http://www.usda.gov/wps/portal/usda/usdahome?navid =PEOPLES_GARDEN (accessed August 1, 2013).

U.S. Department of Agriculture (USDA). 2012g. Food and Nutrition Service. Know Your Farmer–Know Your Food (KYF2) Home Page. http://www.usda.gov/wps/portal/usda /usdahome?navid=KYF_MISSION (accessed December 6, 2012).

U.S. Department of Agriculture (USDA). 2012h. Risk Management Agency. History of the Crop Insurance Program. http://www.rma.usda.gov/aboutrma/what/history.html (accessed December 14, 2012).

U.S. Department of Agriculture (USDA). 2012i. Agricultural Marketing Service. Healthy Food Financing Initiative. Creating Access to Healthy, Affordable Food. http://apps. ams.usda.gov/fooddeserts/Default.aspx (accessed May 4, 2014).

U.S. Department of Agriculture (USDA). 2013a. National School Lunch Program. http:// www.fns.usda.gov/cnd/lunch/ (accessed January 10, 2013).

U.S. Department of Agriculture (USDA). 2013b. Food and Nutrition Service. Summer Food Service Program. http://www.fns.usda.gov/summer-food-service-program-sfsp (accessed July 26, 2013).

U.S. Department of Agriculture (USDA). 2013c. Child and Adult Care Food Program. http://www.fns.usda.gov/cnd/care (accessed January 10, 2013).

U.S. Department of Agriculture (USDA). 2013d. Economic Research Service. Foreign Agricultural Trade of the United States [FATUS]. http://www.ers.usda.gov/data-products/foreign-agricultural-trade-of-the-united-states-(fatus)/calendar-year.aspx. (accessed July 24, 2013).

U.S. Department of Agriculture (USDA). nd. Agricultural Marketing Service, Grant Opportunities. http://apps.ams.usda.gov/fooddeserts/grantOpportunities.aspx (accessed May 4, 2014).

U.S. Environmental Protection Agency (US EPA). 2012a. Ag 101. Demographics. http://www .epa.gov/oecaagct/ag101/demographics.html (accessed December 13, 2012).

U.S. Environmental Protection Agency (US EPA). 2012b. How Do CAFOs Impact the Environment? http://epa.gov/region7/water/cafo/cafo_impact_environment.htm (accessed December 18, 2012).

Wikipedia Commons. Map of the Great Plains2/jpg. http://upload.wikimedia.org/wikipedia /commons/4/49/Map_of_Great_Plains2.jpg. (accessed July 28, 2013).

3 Environmental Injustice Connects Local Food Environments with Global Food Production

Steve Wing

President Dwight Eisenhower warned the nation about the dangers of the military-industrial complex—an unhealthy alliance between the defense industry, the Pentagon, and their friends on Capitol Hill. Now, the agro-industrial complex—an alliance of agriculture commodity groups, scientists at academic institutions who are paid by the industry, and their friends on Capitol Hill—is a concern in animal food production in the 21st century.

Robert P. Martin (2008)

The concept of the local food environment focuses attention on the kinds of groceries and restaurants that are available in people's neighborhoods. It challenges the unrealistic (and potentially detrimental and discriminatory) notion that education about what to eat necessarily improves mass nutrition. Although people with means who live in neighborhoods with healthy foods can change what they eat based on nutrition education (including commercial advertising), many people live where healthy foods are simply not readily available or unaffordable. The concept of the local food environment is an extension of the basic principle of public health that the most effective means for promoting behaviors that prevent disease and promote health are those that create environments in which it is easier for people to make healthy, rather than unhealthy, choices (Milio 1976).

Variability in local food environments can be understood from several perspectives. Stores and restaurants locate where people buy their products. Culture and marketing affect food choices. Wealth and income determine what people can afford. Housing policies, immigration, and discrimination influence racial segregation of neighborhoods and placement of retail stores. Forces that promote exploitation and inequality versus equity affect the distribution of wealth. Agriculture, transportation, energy, and waste disposal affect relationships between urban and rural areas. Variations in local food environments are shaped in this ecological context.

Public health research has focused on social inequalities in local food environments in relation to race and class, and the consequences of that variability for diet and risk of disease (Morland et al. 2002a,b). Although clearly important for health disparities, this heterogeneity of local food environments occurs within an industrial uniformity that is imposed by consolidation and concentration throughout the food system, from agricultural production to product development, to distribution and marketing. For example, the U.S. Department of Agriculture (USDA) estimates that, as of 2012, over 90% of soybeans and over 70% of corn planted in the United States are genetically modified crops (USDA 2012). Herbicide-tolerant and insect-resistant crops developed and controlled by large corporations that also produce companion chemicals establish uniformity in production by replacing conventional seed stocks that farmers could save and plant from one season to the next. Genetically modified corn and soybean products dominate the food supply through their use in grains, oils, and as feed for livestock. This uniformity, created through government policies that promote corporate control of the food supply, is projected to some extent into all local food environments.

The co-occurrence of variability in local food environments with uniformity of the mass food supply has significant public health consequences. One is bifurcation of food consumption. People who are well informed about nutrition, place a high value on health, have sufficient resources, and live in areas with access, can obtain foods that are locally produced, organic, fresh, and unprocessed. They may even choose foods based on other values, such as avoiding exploitation of farm and food-processing workers, animal welfare, or impacts on the environment. However, economic inequalities—for example, the fact that the bottom 80% of U.S. households held 4.7% of nonhome wealth in 2010, whereas the top 1% held 42.1% (Domhoff 2012)—mean that only a small proportion of people can afford to eat in this way. Low-income families must depend on the industrial food supply dominated by highly processed, high-calorie foods that, although available in wealthier neighborhoods, need not dominate diets of the people with means who live in those neighborhoods.

Bifurcation of food consumption, which is connected to differences in local food environments and diet between neighborhoods based on class and race, reflects the fact that consumers pay less for industrially produced foods than for foods produced by small- and medium-sized farmers and distributors. Consumer prices for industrial foods are low relative to historical food prices and to the costs of nonindustrial foods, because corporate producers do not pay for the environmental damages caused by industrial food production. This is the second public health consequence of the uniformity of the mass food supply that occurs together with variability in local food environments—the environmental health impacts of industrialized food production.

ENVIRONMENTAL INJUSTICE AND INDUSTRIAL FOOD PRODUCTION

Environmental injustice occurs when populations benefit from practices that negatively impact the environment of others. Food production always has the potential to create environmental injustice by depleting water supplies and reducing water quality, topsoil and soil productivity, and ecological diversity in agricultural areas that provide food for people in nonagricultural areas. This potential has been vastly expanded with the industrialization of agriculture. Industrialization "refers to the organization of agriculture as an in line, quasi-manufacturing process wherein the energy and materials of production are treated as exogenous to the system of biological productivity, and the primary goal is maximum sustained yield of single commodity items" (Mancus 2007).

Industrialized agriculture requires large inputs of fossil fuels and chemicals, notably inorganic nitrogenous fertilizer. Pollution from the production and refinement of oil, gas, and other petrochemicals impacts nearby communities (Allen 2006) in order to create inputs required by industrial agriculture. Therefore, the burdens of environmental pollution borne by communities in fossil fuel production areas benefit industrial agribusiness by helping to keep profits high and prices of industrially produced foods low. In agricultural areas, heavy chemical inputs can contaminate groundwater with nitrates and pesticides, and can lead to nutrient runoff that promotes eutrophication of surface waters. Furthermore, industrialization of agriculture leads to spatial concentration of production, requiring large-scale transportation of products to remote locations of consumption, with the additional demands for fossil fuels. In turn, spatial concentration of production brings about long-range transport of crops, depleting soil nitrogen and increasing the need for inorganic nitrogenous fertilizers, which (along with mechanical cultivation and monoculture) degrades the plant–soil relationships that make biological fixation of nitrogen possible, increasing further requirements for inorganic nitrogenous fertilizers (Mancus 2007). Large transportation corridors for agricultural products lead to excess local air pollution from ports, rail terminals, road traffic, destruction of housing and community facilities, and reduction of walkability in communities (Hricko 2006, 2008).

Exploitation of labor is rampant in agriculture. Chemical exposures, inadequate housing, and lack of sanitation affect the mental and physical health of many farm workers and their families (Villarejo 2003), while acute and repetitive trauma injuries are hazards in processing plants (Lipscomb et al. 2005, 2006, 2007, 2008). Workers in industrial animal confinements are exposed to bioaerosols, ammonia, and hydrogen sulfide (Donham 1993), and they exchange bacteria and viruses with livestock (Gray et al. 2007; Price et al. 2007). In the United States, agriculture is exempted from labor laws that cover industrial workers.

Industrial agriculture generates environmental injustice by exposing agricultural communities, workers, and urban populations to chemical production and goods movement; these populations suffer dangerous jobs and pollution in the interests of corporate profits and low consumer prices. Ironically, wealthy people can afford to buy from small, more sustainable producers, minimizing their consumption of foods produced in ways that generate the most environmental injustice, whereas low-income people must depend on the mass food supply that is more affordable because the costs of production are not counted. Industrial farm animal production in general, and pork production in particular, illustrates how products that are common to most local food environments create environmental injustices and health damage through the food production system.

INDUSTRIAL FARM ANIMAL PRODUCTION

Until the middle of the twentieth century, most meat, eggs, and milk came from farms that were located not too far from populations that consumed their products. Nonindustrial livestock farms support a diversity of production including pasture and grains used to feed the livestock. Livestock waste is used to fertilize the pastures and grains that become the next year's feed, establishing a feedback loop between animal and plant growth. Free-range animals fertilize soils as they graze, reducing the need for storage of animal wastes.

My experience with nonindustrial farms began in the 1970s when I moved to a rural area of North Carolina. My neighbors raised feed grains, chickens, and hogs. They fed the grain to their hogs. In the fall, after grain harvest, they released the hogs from their pens to roam through the fields where they consumed the remaining grains and plant parts and rooted up the soil, turning it over and depositing their waste.

In 1995, I met Gary Grant, director of the Concerned Citizens of Tillery, a grassroots organization in an area of eastern North Carolina where industrialized hog production was rapidly expanding. Given my experiences with hog farming in my community, I was surprised when Gary told me that his community and others in eastern North Carolina were having serious problems with hog farm pollution, which threatened the aquifers that supplied their drinking water and the air they breathed. This was a different kind of hog production than what I knew about from my neighbors.

Industrial hogs never touch the ground. Hundreds to thousands of hogs are kept in long buildings referred to as confinements, not the barns that my neighbors called pig parlors. Feeding is automated, and large fans help exhaust waste gases and dusts from the buildings. Feces, urine, spilled feed, and residues of pesticides drop below slats and are flushed into open cesspools, euphemistically referred to as lagoons. Gary explained to me that the waste pits in his community were dug into the water tables where rural residents, who lacked connections to municipal water supplies, drew their well water. Industrial producers empty these waste pits by spraying the liquid on nearby fields. Although the lagoons have clay or plastic liners that slow movement of fecal waste into the water table, the spray fields have no barriers to keep the liquid waste from groundwater, and many have subsurface drains, originally installed to make swampy land arable, which act as conduits for hog waste to reach surface waters.

Figure 3.1 shows the three primary components of an industrial hog operation in North Carolina: the confinements, the waste lagoons, and the spray fields. Confinement buildings must be ventilated, which exhausts waste gases and dusts into the surrounding neighborhood. Air and water pollution also come from the open waste pits and spray fields (Figure 3.2). North Carolina hog operations house as many as 20,000 pigs each, producing more waste than a city of 60,000 people, but with no sewer treatment plant.

Tillery is mostly African-American. Gary Grant's organization, Concerned Citizens of Tillery, grew out of civil rights era struggles for political enfranchisement, education, and fair treatment from local, state, and government agencies

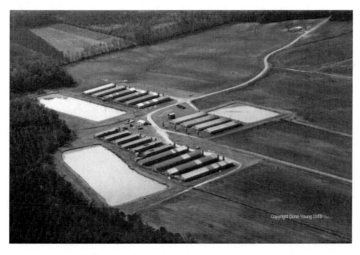

FIGURE 3.1 (See color insert.) Industrial hog operation confinements, waste lagoons, spray fields, and home in the upper right. (Courtesy of Donn Young Photography, DSC no. 9566, Chapel Hill, North Carolina, 2013.)

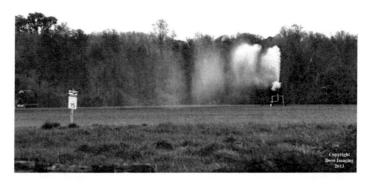

FIGURE 3.2 (See color insert.) Hog waste spray fields aerosolize particles that can drift downwind and soak fields with fecal waste that can run off into surface waters and impact upper aquifers of ground water. (Courtesy of Dove, R., www.doveimaging.com, New Bern, North Carolina, 2013.)

that had favored the white power structure and practiced gross discrimination against people of color (Wing et al. 1996). Concerned Citizens of Tillery, located in Halifax County, North Carolina, had watched as, in the early 1980s, neighboring Warren County was chosen as the site for a toxic waste landfill, giving rise to the term environmental racism and the movement for environmental justice. They viewed industrial hog production as another form of environmental racism and the exploitation of African-American communities. At a meeting in an African-American church near an industrial hog operation in a neighboring county, I heard residents describe respiratory problems, water contamination, and hog odor so strong that they had to keep their houses shut, and their children inside. On the church's meeting room wall they posted a county map with pins of different colors that showed how close hog operations were located to African-American schools and churches. Residents had approached government officials with this evidence of discrimination, but they were told that their observations were anecdotal, not evidence of a systematic problem.

As industrial hog operations expanded in North Carolina from the 1970s into the 1990s, small- and medium-sized producers were driven out of business (Figure 3.3) (Edwards and Ladd 2000). By 1998, when the state adopted a moratorium on new lagoons and spray fields after a hog producer applied for a permit to construct a hog operation near golf courses and country clubs, the state was home to almost 10 million hogs.

As the population of pigs exploded, the geographic distribution of production imploded, concentrating heavily in the eastern part of the state known as the Black Belt (Figure 3.4) (Furuseth 1997). This region of North Carolina, part of the southern coastal plain where agriculture before the Civil War was based on slave labor, is where the majority of rural African-Americans still reside. Figure 3.5 shows that the proportion of nonwhites in North Carolina census block groups mirrors the spatial distribution of industrial hog operations in Figure 3.4.

With funding through a community-driven research and education program created by the National Institute of Environmental Health Sciences following President Clinton's executive order on environmental justice, we analyzed race and poverty statistics for North Carolina census block groups in relation to the presence of industrial hog operations permitted by the state. The study documented the excess of hog operations in low-income communities of color and showed that there were

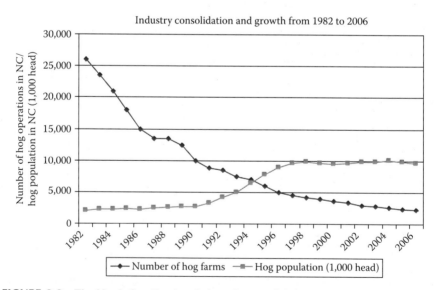

FIGURE 3.3 The North Carolina hog industry's consolidation and growth from 1982 to 2006. Growth is represented by the state hog population, whereas consolidation is exhibited in the number of hog farms in the state. (Edwards, B., *Twenty Lessons in Environmental Sociology*, 2009 by permission of Oxford University Press.)

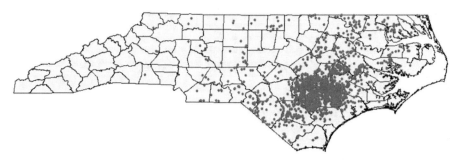

FIGURE 3.4 (See color insert.) The 2407 industrial hog operations permitted by the North Carolina Division of Water Quality. (From Wing, S. et al., *American Journal of Public Health*, 98, 1390–1397, 2008.)

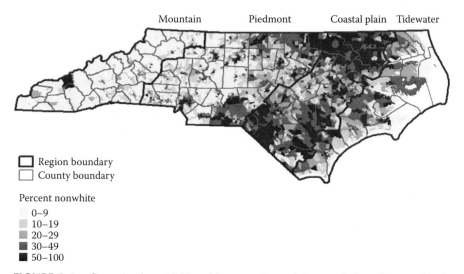

Mountain   Piedmont   Coastal plain   Tidewater

☐ Region boundary
☐ County boundary

Percent nonwhite
  0–9
  10–19
  20–29
  30–49
  50–100

FIGURE 3.5 (See color insert.) Nonwhite percentage of the population of census block groups in North Carolina, 2010. (From Norton, J. et al., *Environmental Health Perspectives*, 115, 1344–1350, 2007.)

almost 10 times as many of these operations located in block groups with higher levels of poverty and people of color compared to the lowest levels, even after adjustment for how rural they are (Wing et al. 2000).

HEALTH EFFECTS OF INDUSTRIAL HOG OPERATIONS

Since the 1970s, researchers have documented the respiratory effects of working in hog confinements. In the 1990s, researchers began to publish results of studies of the mental and physical health of hog operation neighbors (Cole et al. 2000). A study of Iowa residents reported excess frequency of several clusters of symptoms among hog operation neighbors and was cited by eastern North Carolina residents as relevant to their health concerns (Thu et al. 1997). However, some officials said the Iowa study was not relevant to North Carolina. As Gary Grant responded, "They think hog shit smells different in North Carolina than in Iowa."

The Concerned Citizens of Tillery and other community-based organizations supported the idea of conducting similar research in eastern North Carolina. With funding and cooperation from the North Carolina Division of Occupational and Environmental Health and the National Institute of Environmental Health Sciences, we conducted a health survey of residents of three rural areas matched on demographic characteristics (Wing and Wolf 2000). Residents of one area lived within 3200 meter (m) of an industrial hog operation with about 6000 hogs and one lagoon, and in a second area within 3200 m of two adjacent dairy farms with a combined 300 cows and two lagoons. Residents of a third area lived more than 3200 m away from a livestock operation with a lagoon. Following an enumeration of households in each area, university researchers conducted a door-to-door survey of adults that included questions about physical symptoms and quality of life; the questions did not mention livestock or odor. The mostly white researchers were accompanied by members of African-American community organizations who introduced them to residents but were not present for the interviews. More than 90% of the 155 study participants were African-American and 65% were women.

Residents of the area with the hog operation reported more frequent respiratory and gastrointestinal symptoms, and reduced quality of life, compared to residents of the other areas, with adjustment for age, gender, smoking, and work outside the home (Wing and Wolf 2000). After results of the study were presented to community members at a meeting in Tillery, the North Carolina Department of Health and Human Services issued a press release announcing the results. Later that day, lawyers for the North Carolina Pork Council requested the identities of study participants, locations of their homes, responses to the questions we had asked, and copies of all documents produced in connection with the study. They also notified me and my coauthor Susanne Wolf that they were considering whether we had defamed the pork industry. Despite my obligation to keep the identity of research participants confidential, the University of North Carolina at Chapel Hill's response was to direct me to turn over all the documents. Only after I had obtained the assistance of a lawyer who would represent my interests and the interests of the study communities was I able to negotiate an arrangement to turn over documents that were redacted to protect the identity of the individuals and communities in the study. They did not pursue the charge of defamation.

This incident, which I wrote about in more detail in a 2002 article (Wing 2002), is relevant here because it indicates the clout of the pork industry in North Carolina and their willingness to use threat and intimidation against people who question their practices. The primary targets of these tactics are people who have fewest resources to combat them—community residents and workers. Industrial hog production not only exposes people to dusts, gases, bacteria and viruses but also exposes them to social and political infections that parasitize communities and whole societies. I expand on this later.

Results of the symptom survey were released in May, 1999. In September 1999, eastern North Carolina was hit by Hurricane Floyd. Subsequent flooding resulted in the release of massive quantities of hog waste into neighboring communities (Figure 3.6).

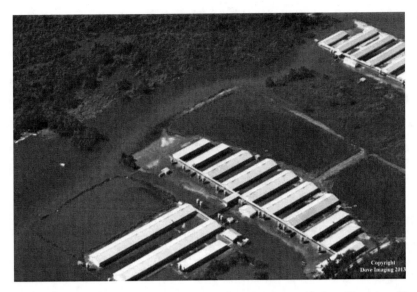

FIGURE 3.6 (See color insert.) Fecal waste pits flooded following Hurricane Floyd. (Courtesy of Dove, R., www.doveimaging.com, New Bern, North Carolina, 2013.)

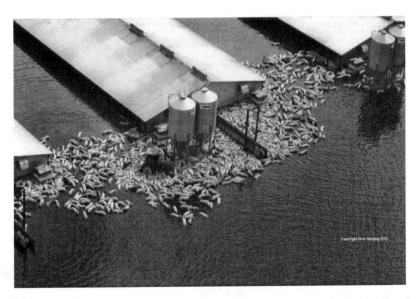

FIGURE 3.7 (See color insert.) Tens of thousands of hogs drowned in the flooding from Hurricane Floyd. (Courtesy of Dove, R., www.doveimaging.com, New Bern, North Carolina, 2013.)

At least tens of thousands of hogs were drowned (Figure 3.7), resulting in serious carcass disposal problems.

We used digital satellite images from approximately 1 week after Floyd hit to estimate the number of hog operations that could have been affected, and found that the coordinates of 237 hog operations, permitted to house over 736,000 hogs, were within the flooded area (Wing et al. 2002). The North Carolina Division of Water Quality, which permits these facilities, reported that 45 hog operations were flooded, more than half of which were not classified as flooded in our analysis based on areas under water 1 week after the rains fell (Figure 3.8).

Although Hurricane Floyd resulted in an unusually large quantity of animal waste entering communities and surface waters of eastern North Carolina, tropical cyclones and locally heavy thunderstorms are routine occurrences in the state. Surveillance of environmental disease from these events, as in the case of routine releases, is hampered by lack of access to medical services.

We subsequently conducted a study of middle-school children who participated in a state-wide asthma survey in 1999–2000 (Mirabelli et al. 2006b). Schools' exposure to air pollutants from industrial hog operations were classified according to their distance to the nearest hog operation and also according to responses of school staff to a survey asking how often they noticed livestock odors inside school buildings. The prevalence of wheezing among 576 children attending three schools where school staff reported livestock odors inside more than two times per week was 23% higher than at schools where no livestock odor was reported, adjusted for 12 potentially confounding personal and environmental factors (Mirabelli et al. 2006b). Schools

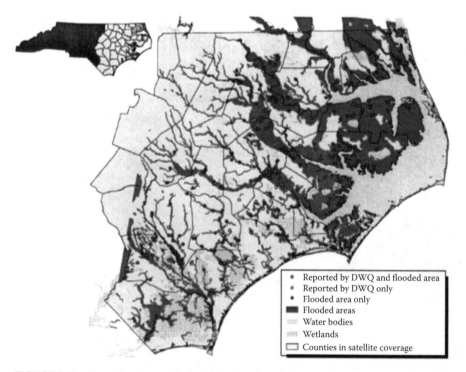

FIGURE 3.8   (See color insert.) Industrial animal production facilities with coordinates in the digital flood image or flooding reported by the North Carolina Division of Water Quality, September 1999. About 98% of these facilities were raising hogs. (From Wing, S. et al., *Environ. Health Perspect.*, 110, 387–391, 2002.)

with lower proportions of white children and more children receiving free and reduced lunch, an indicator of poverty, were closer to industrial hog operations—showing that environmental injustice extends to the educational environment (Mirabelli et al. 2006a). This North Carolina study is just one of a growing number of studies that find evidence of respiratory impacts of airborne emissions from industrial animal operations (Heederik et al. 2007).

These and other studies of the health of hog operation neighbors used information about exposure to pollutants (usually distance from the hog operation) and illness at the same time point. In such cross-sectional studies, it is not clear whether or not exposure occurs before the onset of illness. Distance is a crude measure of air pollution exposure. In addition, people who live near hog operations may differ in many ways, both known and unknown, from people who live in comparison areas, making it difficult to be certain that differences in illness are caused by hog pollution or something else. These limitations led us to conduct Community Health Effects of Industrial Hog Operations, a repeated-measures study of hog operation neighbors (Wing et al. 2008b). As in earlier studies, researchers partnered with the Concerned Citizens of Tillery to conduct the study. We also worked with a predominantly white community-based group, Alliance for a Responsible Swine Industry. Support from these groups was critical for the study because trust in government and research is low in areas impacted by industrial hog production.

Community organizers first talked with residents of neighborhoods near industrial hog operations and told them about the ongoing research (Wing et al. 2008b). They used maps from our prior environmental justice research to inform residents about the large number of hog operations in eastern North Carolina and their disproportionate placement in low-income communities of color. Many of these operations are located off main roads and behind stands of trees, so even local residents were not aware that so many of them were nearby.

People who expressed interest in participating in the study were asked if they would call the researchers or provide a phone number for the researchers to contact them. Nonsmokers aged 18 and above were invited to participate in the study for 2–3 weeks. They attended a training session where they provided consent to participate in research, their odor sensitivity was tested, and they learned to use the study instruments including a digital timer, an automated blood pressure monitor, a peak flow (lung function) meter, tubes for saliva collection, and a diary for reporting odors, health, and quality of life. Participants selected morning and evening times to sit outside on their porches every day for 2–3 weeks. While outside, they reported hourly levels of hog odor during the prior 12 hours in their diaries. Back inside, they recorded the level of hog odor that they noticed during the 10 minutes outside, physical symptoms, mood states including stress and anxiety, and daily activities. They measured their lung function and blood pressure using digital instruments that stored the data, and collected saliva in a tube that they stored in their freezer (Figure 3.9).

While participants collected data, we ran air pollution monitoring equipment on a trailer placed at a central location in the neighborhood (Figure 3.10). We monitored temperature, humidity, wind speed and direction, and hydrogen sulfide, a toxic gas produced by the decomposition of fecal waste that smells like rotten eggs. We also measured several components of particles less than 10 μ in diameter (PM_{10}): hourly

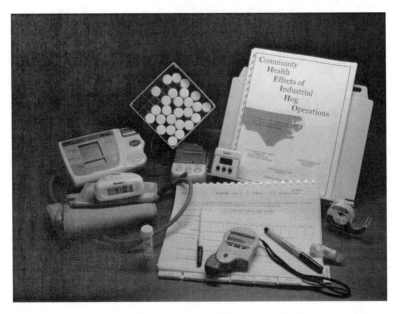

FIGURE 3.9 **(See color insert.)** Instruments used for data collection by participants in the Community Health Effects of Industrial Hog Operations Study. (Courtesy of Denzler, B., University of North Carolina.)

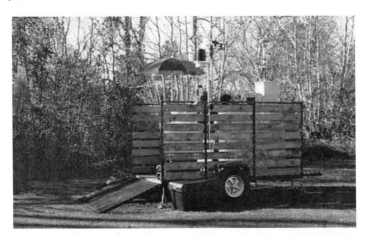

FIGURE 3.10 **(See color insert.)** Monitoring trailer used to house equipment for measuring hourly pollution levels in 16 neighborhoods in eastern North Carolina. (Courtesy of Denzler, B., University of North Carolina.)

PM_{10} and semi-volatile PM_{10}; 12-hour $PM_{2.5}$ (fine) and $PM_{2.5-10}$ (*coarse particles*); and endotoxin (Figure 3.10). The study was conducted sequentially in 16 communities where people lived within 2400 m of between 1 and 16 industrial hog operations (Wing et al. 2008b).

Rather than comparing hog operation neighbors to people who live somewhere else, we compared the health of hog operation neighbors during periods when they were exposed to pollutants from hog operations with their health during times when they were not exposed. Each person served as her or his own control, a design that controls for characteristics such as age, race, sex, medical history, and other factors that do not change during the short time of the study; however, this meant that we were not able to study chronic effects of exposure. Instruments for measuring air pollution and some outcomes were used, in part, to help avoid the potential for bias from self-reporting (Wing et al. 2008b).

Between 2003 and 2005, 102 volunteers completed the study protocol; one person who had trouble following the protocol was excluded from analyses. Among the remaining 101 participants who ranged in age from 19 to 89 years, 66 were women and 85 described themselves as black. They contributed 2949 records, typically two per day. Only two people dropped out before 14 days, and responses to individual diary questions were complete about 98% of the time (Schinasi et al. 2009). Blood pressure was missing in 1.4% of records; however, 34% of records had no valid lung function reading, reflecting the difficulty of performing that measurement (Schinasi et al. 2009).

Even though hydrogen sulfide concentrations were usually below typical odor detection threshold of 5–10 ppb, Figure 3.11 shows that the average hourly hog odor, reported on a nine-point scale from 0 (none) to 8 (very strong), varies in parallel with the hourly average hydrogen sulfide measured at the monitoring trailer (Wing et al. 2008a,b). Hog odor intensity during the 10-minute outdoor times rose, on average, 0.15 units per 1 ppb increase in measured hydrogen sulfide (Wing et al. 2008a). A similar relationship between hydrogen sulfide and odor was observed in a chamber experiment in which naïve volunteers were exposed to air from a hog confinement (Schiffman et al. 2005). Hog odor was related to PM_{10} only when the wind speed was above approximately 3 m/s; this may reflect the longer range transport of particles during higher wind conditions (Wing et al. 2008a). Participants reported disruptions of their daily activities far more often during periods of higher odor than lower odor (Wing et al. 2008a). Figure 3.11 also shows that average levels of hydrogen sulfide and reported hog odor were highest during morning and evening times when people are most often at home and wanting to engage in outdoor activities, especially during

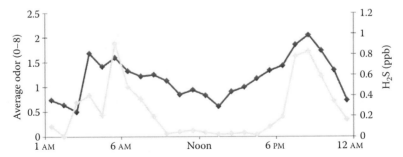

FIGURE 3.11   (See color insert.) Average hourly odor levels (left vertical axis) and hydrogen sulfide (right vertical axis) in 16 eastern North Carolina communities located near industrial hog operations. (Based on Wing, S. et al., *American Journal of Public Health*, 98, 1390–1397, 2008.)

the summer when mid-day temperatures are high. Participants reported hog odor during the 10 minutes outside on 61.3% of study days, and they reported hog odor inside their homes on 12.5% of days (Wing et al. 2008a).

Respiratory symptoms and mucous membrane irritation were also related to pollutant levels. The odds of reporting acute eye irritation immediately following the 10-minute outdoor exposure increased, on average, 16% for each 1 ppb increase in hydrogen sulfide and 43% for each 10 µg/m³ increase in PM_{10} (Schinasi et al. 2011). The odds of reporting nasal irritation, burning eyes, difficulty breathing, and wheezing during the previous 12 hours increased 61%, 84%, 65%, and 132%, respectively, for a 10 µg/m³ increase in $PM_{2.5}$. Endotoxin levels in the coarse particle fraction of PM_{10} were related to reports of chest tightness; however, semi-volatile and coarse particle mass was not related to respiratory symptoms or mucous membrane irritation (Schinasi et al. 2011).

Sensory exposures such as noise, threats, and pain can cause physiological changes and affect mental health. We asked participants to rate the extent to which they felt stressed or annoyed following their 10-minute times outside. The odds of feeling stressed or annoyed increased 18% for every 1 ppb increase in hydrogen sulfide concentration and 81% for each unit increase in hog odor on the 0- to 8-point scale (Horton et al. 2009). Systolic blood pressure, measured after returning indoors after the 10-minute outdoor exposure, rose an average of 0.29 mmHg for every 1 ppb increase in hydrogen sulfide, and diastolic blood pressure rose an average of 0.23 mmHg for a one unit increase in reported hog odor (Wing et al. 2013). The odor–diastolic blood pressure relationship is depicted in Figure 3.12, scaled to represent a participant whose average diastolic pressure was 80.5 mmHg during times of no odor.

After completing data collection in the repeated-measures study, qualitative researchers from our team conducted in-depth interviews with 49 of the participants using an interview guide designed to obtain detailed information about the context, beliefs, experiences, attitudes, and coping mechanisms of hog operation neighbors in relation to pollution from these facilities (Tajik et al. 2008). The interviews also

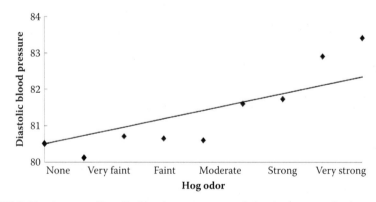

FIGURE 3.12 Average diastolic blood pressure at each level of reported odor, adjusted for time of day, and linear slope estimated by fixed effects regression, scaled to a person with an estimated blood pressure of 80.5 during times of no odor. (Based on Wing, S. et al., *Environmental Health Perspectives*, 121, 92–96, 2013.)

assessed individual and collective actions undertaken by community residents to resist the contamination of their neighborhoods. Each interview was conducted by a pair of interviewers: one academic and one community organizer. The participants were asked what they like and dislike about their community, what it was like growing up, how things had changed, how they responded to hog odor, and what they could do about the odor. Interviews were recorded and transcribed, and themes in the text were coded to identify common threads.

Tajik et al. (2008) summarized the impacts of hog odor in two primary areas that emerged from the interviews: (1) beneficial use of property and (2) quiet enjoyment of life. The theme beneficial use of property was based on statements about how low-income rural residents expect to be able to enjoy outdoor activities around their homes, such as walking, tending livestock, gardening, cooking out, and playing games. They also expect to be able to open their windows for fresh air and to be able to line-dry their clothes. Such activities are especially important for people who cannot afford or access fitness centers, vacation destinations, public facilities, or air conditioning (Tajik et al. 2008).

Participants said, for example, that hog odor prevented them from sitting outside, inviting guests for cookouts and family reunions, working and playing outside, drying clothes, and gardening. They talked about not being able to use their well water and having to buy bottled water. They talked about devaluation of their property and not being able to sleep at night because of the odor. In their own words:

"A lot of my family come and can't stay here. They say, 'God, I can't stand this. How can you live here?'"

"My son has asthma and allergies... he just stays inside."

"I had a rose garden... do you see those weeds there... I haven't done it for the past few years...."

"Sometimes it's so unbearable you couldn't even hardly stand it, not even in the house."

"On a bad day it is not that you can't go outside... but the odor determines how long you gonna stay..."

"When the smell [hog odor] get in, you can't get rid of it."

"... I had stuff here in writing saying that the property has gone down 20–30 percent because you are near a hog farm."

"The water turns everything yellow. If I wash my clothes for a good six weeks in that water, I will have to buy new clothes... I will have to buy new clothes every six weeks."

"I don't drink the ground water no more because of the hog farms... now we have to buy water to drink."

"It [hog odor] woke me up. And I had to get up. I couldn't sleep. I put the covers up over my face and it didn't do any good."

These interviews support findings from the repeated-measures study that hog odor affects people's ability to exercise outdoors, their sleep patterns, and their experience of stress and anxiety. Public health advocates tell people to exercise, get adequate sleep, and avoid social isolation. Neighbors of industrial hog operations report that hog odor interferes with following these basic health recommendations (Tajik et al. 2008).

HEALTH EFFECTS OF INDUSTRIAL ANIMAL PRODUCTION EXTEND
BEYOND LOCAL COMMUNITIES

Eastern North Carolina has the top 10 ranked counties for hog density in the United States. Three of these are the top ranked counties for turkey density. Broiler chicken production is also high in this same area. Although turkey and broiler operations do not use lagoons and spray fields, the confinements, manure storage sites, and spreading of manure on fields also produce air emissions that neighbors find to be offensive. Although industrial animal production has its most direct impacts on neighboring communities, the environment and health effects are not confined to local areas.

Historically, epidemic strains of influenza have emerged from interactions of people, pigs, and poultry in areas where humans are in close domestic contact with their animals. One argument for growing animals in confinement has been that this practice minimizes potential for infectious diseases to be transferred between people and livestock (Graham et al. 2008). However, a study of H1N1 swine flu in Iowa found that the odds of having H1N1 antibodies were 55 times higher in swine workers, and 28 times higher in their spouses, compared to people who did not live near livestock (Gray et al. 2007). Flu virus can be highly infectious and could spread rapidly from high livestock density areas to other populations. There has been concern that the 2010 global pandemic of swine flu originated in Vera Cruz, Mexico, an area of industrial swine production where the first case was identified.

The majority of antibiotics in the United States are used to promote livestock growth in confined growing facilities, not to treat human disease (Silbergeld et al. 2008). Such subtherapeutic administration contributes to the development of antibiotic resistance because bacteria that are susceptible to antibiotics produce fewer offspring than those with genetic resistance. In addition, resistance genes can be transferred directly between bacteria. Antibiotic resistance, which is traditionally identified with hospitals and human medicine, is an important public health problem because resistance makes treatment of human infection more difficult. Antibiotics commonly used to promote livestock growth belong to classes of drugs that are important in medicine; therefore, development of antibiotic resistance in livestock threatens to undermine treatment of human infection (Silbergeld et al. 2008). Several stains of methicillin-resistant *Staphylococcus aureus*, which is responsible for substantial morbidity and mortality, have been linked to livestock production (Smith and Pearson 2011). *S. aureus* sequence type 398 has been shown to be related to livestock density in the Netherlands (Feingold et al. 2012).

Industrial swine facilities typically use several measures to limit spread of pathogens. This is of economic importance due to the potential for animal mortality. Vehicles must have their tires disinfected upon entry, and workers must shower-in, shower-out, and change clothes when they leave confinement buildings. However, bacteria can survive in workers' nasal mucosa (Frana et al. 2013), and animal vectors such as rodents and birds, in addition to flies, can carry bacteria off-site (Graham et al. 2009). In one study, antibiotic-resistant bacteria were found in the feces of migratory geese that land on swine-waste lagoons (Cole et al. 2005). Bacteria resistant to antibiotics that are used in poultry feed have been found in excess behind poultry transport trucks and are carried by flies near poultry operations on Maryland's eastern shore (Rule et al. 2008).

Another animal feed additive of concern is arsenic, a human carcinogen. Arsenical drugs are common in poultry feed and may also be used in swine. Land application of animal wastes distributes arsenic onto land, potentially affecting ground and surface water, as well as food crops. Emphasis on renewable energy for electricity production, combined with the large excess of animal waste in high-density livestock production areas like eastern North Carolina, has led to pressures to burn poultry waste for electricity production, a practice that produces more air pollution than burning coal, which could result in widespread distribution of arsenic in the environment (Stingone and Wing 2011).

Traditional agriculture is based on producing a diversity of species. Because animal wastes are used to fertilize feed crops used to grow the next year's livestock, this system results in a feedback loop wherein wastes are recycled on the farm. Furthermore, in pasture-based operations, livestock play an important role in scavenging crop residues that remain in the fields after harvest, reducing insect populations, and conditioning soil by disturbing the ground and depositing manure. Diversity of production not only creates nutrient feedback loops and symbiotic relationships between multiple species but it also makes agriculture more resistant to periodic problems such as pests, drought, and temperature fluctuations, which usually affect one species more than others.

In contrast, industrial agriculture is designed to minimize diversity by focusing on a single crop (Mancus 2007). In the case of industrial animal production, feed is often produced at distant locations and transported to livestock-growing areas using fossil fuels. In the absence of manure fertilizer from livestock that consume feed grains, feed crops require more chemical fertilizers that require large fossil fuel inputs and increase levels of reactive nitrogen in the biosphere (Mancus 2007). Nitrogen pollution presents a myriad of health concerns due to respiratory impacts of air pollution, ingestion of nitrate-contaminated groundwater, and impacts on algal blooms and eutrophication of surface waters. Nitrogen pollution results not only from production of feed grains in the absence of animal manure but also from disposal of animal manure in the absence of adequate capacity for uptake by crops. Dense livestock-producing areas such as eastern North Carolina have large excesses of nitrogen and phosphorus from animal manures, which impact ground and surface waters in those locations and downstream coastal waters (Burkholder et al. 2007).

Livestock production is also an important source of methane, which is 25 times more potent than carbon dioxide as a greenhouse gas (Pew Commission on Industrial Food Animal Production 2008). Methane's half-life in the atmosphere is less than that of carbon dioxide, but it converts to carbon dioxide. Industrial livestock production's contribution to climate change shows that it affects environmental health over spatial scales from the local to the global.

ECONOMIC, SOCIAL, AND POLITICAL IMPACTS OF INDUSTRIAL ANIMAL PRODUCTION

Public health is affected not only by food quality but also by access to clean air and water, safe working and living conditions, quality education, medical and health services, and opportunities for physical activity. The extent to which these needs are met depends on the organization of social systems, the collective aspect of public health that determines individual exposures, choices, opportunities, and health inequalities. Industrialization of agriculture not only impacts environmental and occupational exposures in rural communities but also affects the political and food environments in both rural and urban communities.

Industrial animal agriculture is vertically integrated (Pew Commission on Industrial Food Animal Production 2008). This means that one company controls the production process from basic inputs to retail sale. Livestock producers either own animal production facilities or, more commonly, use contract growers, typically former family farmers, to raise the animals. In the case of hogs, the integrator owns the animals, animal feed, veterinary supplies, trucks, rendering plants, and processing plants. The contract grower owns (and has liability for) the buildings and the waste and must follow the integrator's terms for raising the animals. Most hog producers are unable to remain independent because they cannot get access to processing plants without a contract, and integrators control the processing plants (Pew Commission on Industrial Food Animal Production 2008).

Family farmers buy feed, equipment, and supplies from local retailers and spend their profits in their communities. In contrast, with industrial food animal production, corporations that integrate all aspects of production do not need to support local communities. In fact, corporations are legally responsible to maximize returns for their shareholders. Unlike businesses that support local communities, corporations syphon profits from rural communities for the benefit of distant shareholders. Their ability to impact rural communities is enhanced by campaign contributions and representation of business interests at all levels of government from local commissions and health boards to state legislatures, environmental agencies, and agriculture departments (Thu 2001). This political contamination, as detrimental to social and economic organization as toxins are to the health of individual humans, promotes economic inequalities and exploitation of workers while it prevents adoption of environmental and occupational protections that could be implemented to reduce impacts on rural communities. Perhaps most importantly, economic and political control of communities by national and global corporations prevents democratic participation and local control (Thu 2001, 2003).

The influence of corporate agribusiness at the state and national level inhibits the adoption of food safety regulations that could reduce the presence of pathogens, antibiotic-resistant bacteria, arsenic, and other contaminants in retail foods consumed by the general population. As in other areas such as pharmaceuticals, energy, and transportation, corporate influence helps direct government funds to university research that is more oriented toward industry profit than protection of the health of workers, residents exposed to pollutants, and consumers. Public land-grant universities are particularly harnessed in service to industrialized agriculture (Food and Water Watch 2012).

Industrialization of agriculture and the entire food system has promoted homogenization of food environments. Highly advertised packaged foods and chain restaurants result in the same foods being available in retail outlets across the country, and to some extent the world. Sugar, salt, fats, and flavorings, as well as appearance of foods and packaging, are manipulated to increase sales and consumption.

The convenience of packaged, prepared foods is not only attractive to people who work long hours in addition to caring for family members but makes it easier for everyone to eat more and more often. Resulting mass obesity, although it is often viewed as a problem of the obese person who lacks self-control, is an engine of profits, not only for food companies but for companies that sell clothes; exercise equipment and club memberships; diet pills; drugs for hypertension, hypercholesterolemia, and diabetes; and ultimately medical and surgical treatment of victims of ischemic heart disease, stroke, and other obesity-related conditions. Because changing the environment that promotes mass obesity will reduce industry profits, corporate control of the political system will need to be challenged if major changes are to occur.

Most pork, chicken, beef, dairy, and egg production occurs in concentrated animal feeding operations; for example, in 2007, 97% of hogs in the United States were housed in units with over 500 heads. This system is organized to produce profits for global corporations, and it results in cheap food because the environmental and human costs entailed by the system are not reflected in retail prices. Workers are sickened in factory farms and processing plants. Neighbors are exposed to air and water pollution that degrades their health, quality of life, and property values, and increases the cost of basic needs such as water and energy. Aquifers are contaminated, and surface waters suffer pollution that affects aquatic life and increases costs of water treatment in downstream communities. Retail meats are contaminated with antibiotic-resistant bacteria. These costs of industrial agriculture are not reflected in the price of food, which is in this way subsidized by loss of human and environmental health. Health disparities are fueled by the relatively higher dependence on these foods of low-income people compared to wealthier people.

How has this happened? The system is highly complex, but one feature has been key: environmental and social injustice. If workers and residents in rural communities that are most directly impacted had basic political and human rights, industrial agriculture would not have developed with such destructive force because those affected by its side effects would have been able to protect themselves. However, racism, classism, and political disenfranchisement of rural communities make it possible for the entire population to suffer detrimental health effects.

Addressing these problems will require many different strategies and struggles. Some may be taken by public health authorities acting as social engineers who, upon identifying pathological aspects of our food system, intervene to improve matters. Government interventions including environmental regulations, occupational safety and health rules, prohibitions on misuse of antibiotics and agricultural chemicals, and food safety regulations, are important. However, more fundamental changes in public health have been brought about not just by benevolent managers, but by mass movements such as the anti-slavery, women's rights, civil rights, peace, environmental, and human rights movements (Wing 2005). Such movements provide people who are most negatively impacted by exploitation with opportunities for self-preservation and increased protections, and in doing so improve conditions for the general population. Transformation of the food system, which can improve local food environments for all, depends on such basic social changes.

REFERENCES

Allen, B. 2006. Cradle of a revolution? The industrial transformation of Louisiana's lower Mississippi River. *Technol Cult* 47:112–119.

Burkholder, J., B. Libra, P. Weyer, S. Heathcote, D. Kolpin, P.S. Thorne, M. Wichman. 2007. Impacts of waste from concentrated animal feeding operations on water quality. *Environ Health Perspect* 115:308–312.

Cole, D., D.J. Drum, D.E. Stalknecht, D.G. White, M.D. Lee, S. Ayers, M. Sobsey, et al. 2005. Free-living Canada geese and antimicrobrial resistance. *Emerg Infect Dis* 11:935–938.

Cole, D., L. Todd, S. Wing. 2000. Concentrated swine feeding operations and public health: A review of occupational and community health effects. *Environ Health Perspect* 108:685–699.

Domhoff, G. 2012. Who Rules America? Wealth, Income, and Power. Available at http://www2.ucsc.edu/whorulesamerica/power/wealth.html; accessed December 27, 2012.

Donham, K. 1993. Respiratory disease hazards to workers in livestock and poultry confinement structures. *Sem Resp Med* 14:49–59.

Edwards, B., A. Driscoll. 2009. From farms to factories: The environmental consequences of swine industrialization in North Carolina. In *Twenty Lessons in Environmental Sociology*, eds, Gould K.A., T. L. Lewis, pp. 153–175. New York: Oxford University Press.

Edwards, B., A. Ladd. 2000. Environmental justice, swine production and farm loss in north carolina. *Socio Spec* 20:263–290.

Feingold, B.J., E.K. Silbergeld, F.C. Curriero, B.A.van Cleef, M.E. Heck, J.A. Kluytmans. 2012. Livestock density as risk factor for livestock-associated methicillin-resistant *Staphylococcus aureus*, the Netherlands. *Emerg Infect Dis* 18:1841–1849.

Food and Water Watch. 2012. Public Research, Private Gain: Corporate Influence Over University Agriculture. Available at http://www.foodandwaterwatch.org/reports/public-research-private-gain/; accessed March 31, 2013.

Frana, T.S., A.R. Beahm, B.M. Hanson, J.M. Kinyon, L.L. Layman, L.A. Karriker, A. Ramirez, et al. 2013. Isolation and characterization of methicillin-resistant *Staphylococcus aureus* from pork farms and visiting veterinary students. *PloS One* 8:e53738.

Furuseth, O. 1997. Restructuring of hog farming in North Carolina: Explosion and implosion. *Prof Geog* 49:391–403.

Graham, J.P., J.H. Leibler, L.B. Price, J.M. Otte, D.U. Pfeiffer, T. Tiensin, E.K. Silbergeld. 2008. The animal-human interface and infectious disease in industrial food animal production: Rethinking biosecurity and biocontainment. *Pub Health Rep* 123:282–299.

Graham, J.P., L.B. Price, S.L. Evans, T.K. Graczyk, E.K. Silbergeld. 2009. Antibiotic resistant enterococci and staphylococci isolated from flies collected near confined poultry feeding operations. *Sci Total Environ* 407:2701–2710.

Gray, G.C., T. McCarthy, A.W. Capuano, S.F. Setterquist, C.W. Olsen, M.C. Alavanja. 2007. Swine workers and swine influenza virus infections. *Emerg Infect Dis* 13:1871–1878.

Heederik, D., T. Sigsgaard, P.S. Thorne, J.N. Kline, R. Avery, J.H. Bonlokke, E.A. Chrischilles, et al. 2007. Health effects of airborne exposures from concentrated animal feeding operations. *Environ Health Perspect* 115:298–302.

Horton, R.A., S. Wing, S.W. Marshall, K.A. Brownley. 2009. Malodor as a trigger of stress and negative mood in neighbors of industrial hog operations. *Am J Pub Health* 99 Suppl 3:S610–615.

Hricko, A. 2008. Global trade comes home: Community impacts of goods movement. *Environ Health Perspect* 116:A78–81.

Hricko, A.M. 2006. Ships, trucks, and trains: Effects of goods movement on environmental health. *Environ Health Perspect* 114:A204–205.

Lipscomb, H.J., K. Kucera, C. Epling, J. Dement. 2008. Upper extremity musculoskeletal symptoms and disorders among a cohort of women employed in poultry processing. *Am J Ind Med* 51:24–36.

Lipscomb, H.J., R. Argue, M.A. McDonald, J.M. Dement, C.A. Epling, T. James, S. Wing, et al. 2005. Exploration of work and health disparities among black women employed in poultry processing in the rural south. *Environ Health Perspect* 113:1833–1840.

Lipscomb, H.J., D. Loomis, M.A. McDonald, R.A. Argue, S. Wing. 2006. A conceptual model of work and health disparities in the United States. *Int J Health Serv* 36:25–50.

Lipscomb, H.J., J.M. Dement, C.A. Epling, B.N. Gaynes, M.A. McDonald, A.L. Schoenfisch. 2007. Depressive symptoms among working women in rural North Carolina: A comparison of women in poultry processing and other low-wage jobs. *Int J Law Psych* 30:284–298.

Martin, R.P. 2008. Preface, p viii, in: National Commission on Food Animal Production, Putting Meat on the Table: Industrial Farm Animal Production in America. Baltimore, MD: Pew Commission

Mancus, P. 2007. Nitrogen fertilizer dependency and its contradictions: A theoretical exploration of social-ecological metabolism. *Rural Soc* 72:269–288.

Milio, N. 1976. A framework for prevention: Changing health-damaging to health-generating life patterns. *Am J Pub Health* 66:435–439.

Mirabelli, M.C., S. Wing, S.W. Marshall, T.C. Wilcosky. 2006a. Race, poverty, and potential exposure of middle-school students to air emissions from confined swine feeding operations. *Environ Health Perspect* 114:591–596.

Mirabelli, M.C., S. Wing, S.W. Marshall, T.C. Wilcosky. 2006b. Asthma symptoms among adolescents who attend public schools that are located near confined swine feeding operations. *Pediatrics* 118:e66–75.

Morland, K., S. Wing, A.Diez Roux. 2002a. The contextual effect of the local food environment on residents' diets: The atherosclerosis risk in communities study. *Am J Pub Health* 92:1761–1767.

Morland, K., S. Wing, A. Diez Roux, C. Poole. 2002b. Neighborhood characteristics associated with the location of food stores and food service places. *Am J Prev Med* 22:23–29.

Pew Commission on Industrial Food Animal Production. 2008. Putting Meat on the Table: Industrial Farm Animal Production in America. Available at http://www.ncifap.org/; accessed March 23, 2009.

Price, L.B., J.P. Graham, L.G. Lackey, A. Roess, R. Vailes, E. Silbergeld. 2007. Elevated risk of carrying gentamicin-resistant *Escherichia coli* among U.S. poultry workers. *Environ Health Perspect* 115:1738–1742.

Rule, A.M., S.L. Evans, E.K. Silbergeld. 2008. Food animal transport: a potential source of community exposures to health hazards from industrial farming (cafos). *J Infect Pub Health* 1:33–39.

Schiffman, S.S., C.E. Studwell, L.R. Landerman, K. Berman, J.S. Sundy. 2005. Symptomatic effects of exposure to diluted air sampled from a swine confinement atmosphere on healthy human subjects. *Environ Health Perspect* 113:567–576.

Schinasi, L., R.A. Horton, S. Wing. 2009. Data completeness and quality in a community-based and participatory epidemiologic study. *Prog Community Health Partnersh* 3:179–190.

Schinasi, L., R.A. Horton, V.T. Guidry, S. Wing, S.W. Marshall, K.B. Morland. 2011. Air pollution, lung function, and physical symptoms in communities near concentrated swine feeding operations. *Epidem* 22:208–215.

Silbergeld, E.K., J. Graham, L.B. Price. 2008. Industrial food animal production, antimicrobial resistance, and human health. *Ann Rev Pub Health* 29:151–169.

Smith, T.C., N. Pearson. 2011. The emergence of *Staphylococcus aureus* st398. *Vector Borne Zoonotic Dis* 11:327–339.

Stingone, J.A., S. Wing. 2011. Poultry litter incineration as a source of energy: Reviewing the potential for impacts on environmental health and justice. *New Solut* 21:27–42.

Tajik, M., N. Muhammad, A. Lowman, K. Thu, S. Wing, G. Grant. 2008. Impact of odor from industrial hog operations on daily living activities. *New Solut* 18:193–205.

Thu, K., K. Donham, R. Ziegenhorn, S. Reynolds, P. Thorne, P. Subramanian, P. Whitten, et al. 1997. A control study of the physical and mental health of residents living near a large-scale swine operation. *J Agr Safe Health* 3:13–26.

Thu, K. 2001. Agriculture, the environment, and sources of state ideology and power. *Cult Ag* 23:1–7.

Thu, K. 2003. Industrial agriculture, democracy, and the future. In *Beyond Factory Farming: Corporate Hog Barns and the Threat to Public Health, the Environment, and Rural Communities*, eds, Ervin A., C. Holtslander, D. Qualman, R. Sawa. Saskatoon, Saskatchewan: Canadian Centre for Policy Alternatives.

USDA. 2012. Adoption of Genetically Engineered Crops in the U.S. Available at http://www.ers.usda.gov/data-products/adoption-of-genetically-engineered-crops-in-the-us/recent-trends-in-ge-adoption.aspx; accessed December 19, 2012.

Villarejo, D. 2003. The health of U.S.-hired farm workers. *Ann Rev Pub Health* 24:175–193.

Wing, S., G. Grant, M. Green, C. Stewart. 1996. Community based collaboration for environmental justice: South-East Halifax environmental reawakening. *Environ Urban* 8:129–140.

Wing, S., D. Cole, G. Grant. 2000. Environmental injustice in North Carolina's hog industry. *Environ Health Perspect* 108:225–231.

Wing, S., S. Wolf. 2000. Intensive livestock operations, health, and quality of life among Eastern North Carolina residents. *Environ Health Perspect* 108:233–238.

Wing, S. 2002. Social responsibility and research ethics in community-driven studies of industrialized hog production. *Environ Health Perspect* 110: 437–444.

Wing, S., S. Freedman, L. Band. 2002. The potential impact of flooding on confined animal feeding operations in Eastern North Carolina. *Environ Health Perspect* 110:387–391.

Wing, S. 2005. Environmental justice, science and public health. *Environ Health Perspect* Special Issue: 54–63.

Wing, S., R.A. Horton, S.W. Marshall, K. Thu, M. Tajik, L. Schinasi, S.S. Schiffman. 2008a. Air pollution and odor in communities near industrial swine operations. *Environ Health Perspect* 116:1362–1368.

Wing, S., R.A. Horton, N. Muhammad, G.R. Grant, M. Tajik, K. Thu. 2008b. Integrating epidemiology, education, and organizing for environmental justice: Community health effects of industrial hog operations. *Am J Pub Health* 98:1390–1397.

Wing, S., R.A. Horton, K.M. Rose. 2013. Air pollution from industrial swine operations and blood pressure of neighboring residents. *Environ Health Perspect* 121:92–96.

Section II

Local Food Environments
Research, Methods, and Analytical Issues

4 Geography of Local Food Environments

People and Places

Kimberly B. Morland

Residential segregation lies beyond the ability of any individual to change; it constrains black life chances irrespective of personal traits, individual motivations, or private achievements.

Douglas S. Massey and Nancy A. Denton (1993)

The area of public health research that aims to investigate the health effects associated with disparities between local food environments stems from earlier epidemiology* investigations that have identified difference in disease rates by geographic regions. Within these studies, researchers have found geographic clustering of diseases. For instance, it is well documented that the highest mortality resulting from stroke is clustered in the Southeast region of the United States, known as the Stroke Belt (Figure 4.1). Black Americans are also concentrated in the Southeast region of the United States. Furthermore, although the incidence of stroke is higher among African-Americans and Hispanic Americans compared to Caucasians, the geographic difference in rates cannot be fully explained by traditional risk factors for stroke among these groups of Americans (National Institutes of Health 2009).

In addition to race, areas in the United States are segregated by income brackets of residents. For example, differences in household incomes can be observed across the United States using 2010 U.S. Census Bureau data (Bloch et al. 2013). The geographic tool demonstrates household income differences between small and large geographic areas (http://projects.nytimes.com/census/2010/explorer). For instance, using the New York City area as just one example, the household income distribution of the borough of Manhattan compared to the outer boroughs, such as Brooklyn, is quite striking. Investigators have identified the clustering of people by socioeconomic factors to be predictive of disease (Acevedo-Garcia and Lochner 2003). Many early studies focused on the disease distributions across countries, which vary considerably where those countries with higher gross national products have better health outcomes for their populations (Marmot and Bell 2006). Investigators have

---

* Epidemiology is a field of science where determinants of human disease are investigated. Unlike clinical studies that focus on individual patients, epidemiology is the study of population health and measures risk of disease for groups of people. This area of science contributes to public health by identifying modifiable risk factors that can affect groups of people and hence shift distributions of disease.

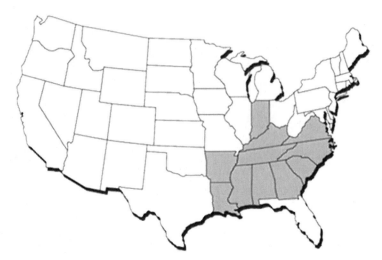

FIGURE 4.1 United States stroke belt. (From National Institutes of Health, National Heart, Lung and Blood Institute, Stroke Belt Initiative. http://www.nhlbi.nih.gov/health/prof/heart /other/sb_spec.pdf.)

argued that the underpinnings of geographic difference pertain to socioeconomic disadvantages experienced by some groups of people and, moreover, that these disadvantages are broader than simply the classification of low income. Rather, it is *poverty* that places individuals within a social class that affects opportunities for reaching their potential and meeting basic needs. Some have argued that the perpetuation of these economic strata in societies create social injustices associated with poor health conditions (Levy and Sidel 2006). Many public health investigators have conducted studies focused on determining how physical and social features of neighborhood environment influence health behaviors and outcomes (Kawachi and Berkman 2003). Within this specific area of social epidemiology, a number of area characteristics that disproportionally affect low income and communities of color have been investigated to identify specific features of geographic distribution that place people living in poverty at increased risk for disease.

Poverty is estimated to affect 15.1% of the U.S. population, or 46.9 million people, and those rates affect people of color to a greater extent. In 2010, 27.4% of black Americans and 26.6% of Hispanics experienced poverty (DeNavas-Walt et al. 2011). Poverty has largely driven people to settle in specific regions of the United States that are more affordable, resulting in a culture of inequality and the segregation of neighborhoods (through the concentration of groups of people into geographical areas). In the United States, geographic distribution of residents has historically been characterized by segregation based on race/ethnicity and/or income. In turn, as segregated environments have developed over time, individuals have not only shared social customs, attitudes, and beliefs, but regional resources as well. The identification of geographic areas where disease prevalence is higher compared to other areas is a necessary first step toward understanding health inequalities. The second step, which can encompass health promotion efforts and targeted interventions to rectify these inequities, is to better understand what specific mechanisms actually influence these differences in disease rates among residents residing across geographic locales.

The success of ecological studies has led investigators toward the development of more rigorous research designed to identify mechanisms for these differences. Aiming to identify personal traits, behaviors, and individual-level attributes as causal factors for these geographic distributions of disease, the methods of modern epidemiology have shifted almost entirely away from considering environmental and exposure-related experiences as causal agents.

For those studies that do investigate the health effects associated with environmental exposures, epidemiologists generally focus on single toxins found in air, water, or subsequently the food chain. Toxins are generally measured as indoor or outdoor exposures and sometimes in relation to the environmental source of contamination. Mechanisms of biological action are modeled though pathways such as ingestion or inhalation, and these investigations lend themselves well for validation by toxicology studies. In other words, the focus of disease causation within environmental epidemiology pertains to the effects of a single environmental toxin on endocrine function, cellular function, epigenetic,* or other individual-level response systems that may directly disrupt biological processes. Fewer studies have measured the effects of area resources and infrastructure on human health. Although John Snow attributed the higher rates of cholera in England to the contamination of one specific water pump in 1854, differences in area infrastructure as causal mechanisms of disease are rarely considered in modern epidemiology (BBC History 2013).

ENVIRONMENTAL VERSUS INDIVIDUAL CAUSES OF DISEASE

This paradigm shift affects the interpretation of the statistical models that aim to investigate disease causation. For example, the clustering of stroke in regions where black Americans live has led to many studies aimed at measuring the causes of this higher disease rate among blacks. Risk factors for stroke include hypertension, heart disease, atrial fibrillation, diabetes, fibrinogen, family history of stroke, and race, as well as behavioral factors such as cigarette smoking, alcohol consumption, and low physical activity (Wolf 1994). To note, no direct environmental causes are included, except possibly the variable *race*. Epidemiologists have come to interpret effects associated with race in their statistical models as measures of individual's biological makeup. Rarely considered in the explanation of effects are the social and physical experiences of groups of people. Take, for example, preterm birth in the United States. Higher rates of preterm birth among black women have been documented repeatedly with statistical models such as the one given here:

$$\text{Model 1: } Y = a + b_1 (x_1)$$

where x_1 is black women and Y is preterm birth.

---

* Epigenetics is a field of science that investigates how environmental influences affect genetic programming. In other words, researchers are investigating how genes can be "turned on and off" by experiences and the environment. These modifications of gene function disrupt biological processes that may be responsible for the initiation of disease.

The beta coefficient (b_1) will tell the investigator three things: (1) if the risk of preterm birth is higher or lower than the comparison group, (2) how much higher or lower the risk is, and (3) the precision and statistical significance of that effect (with the standard error associated with the beta coefficient). Effects are then reported as *black women have a higher risk of preterm birth* without answering the question *why?* At face value, the effect of race might be interpreted as there is a biological mechanism within black women that causes their babies to be delivered early. Note that the explanation is not directly measured; rather, it is assumed to be what the variable, *race*, represents.

Some of the narrow interpretation of race variables may stem from a misunderstanding of the inheritability of genes among groups. The interpretation mentioned previously assumes that black women share genetic traits that put them at risk for preterm delivery. But in fact, there are no genetic traits or single gene that is shared in one population. Investigators sometimes assume that skin color is a marker for similarities in genetic heritability or ancestry. But, for example, the skin color of sub-Saharan Africans and Aborigines in Australia share a trait of dark skin but are thought to be of different races (Smedley 2008). Moreover, if DNA markers are predictive of disease outcomes, then black Americans should share disease rates with ancestry in Western Africa. Black Americans do have high rates of hypertension: Western Africans have some of the lowest rates worldwide (Cooper et al. 2005). Furthermore, studies that have shown that the dietary patterns and disease rates of U.S. immigrants are affected by assimilation into American culture documents the influence of environment on behaviors (Jonnalagadda and Diwan 2002; Davies et al. 2006; Akresh 2007).

The problem stems from an underappreciation of how human biology and behaviors are influenced by the places we inhabit. Ecological models of human development have been developed by Bronfenbrenner (1994), who has argued that human development is a function of the environmental conditions in which human beings live and that these environments affect the life course. In other words, individual-level risk factors are not independent from the environments that contribute to disease progression. Therefore, the interpretation of the beta coefficient in Model 1 has to consider the variable *race*, not strictly as a measurement of individual's biology, but as a measurement of the environmental exposures and experiences that may have shaped that biology.

RACIAL SEGREGATION IN THE UNITED STATES

As we delve further into understanding how to develop statistical models that will address *why* certain groups of people who share environments may be at higher risk for disease development, we first need to describe how geographic concentrations of populations have developed in the United States. Segregation is the concentration of groups of people into geographical areas. Many groups of people have historically, and to current day, lived in areas segregated by socioeconomic factors. Within concentrated environments, individuals often share customs, attitudes, and beliefs, as well as resources.

However, there may be differential effects of segregation depending on the factors that may influence the relationship between environment and health. First, there is variance of isolation between segregated neighborhoods. For example, although there are individuals from any number of racial/ethnic backgrounds (e.g., Italian, Polish, Chinese, Mexican) concentrated into neighborhoods across the United States, it is argued that no group in American history has experienced the systematic segregation on par with that experienced by black Americans (Massey and Denton 1993). The differential experience of black Americans is rooted in the history of slavery with a sustained social and institutional racism levied against this population from white Americans in particular. Distinctions between racially segregated black neighborhoods and that of other ethnic groups have been described to be more concentrated and more permanent (Massey and Denton 1993). For instance, as early as 1910, only a few cities had areas of isolation for groups such as Italian or Jewish, whereas concentrated black neighborhoods were prominent in more than 10 cities. The area concentrations were supported in cities such as Baltimore, Richmond, and Atlanta by the legal institution of segregation in housing through the establishment of clear delineations between black and white areas within these cities (Rice 1968). Furthermore although residents living in immigrant communities were typically transient, and segregation in these areas fell after 1910 for most racial/ethnic groups, the experience of black Americans was shaped by different sociopolitical factors; the result of which only led to further development of segregated black neighborhoods over the next several decades throughout the country (Lieberson 1963).

As early as the 1920s, racial homogeneity of neighborhoods was garnered with the institution of restrictive covenants by real estate boards and homeowner associations, targeting black Americans in particular. Under these covenants, property owners would sign agreements to not allow black Americans to own, occupy, or lease their properties (Drake and Cayton 1970). These types of contracts were used in the United States until 1948 when the U.S. Supreme Court finally declared they were unenforceable (Helper 1969). However, up until this time, these restrictive covenants were commonplace and supported by the official policies of the National Association of Real Estate Brokers in their code of ethics which stated: "A Realtor should never be instrumental in introducing into a neighborhood … members of any race or nationality … whose presence will clearly be detrimental to property values in that neighborhood" (Helper 1969). These policies were also supported by bankers who would not grant loans to black applicants for home financing and other financial assistance. This persistent discrimination across communities ultimately relegated black Americans to living within specific regions of the United States (Massey and Denton 1993).

Policies and practices that supported the racial segregation of black Americans in the United States continued after World War II. For example, new construction of homes developed due to the administration of new government loan programs through the Federal Housing Administration (FHA) and the Veterans Administration. These programs made homeownership affordable and contributed to the selective migration of the white middle class from cities to suburbs. The migration of black Americans was made more difficult as these individuals were still being subjected to discriminatory lending and housing practices. In 1930, the federal government began the Home Owners' Loan Corporation (HOLC) and rating system, which was a program developed to assist Americans with refinancing mortgages and creating low-interest loans to support neighborhood development. To assess the risk of the borrower for loan repayment and to evaluate areas worthy of capital investment, the program relied on a rating system based on the residential neighborhood quality of the applicant. Within this system, four categories ranked from lowest to highest risk were developed and the highest risk was coded in red. Maps were then created using the rating procedures and lines were drawn to partition area risk by the four categories. In general, homes located in inner cities and within black neighborhoods were undervalued and hence *redlined* (Helper 1969).

The policies of the FHA followed those of the HOLC and perpetuated the segregation of American neighborhoods with an underwriting manual that stated: "If a neighborhood is to retain stability, it is necessary that properties shall continue to be occupied by the same social and racial classes" (Hays 1985). In addition, FHA loans favored single-family homes, therefore placing residents of attached dwellings and row housing (common in inner cities) at a disadvantage for benefiting from this federal program. The trend to support the growth of the suburbs continued through the 1970s to such an extent that private and government lending to inner city residents lead to the depreciation of homes in predominately black and low wealth areas. Although these federal initiatives focus on housing, the disinvestment of these areas by the federal government was also supported by a disinvestment by commercial entities.

SEGREGATION AND AREA RESOURCES

Although much has been written regarding where groups of people live in the United States, less has been described about how economic and racial structures of neighborhoods effect the commercial establishments in those areas. Although it can be assumed, based on discussion in Chapters 1 through 3, that because commercial establishments are in the business of making money, they would locate stores and services in areas where mass merchandising would work best. In brief, mass merchandising requires a large number of products to be offered to customers to offset profit margins, as well as a large enough volume of customers to purchase these high levels of stock. Certainly, business practices are proprietary, but it can be safely assumed that retailers are attracted to expansive, inexpensive spaces to locate these types of large-scale businesses—areas that are typically located away from inner cities in increasingly suburban and rural environments. While the motivations of business retailers are protected, the empirical observations of the geographic differences in the availability of stores, services, and other resources can be measured.

Interestingly, there were a very limited number of these types of studies within the health literature prior to the local food environments disparities studies. However, the West Coast Regional Office of Consumers Union in San Francisco published a report in 1993 that did compare the presence of basic goods and services between three areas of Los Angeles and four areas of Oakland, California (Troutt 1993). The report was intended to help low-income consumers obtain affordable housing, quality foods, health care, as well as banking and credit needs. The spatial analysis was intended to demonstrate differences in the local availability of resources by neighborhood wealth with a comparison of low- and middle-income areas in each region of California. The author concludes that the "Red line of economic discrimination extends throughout the low income consumer infrastructure, with dramatic effects on low income consumers and their neighborhoods" (p. 8). It is argued that, because low-income consumers spend their money for goods and services outside their immediate neighborhood (because of the lack of availability), these local areas also miss opportunities for economic growth, thus perpetuating a cycle of redlining and poor credit in these neighborhoods.

As part of this study, areas were surveyed for the presence of places that provided goods and services. For instance, in Oakland, California, the middle-class neighborhood Rockridge was compared to West Oakland, Fruitvale, and Elmhurst, all of which were distinctly low-income neighborhoods. Areas varied by racial composition and median household income, as well as homeownership. Maps were developed denoting the location of types of businesses within those areas showing that the neighborhoods were distinctly different. For instance, the number of restaurants, grocery stores, and supermarkets located along College Avenue, a major retailing artery in the area, were much higher in Rockridge as compared to the other three low-income neighborhoods, all of which were characterized by a dearth of stores (despite the preponderance of liquor stores). Supermarket density at that time in Rockridge was 4333 people per supermarket with densities nearly four times greater in other Oakland neighborhoods, documenting the disproportionate availability of this type of food store within the region of California (West Oakland: 16,445; Fruitvale: 14,971; and Elmhurst: 18,256).

According to the report, these area differences in amenities caused residents to conduct activities of daily living differently. Participants in this study were asked how they were able to accomplish basic needs within their neighborhoods and unequivocally, in all types of purchases, people in low-income area met needs outside their neighborhoods more often. Reasons for shopping outside local neighborhoods included the higher prices of foods, the lack of availability, and the absence of major chain supermarkets.

The report also documented price differences between supermarkets located in the different areas and in fact sometimes within the same supermarket chain. A market basket survey* of seven supermarkets located in the four areas of Oakland was also conducted as part of the West Coast Regional Office of Consumer Union evaluation. The aim was to compare the monthly cost of purchasing U.S. Department of Agriculture (USDA)-recommended diets for a single parent and three children across these areas. For instance, the report demonstrated that the lowest monthly costs were $239.77 in Elmhurst at the Lucky Supermarket. Prices were 10% higher at the Lucky Supermarket in Rockridge and 16% higher at the Lucky Supermarket in Fruitvale. The other supermarkets had prices that were proportionally higher with the greatest differences at the only supermarket in West Oakland (Acorn) where shoppers would pay 41% more for the same foods that could be purchased at the Lucky Supermarket in Elmhurst. Interestingly, the proportion of monthly costs of produce

---

* A market basket survey is a type of study where the same number and types of foods are purchased at more than one food store in order to compare prices.

was similar across neighborhoods and ranged from 8.9% to 10.1% of market basket expenses. Moreover, the discrepancies of prices between stores and neighborhoods were more stable for produce. Nevertheless, shoppers at the Acorn Supermarket in West Oakland would pay 36% more for produce compared to the lowest price found at the Lucky Supermarket in Rockridge.

DEVELOPING A CONCEPTUAL MODEL

The previous sections are intended to reveal how residential disparities of resources, amenities, and other aspects of neighborhoods might be responsible, at least in part, for the geographic distribution of diseases. The fact that people who live in places concentrated with poverty have a greater burden of disease in the United States is well documented. Now, considering how people of color and low income communities are concentrated into certain areas of the United States, hypotheses of the pathways by which this concentration may lead to specific health outcomes can be developed, thereby moving away from studies that describe the aggregate distribution of disease by area characteristics toward *mechanistic* studies that aim to determine specific individual and environmental factors that may contribute to disease development.

Local food environment research stems from these principles. This area of research aims to identify factors in the environment, specifically food availability,* to better understand how differences in food availability are associated with variability in dietary intake (Chapter 5) and also diet-related health outcomes (Chapter 6). Disparities in the availability of food stores and food prices were identified by the West Coast Regional Office of Consumers Union in Oakland and Los Angeles, and the studies that are summarized within this chapter aim to build on this report, published two decades ago, by measuring current disparities in other areas of the United States. In addition, this field of research also intends to empirically measure the effects of these disparities on behaviors (e.g., food purchasing, dietary intake) and health (e.g., obesity), which are described in Chapters 5–8.

MEASURING THE EFFECTS OF LOCAL FOOD ENVIRONMENT TO TARGET INTERVENTIONS

Barriers to developing interventions to local food environments remain because of several unanswered questions regarding: (1) the mechanisms by which the food environment may be influencing the health behaviors and health outcomes of residents, (2) how the food environment may affect different subsets of the population differently, and (3) what population or neighborhood characteristics are determinates of neighborhood dependency. Statistical models and research designs aimed to understand how behaviors may be influenced by exposure to local food environments can benefit from the development of simple visual depictions of pathways hypothesized to be involved in the development of disease. Certainly, the pathways of how such factors as racial segregation affect health can be quite complicated. For this reason,

---

* Note, food availability has been defined specifically for local food environment research in Chapter 1. In brief, food availability is defined as the retailing of food within local areas and specifically focuses on the routine availability of food store outlets and the variety and cost of foods sold at those outlets.

developing very specific depictions of environmental and individual-level factors and the directions of the hypothesized relationships is a critical next step. To that end, simpler visual descriptions can be useful in creating protocols for measuring factors within studies and also in building statistical models, as causes for human behavior and disease development are complicated multifactorial processes; therefore, it is important that the figure is as specific as possible. Other factors that may be effect modifiers of the associations between local food environments and health also need to be considered. These issues will be discussed in more detail in Chapter 7.

SIMPLIFIED CAUSAL PATHWAYS

As a point of departure, Figure 4.2 presents a basic diagram describing the direction of the proposed relationships. This schematic, although admittedly simplistic, can be further developed as specific hypotheses are addressed in Chapters 5 and 6. The figure is based on the hypothesis that local food environments influence dietary intake through the local purchasing of food. The direction between local food environments and diet is hypothesized here to be unidirectional, from the environment to behavior. This may, in fact, be an oversimplified representation, as it is possible that people with better diets locate into areas where local food environments are less restricted. Unfortunately, the direction of the relationship between local food environments and diet requires longitudinal and experimental study designs that are generally rather expensive to conduct. Therefore, early research aimed to measure any association between local food environments and dietary intake with the rationale that if there are no associations, then the direction of those associations becomes a moot point. Furthermore, local food environments may influence diet-related health outcomes, such as obesity, through a pathway of difference in dietary intake. Here, the schematic hypothesizes a bidirectional relationship from diet to obesity, whereby dietary choices influence weight gain and individuals' personal weight status influences their dietary choices. Note that the relationship between the diet-related health outcomes and the local food environment is not independent, but instead dietary intake (and food purchasing) is presented as an intermediate of that relationship.

Taken in its entirety, this schematic identifies several important factors that may be influencing the association between local food environments and the main effects

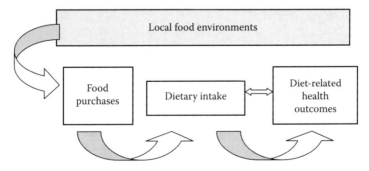

FIGURE 4.2 Simplified model of the relationship between local food environments, diet, and diet-related health outcomes.

(diet and disease). However, within this chapter, the focus rests on the local food environments (Figure 4.2), which considers whether or not there is variability between local food environments. Simply stated, if there is no variability, then we cannot expect differences in dietary intake or diet-related health outcomes to be attributed to this environmental factor. In the event that variability does exist, then it is important to know if any observed differences in local food environments follow economic distributions of residents, racial compositions, and/or other characteristics of areas.

As with any area of science, the precision of measurement is paramount to the success of detecting associations. Subsequently, the initial challenge for investigators who embarked on these types of analyses was to develop assessments of local food environments that were specific enough to detect any true variability between local food environments. There are two main components to the measurements of local food environments: (1) determining the appropriate geographic boundary to use to represent *local or convenient* and (2) creating a measureable definition of healthy food availability.

MEASUREMENT OF GEOGRAPHIC BOUNDARIES OF LOCAL FOOD ENVIRONMENTS

One of the most challenging issues related to local food environment research is determining the appropriate geographic area that represents an individual's *local food environment*. There are several reasons for this difficulty. The first challenge is that Americans do in fact live in a variety of urban, suburban, and rural areas across the United States, and therefore differences in the size and scale of a local food environment are expected across these types of residential environments. For instance, within densely populated urban environments, commercial business is likely to be more tightly packed, resulting in smaller local food environments that support the population density. Alternatively, within rural areas, local food environments may be defined by larger geographic areas to gain enough density of people and food retailers. In other words, the geographic size of the local food environment is dependent on the population being studied. The second challenge pertains to the concept of how to define when retail establishments are *conveniently located*. Even within urban areas where there is a large density of commerce, researchers still contend with defining geographic areas that represent a reasonable density of food purveyors. For example, there may be commerce on many city blocks in urban areas such as New York City or Los Angeles, but when is a city block too small? Is it important to look for variation in the availability of food block to block, or is food availability within a larger geographic region still considered convenient? The third challenge relates to the necessity of defining boundaries that are visually apparent to the community members who reside within those areas. The West Coast Regional Office of Consumers Union chose to conduct their study by neighborhood, but the question remains as to whether or not it is necessary to have the unit of measurement at this level. The specific challenge in this example is that neighborhood boundaries are constantly shifting and in flux, rather than static. Complicating matters is the fact that residents do not always agree about what boundaries define their neighborhood in the first place. On the other hand, thinking about areas in terms of neighborhood classification is arguably logical; for instance, real estate brokers still rely on neighborhood concentration of people to maintain home values. Defining measurable local food environments is as critical as it is difficult, and will continue to require careful examination of how individuals tend to perceive and interact with the built characteristics of their own neighborhoods, as well as the amenities and resources within and surrounding those neighborhoods. Even when we do not live near certain areas, neighborhoods across the United States are familiar to Americans, such as Watts in Los Angeles, the South Side of Chicago, the 8th Ward of New Orleans, and Harlem in New York City. All of these issues become relevant for determining the best geographic boundaries to use in these studies to measure the residential experience with enough specificity and internal validity that any true effect is detected.

ASSIGNING EXPOSURE AND TYPES OF BOUNDARIES

Using principles from environmental epidemiology, environmental exposure affects groups of people, but individual exposures may be mitigated by individual-level behaviors and resources. For instance, in studies of the effect of air pollution and lung disease, regional air monitors have been used to assign exposure. Individual differences in exposure, modeled as effect modifiers, may be due to distance from plume, wearing protective mask, time spent inside one's home, or other factors. Despite individual variability, however, all individuals within a geographic area are exposed to air pollution. Similarly, it can be thought that all people within a certain geographic area are *exposed* to a certain local food environment. As learned from the examples in Oakland highlighted earlier, in areas where there are fewer food retailing options, people may travel further for food shopping. This type of modification of exposure could and should be incorporated into statistical models, or else results may not accurately describe the relationship between local food environments and outcomes of interest. For instance, the ability to transport oneself via car ownership, availability of public transit, or ride shares to another area becomes a component of local food environment utilization. These types of resources become effect modifiers of the associations between local food environments and diet or health. For instance, one might consider the age of the population being studied. With middle-aged adults, residential local food environment may or may not be the primary source of food procurement for individuals and their families because they are typically employed and their jobs may be located far away from home. Therefore, these individuals may purchase and consume the food available within the local food environment surrounding their places of employment. Alternatively, older adults are thought to rely on local amenities more than other age groups because they are generally retired and may have mobility issues that restrict the utilization of neighboring areas for food purchases (U.S. Administration on Aging 2002). Another example is children, whose parents and caregivers almost exclusively control and modify the influence of their local food environments. Especially for very young children, few food decisions are made without parent supervision and certainly, no food purchases are made from retailers that are not by parents or other supervising adults. For adolescents, there may be more independence in food choices outside the home and certainly, like adults, car ownership and other transportation amenities may affect the relationships between local food environments and diet/health of this age group. Nevertheless, even for adolescents, the relationship between local food environment and diet/health is controlled at some level by parental/adult supervision. These issues become particularly important in Chapters 5 and 6, where the studies that measure the effects of local food environments on diet and health are reviewed in greater detail.

The key here is to keep the main research question in mind, which is to measure how geographic patterns of disease may be attributed to disparities between local food environments. The effect modifiers mentioned earlier, as well as others, may explain differences in effects between local food environments and diet/health for some groups of people. People are resilient and must eat to survive. So, if residents of West Oakland are traveling to Rockridge to purchase healthier food options, then it may appear in our statistical models that the local food environment in West Oakland is not predictive of poor diets. But the reason for this finding would be that individuals have modified their neighborhood experience. The counterfactual experience of shopping solely within the restricted food environment of West Oakland would remain unknown. Therefore, appreciating these effect modifiers and incorporating them into our studies strengthens our understanding of the mechanisms by which local food environments affect behaviors and health.

Researchers have used numerous types of geographic boundaries to investigate disparities between local food environments. The geographic boundaries include U.S. Bureau of the Census-defined borders, zip codes, urban and rural boundaries, and distance measurements. Each type of measurement is described in the following subsections.

Census-Defined Boundaries

The U.S. Census Bureau conducts an enumeration of the American population every decade, whereby trends in population density, demographics of Americans, and other information can be used publically (U.S. Bureau of the Census 2013). The U.S. Census Bureau presents data within a number of different geographic boundaries that fall within a standard hierarchy, beginning with the *nation*. The nation is subdivided into *regions* (e.g., the Southeast), then subdivided into *divisions*, and then further subdivided into *states*. Within states, there are *counties*, which contain *census tracts*, *block groups*, and *blocks*. Importantly, the geographic boundaries of each one of these entities do not cross the hierarchy of borders. In other words, there are a certain number of census tracts with a certain county and those tracts do not cross county lines. The attractive feature of U.S. Census-defined borders from a research perspective is that the information about the racial distribution and income of the populations that reside within those borders has already been collected. Therefore, for the studies that are aiming to look for disparities between local food environments and characterize area differences, Census-defined borders are extremely useful. In addition, using this type of secondary dataset is similar to how research is conducted when looking for geographic differences in disease rates, making the method one that is familiar to most researchers interested in this area of study. That being said, there are very large differences in the sizes of Census geographic entities, and it is therefore important to remember that local food environment disparities are conceptualized to take place at the neighborhood level (U.S. Bureau of the Census 2013). Also noteworthy is the fact that U.S. census-defined boundaries can change at each new decennial of investigation.

Counties

Counties are the first level of geographic unit smaller than states. The population of the United States, based on the 2010 Census, is presented by county in Figure 4.3. First, county borders do not cross state lines. Second, the size of counties varies within states and across the nation, as does the population size within counties. The sizes of these geographic boundaries vary quite considerably. For instance, Brooklyn is one of the five boroughs of New York City and the entire borough is one county—Kings County. In 2010, Kings County contained 2,504,700 people within a landmass of 71 square miles. Comparatively, Fresno County, California, contained 930,450 people within 5,958 square miles in 2010. Difference in landmass and population characteristics of counties can be viewed interactively through the U.S. Census Bureau website: http://quickfacts.census.gov/qfd/index.html.

Tracts

Census tracts are the next unit of measurement smaller than counties that are measured by the U.S. Census Bureau. Tracts are smaller geographic units of measurement containing roughly 3000–5000 people. Census tracts also vary in size and although they do not cross county borders, they do sometimes cross neighborhood boundaries, limiting the use of census tracts as direct measurements of actual neighborhoods. As an example in Figure 4.4, the neighborhood of Bay Ridge in Brooklyn, New York, is presented overlaid with census tracts, demonstrating the comparative size of the census tracts to the neighborhood and the variation in size and shape of the tracts.

Blocks and Block Groups

The census blocks are located within census tracts and are noted in Figure 4.4 with light gray lines. These geographic boundaries generally represent city blocks and hence also vary in size and shape. Block groups are another census geographic boundary, in size, between blocks and tracts where several blocks within a tract are grouped (not shown in Figure 4.4).

Zip Code Tabulation Areas/U.S. Postal Service
Defined Boundaries: Zip Codes

Zip codes are geographic boundaries defined by the U.S. Postal Service for the purpose of delivering mail. Unlike the census-defined boundaries, the intention of these boundaries was not to enumerate Americans. However, zip code tabulation areas are created by the U.S. Census Bureau, which marries the U.S. Postal Service zip code boundaries with U.S. Census data.

Geographic Information Systems-Defined Boundaries

Geographic information systems (GIS) is software (e.g., ArcGIS) that has been used by geographers, urban planners, and other professionals for years. This software is used to develop maps. Some base maps of areas are publicly available and then information is *layered* onto other maps. For instance, the New York City Department of

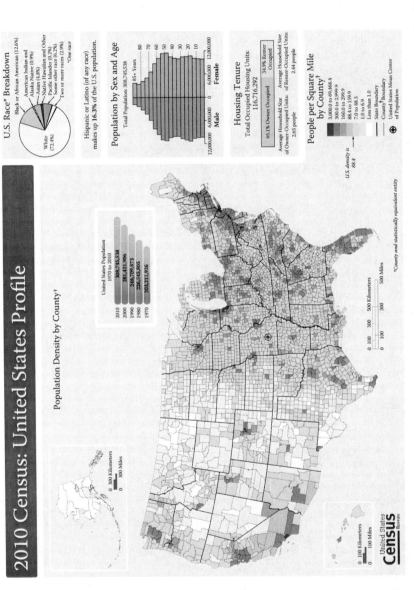

FIGURE 4.3 **(See color insert.)** 2010 Census: United States profile. (From U.S. Department of Commerce Economics and Statistics Administration, U.S. Census Bureau.)

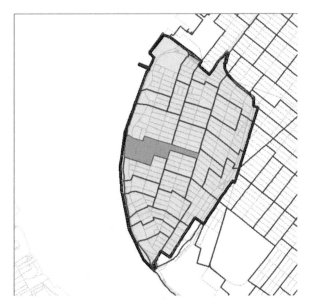

FIGURE 4.4 Bay Ridge, Brooklyn, New York, neighborhood, Census tracts and blocks.

City Planning provides several maps of the city that can be used with GIS software. The DCPLION is a base map of New York City streets and includes other geographic features such as shorelines, surface rail lines, and boardwalks. Because this type of data is publicly available for most of the United States, there has been an increase in secondary data analyses using these types of techniques within public health research. Once the base maps are in place, many types of data can be layered onto the maps by geocoding the latitude and longitude of an address for placement on the map. The geocoding of addresses is commonly used by researchers to place individuals and/or the locations of food retailers onto maps. If addresses are not complete or not known, geographic positioning system devices can be used to collect that information. These devices are now common in motor vehicles, but can also be used in handheld devices where the latitude and longitude of a specific place will be stored when standing in front of the business or place of residence. Finally, because this area of public health is continuing to grow, agencies are providing more prepared maps that may be useful in public health research. For instance, NYC provides the geographic boundaries for the FRESH program, where zoning and discretionary tax incentives are available for the development, expansion, and renovation of full-line grocery stores and supermarkets. This is a geographic file created by the New York City Department of City Planning, showing eligible areas for the zoning incentives adopted May 11, 2009 and eligible areas for tax incentives through the New York City Industrial Development Agency.

Buffer Zones

Buffer zones of many sizes have been used to characterize the geographic space surrounding a specific address, such as a home address. In Figure 4.5, a 300-m radius buffer zone has been drawn around a residential address using ArcGIS. These types

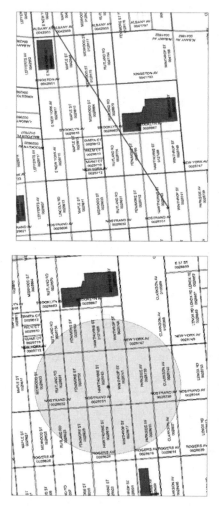

FIGURE 4.5 GIS-derived measurements of local food environments: (1) 300 m buffer zone around a residential address; (2) straight line (Euclidian) distance between two addresses.

of measurements have the advantage of placing an individual in the middle of the geographic area, eliminating some of the concern with the census-defined boundaries where exposure is assigned to an individual regardless of where they may be located within that geographic area.

Distance Measurements

In addition to buffer zones, instead of using geographic boundaries, distance can also be used as a measurement. Distance measurements are calculated using GIS tools as a straight line between two points, a *Euclidian distance*, sometimes called a *crow flies distance* (Figure 4.5). This type of measurement does not take the roadways, sidewalks, or other street features such as dead ends or traffic volume into account. These factors would affect the utilization of the distance between the two points for an individual; however, it is a simple and direct measurement. GIS systems also offer application for more complicated *network distances* to be calculated where the fastest, shortest route, or a path described by a person can be measured.

Neighborhoods

Finally, although uncommonly used in local food environment research, it is possible to utilize the geographic boundaries of neighborhoods as boundaries of local food environments. The geographic boundary of the neighborhood Bay Ridge is shown in Figure 4.4. These types of geographic boundaries may be available from city agencies, and may or may not be associated with demographic data.

Summary of Limitation to Each Type of Boundary

Census-defined borders have been criticized primarily because an individual may live anywhere within that boundary, perhaps even on the perimeter of two adjacent boundaries, thus introducing misclassification. Moreover, because the size and shape of these boundaries vary, there is inconsistency in the definition of local food environments within and between studies. Further, any given census-defined boundary may be a moderate-to-poor proxy of actual neighborhood availability of food with some boundaries possibly being too small (e.g., blocks) and others being too large (e.g., counties). Although the GIS-defined borders have addressed some of these concerns, these boundaries have also been criticized because the GIS boundaries are by definition an individual-level measurement, which conflicts with the concept of the shared environments inherent to neighborhoods. Moreover, the size and shape of the GIS-defined boundaries are not based on any empirical evidence or public health-defined standards. The presentation of multiple sizes within the same study confounds effects due to availability with effects related to utilization. Further, distance measures are limited by the need to determine distance to what specific establishment is of interest. Is the distance to the primary food store reported by the study participant the best definition of local food environments? If so, this store may be far away from a person's home and would more accurately be describing utilization rather than the effects of the restricted nature of the food environment that is closer to home (Morland and Filomena, 2008). Also, this type of measurement focuses on a single food retailer, and therefore does not account for the interdependencies between area features.

MEASUREMENT OF FOOD AVAILABILITY

There are several ways in which investigators have quantified the *availability* of food. This includes the placement of food stores, considering the type of store, such as chain supermarket versus a convenience store. Investigators have also aimed to measure differences in the types of food carried within stores, as well as the quality of those foods and variability in cost. A description of methods for each of these types of food availability measurements are described in the following subsections.

PRESENCE OF STORES/RESTAURANTS

The location of food stores, as a density measure or a distance between two points, is accomplished with the use of GIS. The latitude and longitude of a store address can be determined by geocoding its address, hence the location of that establishment can be placed on a map. Once addresses have been geocoded, density measurements (number of stores within the geographic boundary) or distance measurement, as described previously, can be calculated and used in statistical models as predictors of health behaviors and health outcomes, as well as outcome variables in studies aimed to determine disparities in access to healthy foods.

There are several ways by which investigators have determined the location and types of food stores and restaurants, but the three main avenues include (1) government sources, (2) private companies that compile lists, and (3) primary data collection. All of the sources have strengths and limitations. The first two are convenient and used in most studies as secondary sources of information. Food stores can be easily obtained through government sources, and restaurants are regularly inspected by government public health agencies (tax records can also be used). The disadvantage is that data collected in this way is usually cross-sectional and generally no historical data are kept by these agencies. The reality of this fact is that it hinders the development of retrospective cohort analyses. Also, the type of store is not usually coded (e.g., supermarket, convenience store) and the food service and food store data are regulated by different agencies, sometimes making the acquisition of these data rather cumbersome. A second option is private firms, such as InfoUSA, that track all types of business and their lists can be used to obtain the name and addresses of food retailers, usually for a fee. These agencies often provide additional information about the businesses, such as the type of retailer. However, businesses sometimes need to register to be listed, and therefore information regarding some of the smaller, independent stores may not be captured. Third, because of the limitations of the secondary datasets, some investigators have conducted primary data collection to determine the locations and types of food stores within geographic areas. Several studies have enumerated the placement of food stores by conducting walking or driving audits of specified areas. For instance, in the National Institute of Health–funded study called the Cardiovascular Health of Seniors and the Built Environments, all streets within a 300-m radius buffer zone of each participant have been studied repeatedly, resulting in the longitudinal evaluation of 23,667 streets located in all areas of Brooklyn. A detailed description of the protocol is described in Box 4.1.

BOX 4.1   PROTOCOL OF OBJECTIVE MEASUREMENT OF LOCAL FOOD ENVIRONMENTS: EXAMPLE FROM THE CARDIOVASCULAR HEALTH OF SENIORS AND THE BUILT ENVIRONMENT STUDY

Once enrolled, buffer zones with a radius of 300 m around participants' residential addresses were created using ArcGIS. NYC Department of Planning (DCPLION-2009) street segment files were layered onto the buffer zones, resulting in maps of whole and partial street segments located within buffer zones for each participant. Street segments are typically road length between two adjacent intersections; however, continuous roads (such as freeways) are also segmented without intersections. For simplicity, street segments are referred to as streets.

In 2009 there were at total of 82,907 streets located in Brooklyn ($n = 30,484$) and Queens ($n = 52,423$). Study participants' buffer zones included streets located in all 18 Brooklyn Community Districts and 3 Queens Community Districts (QCD-5, QCD-9, QCD-10), resulting in the evaluation of 66% of all Brooklyn streets and 5% of Queen streets. Community districts, on an average, cover 3.9 square miles, and the populations within districts vary by race/ethnicity and wealth.

Streets identified within buffer zones were highlighted on paper maps and assigned to trained auditors who walked each street to document the types of food stores, physical activity resources, and other neighborhood infrastructure located on each street. Auditors were instructed to document the entrances of specific types of places on both sides of the streets. Most features were assigned to one street only, where the main entrance was found and coded as only one feature. However, features such as parks, with entrances on more than one street, were documented on all buffering streets. All decisions about the type of establishment or land use were made based on observations from the street.

Some streets were excluded from the walking audit because they were either vehicular only, such as the highways (e.g., Brooklyn–Queens Expressway) or another type of street where features of interest were not likely to be located (e.g., the Brooklyn Bridge). Exclusions were made based on street names, feature type codes (railroad, private street, alley, and path), segment type codes (connector, exit/entrance ramp, and faux street), and when coded as vehicular only in the DCPLION file. During the walking audits, additional streets containing no features were identified, resulting in a total of 4,330 streets assumed to contain no features of interest, and therefore excluded from the list of streets for the walking audit. Of the 82,907 streets, 16,047 Brooklyn and 2,362 Queens streets were audited where study participants lived.

The walking audit protocol called for documenting all buildings and land use within each buffer zone, resulting in a complete census of all types of places and land use. Thirty-four different component features of the neighborhoods

(Continued)

BOX 4.1 *(Continued)*

were used to characterize area resources hypothesized to be involved in the causal pathway leading to diet-related health outcome by promoting or preventing good nutrition and/or physical activity for adults. For instance, it is hypothesized that area infrastructure such as the presence of banks and post offices within walking distance will promote physical activity for adults because activity of daily living can take place within the immediate neighborhood. Food environment features include both food stores (supermarkets, grocery stores, bodega, convenience stores, specialty food stores, and liquor stores) and food service places (full-service restaurants, fast-food restaurants, food vendors). The protocol called for all streets to be audited within a 6-month window of the collection of participant health and behavior information. All audit maps were then coded to street segments and entered electronically. Street segments were linked back to participants by assigned buffer zones such that density of each type of food stores could be assigned by buffer zone. Other area features measured included public transportation, park entrances, gyms, and other physical activity resources, as well as general area resources including general retail and services, places of worship, medical facilities, schools, banks, libraries, and post offices.

TYPES OF FOOD STORES/RESTAURANTS

Quantifying types of food stores has also been a challenge in this area of public health research. Often, secondary datasets will not contain detailed classification information about food stores, so investigators will have to make assumptions about the type of venue. The rationale for coding the type relates to the concept that different food stores and restaurants sell different varieties of healthy food options at different prices. For instance, price differences between large-scale supermarkets that can benefit from mass merchandising versus smaller food stores have been documented prior to the genesis of local food environment research (Cotteril and Franklin 1995). Nevertheless, many studies using secondary data to evaluate the placement of food stores rely on name recognition to determine the types of food stores and restaurants. These methods can provide relatively good specificity for determining supermarkets and fast-food establishments, such as Kroger or McDonald's, because most chains are well recognized. However, misclassification is a concern for smaller types of stores and restaurants where the content of the stores cannot be determined from the name. Therefore, some investigators have utilized other information provided about the business such as the amount of retail space, the number of cash registers, or sales to distinguish the larger stores from the smaller stores. In the end, the aim has been to distinguish the types of food sold and the pricing of those goods.

Studies that focus solely on the placement of different types of food stores and restaurants rely on two inherent assumptions—that mass marketing requires a large volume of goods to be available for sale to customers and that this, in turn, will allow customers to benefit from lower prices. It is further inferred that with the larger volume of goods sold, there will be a greater proportion of healthy food items sold in large chain food stores compared to smaller ones. In general, most U.S. investigators have utilized the definitions of food stores and restaurants provided by the U.S. government as the North America Industry Classification System (NAICS), previously known as Standard Industrial Classification, whereby the definitions of each type of industry conducting business in the country has been defined. A summary of the NAICS codes for food stores and food service places has been provided in Chapter 1 (Table 1.1).

CONTENT OF STORES/RESTAURANTS

Given the set of assumptions related to studies that have measured the presence of food stores only, investigators have also conducted studies to measure the availability, prices, and quality of foods sold at food stores, in particular. These studies have been conducted using a variety of research methods. The first example is the measurement of the availability of particular food types and surveys such as the NEMS-S (Glanz et al. 2007), which aims to measure food availability of different types of healthy food items and can be viewed on the following website: http://www.med.upenn.edu/nems/publications.shtml. This survey results in a composite score for surveyed stores that accounts for the availability, cost, and quality of selected health food options. Second, several studies have focused on the Thrifty Eating Plan, where market basket surveys have been used to measure the availability and cost of food recommended to low-income Americans to achieve a healthy diet (USDA 2007). With this measure of food availability, investigators are able to measure differences in the availability and prices of specific food groups such as grains, milk, and meat that are recommended for consumption by the USDA to be nutritious and affordable. Finally, others have focused on key food items important for disease management, such as diabetes (Horowitz et al. 2004) or specific food groups, such as fruits and vegetables (Cole et al. 2010; Morland and Filomena 2007). Overall, there is little consistency between local food environment studies in the measures of within-store availability, affordability, and quality, primarily because it is difficult to quantify *healthy food availability* in such a way that can be a sensitive measure across all populations of Americans. Moreover, the measurement of in-store foods is expensive and impractical for large-scale studies. Nevertheless, the disparities in the accessibility of affordable, healthy food options have been detected using these measures and will be described in the following section.

EVIDENCE OF DISPARITIES IN ACCESS TO HEALTHY FOODS IN THE UNITED STATES (1997–2013)

Although the measurement of local food environments and their impact on health began in the late 1990s, consumer advocate groups such as the Consumers Union had conducted studies to measure disparities in retail environments between neighborhood prior to this time. Others have also documented the influence of economic decline and the decrease of low-cost retailers within American inner cities during the 1960s and 1970s (Anderson 1978). The urban grocery gap during the late 1980s and early 1990s was captured with the Food Marketing Policy Center of the Department of Agriculture and Resources Economics of the University of Connecticut, where Cotterill and Franklin (1995) published a report on 21 American cities and the associations between low-income areas and the presence of supermarkets. The authors report that there were serious distribution problems in some U.S. cities in terms of food delivery and stated that: "Given the recent cuts at the Federal level in food programs and the clear-cut need to improve the efficiency of distribution of federal food program dollars, the focus on the ability of the supermarket food distribution system to deliver food in an efficient, i.e. reasonably priced fashion, to low income urban neighborhoods is extremely timely." These findings were supported by the work conducted by the U.S. House of Representatives Select Committee on Hunger where the migration of supermarkets to the suburbs and lack of transportation was determined to contribute to the malnutrition among low-income Americans (U.S. House of Representatives Select Committee on Hunger 1987, 1992). Other economic experts have investigated issues related to attracting supermarkets to inner cities, noting that citywide grocery initiatives are rare within the 32 U.S. cities investigated (Pothukuchi 2005).

This earlier work guided the development of new investigations within the public health and medical community to investigate how these population and retail shifts, which continue to this day, have impacted Americans' health. The following summarizes 25 studies, published between 1997 and 2013, that document current disparities in access to healthy foods. The studies that measure the impact of local food environment disparities on dietary intake and health of Americans are summarized in Chapters 5 and 6.

The majority of the public health studies included in this summary were conducted between 2005 and 2008, and most have been conducted within urban areas ($n = 23$), particularly New York ($n = 9$) and Los Angeles ($n = 4$). Fewer studies have investigated disparities in access to healthy affordable foods for rural consumers ($n = 4$). Among these studies, most investigators aimed to measure the differences in the placement of food stores (or food items) by economic measures, as had been done in the earlier studies, but also by racial composition of areas. A summary of these studies can be found in Table 4.1 and are ordered by size of the geographic boundary used in the investigations. The majority of the studies measured food availability based on the presence of types of food stores, such as supermarkets ($n = 16$); although several studies have measured the availability of specific types of foods ($n = 9$) and related costs for those purchases ($n = 7$). Fewer studies have focused on the quality of foods ($n = 1$), eating away from home specifically ($n = 2$), or perceptions and utilization patterns ($n = 1$). The specific methods and findings for each study can also be found in Table 4.1.

Overall, investigators have consistently documented disparities in the placement of large-scale food stores, such as supermarkets, by either the wealth of areas investigated or the racial composition of area residents (Alwitt and Donley 1997; Morland et al. 2002; Zenk et al. 2005; Baker et al. 2006; Block and Kouba 2006; Moore and Diez Roux 2006; Morland and Filomena 2007; Powell et al. 2007; Sharkey and Horel 2008; Filomena et al. 2013). Some have shown that the lack of availability of healthy food options is also associated with inequality in the presence of supermarkets within

TABLE 4.1
Summary of Studies Aimed to Measure Disparities between Local Food Environments in the United States

First Author (Year)	Target Area(s)	Population Density	Neighborhood Characteristic	Geographic Unit	Target in LFE	N	Findings
Galvez (2007)	East Harlem, New York City (NYC), New York	Urban	Race/ethnicity	Census block	Presence of supermarkets; grocery stores; convenience stores; specialty food stores; full-service restaurants; and fast-food restaurants by predominately black, predominately Latino, and racially mixed areas	N = 405 food stores and restaurants (objective measurement)	Latino areas had greatest prevalence of all food stores and restaurants except grocery stores
Horowitz (2004)	East Harlem and Upper East Side of Manhattan (NYC), New York	Urban	Race/ethnicity and wealth: East Harlem (predominately Latino and lower income) vs. Upper East Side (predominately white and high income)	Census block group	Food relevant for people with diabetes: diet soda; 1% or fat-free milk; high-fiber bread; low-carbohydrate bread; fresh fruits; fresh green vegetables; tomatoes. Presence of these foods by neighborhood	N = 324 food stores identified from New York State Agriculture and Market Database (objective in-store survey)	Fewer stores located in the Upper East Side, but a greater proportion contained healthy foods surveyed
Hosler (2006)	Downtown Albany, Columbia, and Greene Counties, New York	Urban and rural	Race/ethnicity and wealth; rural	Census block group	Foods within food store retailers: milk, bread, fresh fruits, and vegetables. Comparison of presence of low-fat milk and high-fiber bread between urban and rural areas	N = 256 food stores identified from online business directory and farm fresh products and list of inspected stores (objective in store survey)	A higher proportion of rural area stores stock low-fat milk and high-fiber bread

(Continued)

TABLE 4.1 *(Continued)*
Summary of Studies Aimed to Measure Disparities between Local Food Environments in the United States

First Author (Year)	Target Area(s)	Population Density	Neighborhood Characteristic	Geographic Unit	Target in LFE	N	Findings
Filomena (2013)	Brooklyn, New York	Urban	Race and wealth	Census tract	Change in presence of supermarkets and other food stores over a 5-year period	N = 4311 (2007); 4333 (2008); 4417 (2009); 4425 (2010); 5431 (2011) identified from the New York State Agriculture and Market Database	An overall increase in supermarkets was observed, but stability of stores was greater in higher wealth and predominately white areas
Cole (2010)	Brooklyn Community Districts (BCD) 6 and 9, Brooklyn (NYC), NY	Urban	BCD 6 (predominately white) compared to BCD 9 (predominately black)	Census tract	Evaluation of cost and quality of produce between predominately white, black, and mixed race areas.	N = 45—A 50% sample of any food stores was selected randomly from NY State Agriculture and Market database (objective in-store survey)	The cost of fresh produce was generally lower in predominately black areas although findings are limited by the number of stores that carry fresh produce in these areas. No pattern in quality emerged
Morland (2007)	Brooklyn Community Districts (BCD) 6 and 9, Brooklyn (NYC), NY	Urban	BCD 6 (predominately white) compared to BCD 9 (predominately black)	Census tract	Presence of 39 different types of fresh, 13 types of canned, 9 types of frozen, and 14 types of prepared fruits and vegetables	N = 45—A 50% sample of any food stores was selected randomly from NY State Agriculture and Market database (objective in-store survey)	A lower proportion of black area stores carried fresh produce; supermarkets carried the largest variety of produce and white areas had the highest prevalence of supermarkets

Baker (2006)	St. Louis and eastern part of St. Louis County, Missouri; and area between the Missouri River on the east and Interstate 270, MO	Race/ethnicity and income	Urban	Comparison of availability of healthy foods located in supermarkets and fast food restaurants, area racial and poverty distributions. Foods include: fruits and vegetables; lean, low-fat or fat-free meat, poultry, and dairy products	Census tract	$N = 81$ supermarkets and 355 fast food restaurants (objective in-store survey and survey of corporate menus)	Race and income levels of area are not only associated with the location of food outlets, but also the section of food available that enables individuals to follow dietary recommendations
Moore (2006)	Forsyth County, NC; parts of the city of Baltimore and Baltimore County, MD; northern Manhattan and the Bronx (NYC), NY	Race/ethnicity and wealth	Urban/ suburban	Type of food stores located in predominately black, white, Hispanic, and racially mixed census tracts	Census tract	$N = 2860$ food stores and 477 liquor stores identified from InfoUSA (a commercial database of businesses). Secondary data collection	Predominately white and wealthier areas were found to have more supermarkets than predominately minority and poorer areas. Smaller grocery stores were more prevalent in predominately minority and low-income areas
Morland (2002)	Jackson City, MS; Forsyth County, NC; Washington County, MD; selected suburbs of Minneapolis, MN	Race/ethnicity and wealth	Urban/ suburban	Types of food stores and restaurants located in predominately black; racially mixed and predominately white areas, and types of food stores and restaurants in quintiles of neighborhood wealth	Census tract ($n = 216$)	$N = 2437$ food stores and food service places identified from local departments of Environmental Health and State Department of Agriculture	Four times as many supermarkets were located in white compared to black areas. A greater proportion of supermarkets also located in wealthier areas compared to lower-income areas. The proportion of households with a vehicle is associated with area race and wealth

(Continued)

TABLE 4.1 (Continued)

Summary of Studies Aimed to Measure Disparities between Local Food Environments in the United States

First Author (Year)	Target Area(s)	Population Density	Neighborhood Characteristic	Geographic Unit	Target in LFE	N	Findings
Moore (2008)	Forsyth County, NC, parts of the city of Baltimore and Baltimore County, MD; northern Manhattan and the Bronx (NYC), NY	Urban/ suburban	Race/ethnicity and wealth	Census tract	Perceived vs. objective availability of food stores	N = 2860 food stores identified from InfoUSA (a commercial database of businesses). Secondary data collection. 5774 adult MESA study participants	Perceived availability of healthy foods was positively associated with density of supermarkets. Findings were less consistent with smaller food stores
Liese (2007)	Orangeburg County, SC	Rural	Rural	Census tract	Presence of types of places that sell foods; foods sold and cost of food items between types of stores	N = 77 food stores, identified by South Carolina Department of Health Statistics and Information Services	Healthier food options and lower costs were available at supermarkets and grocery stores compared to convenience stores. Convenience stores were most prevalent
Cassady (2007)	Sacramento and Los Angeles, CA	Urban/ suburban	Low vs. high income areas	Zip codes and 5-mile distance (buffer zone)	Cost differences in Thrifty Food Plan market basket by neighborhood income level and store type. FOCUS ON PRODUCE ONLY	N = 25 food stores sampled three times	Costs of produce was lower in lower income strata and lower at bulk stores compared to traditional supermarkets
Jetter (2005)	Los Angeles and Sacramento, CA	Urban/ suburban	Low vs. high income areas	Zip codes and 5-mile distance (buffer zone?)	Cost differences in Thrifty Food Plan market basket versus "healthier market basket" by neighborhood income level and store type	N = 25 food stores sampled 3 times	Chain and bulk supermarkets had a wider range of healthy options. The healthier MB was more expensive in all stores and areas

Powell (2007)	U.S. National Sample	Urban/rural/ suburban	Race/ethnicity, income	Zip codes using aggregate block group and block census data	Association between the number of available food store outlets and the racial and SES composition of zip codes.	N = 28,050 zip codes	Fewer supermarkets in low-income areas; fewer supermarkets in areas with a dense population of African-Americans
Lewis (2005)	South vs. West Los Angeles, CA	Urban	Proportion of African-Americans and income	Zip codes/zip code tabulation areas	Availability of healthy food and advertising in selected restaurants by type of restaurant and area characteristic	N = 678 restaurants from 19 zip codes	Lower income areas with dense African-American populations had fewer healthy food options at restaurants and a greater proportion of unhealthy food promotion
Sloane (2003)	South vs. West Los Angeles, CA	Urban	Proportion of African-Americans and income	Zip codes/zip code tabulation areas	Comparison of the availability of selected foods from two areas within type of food store	N = 330 food stores from 23 zip codes	Lower income areas with dense African-American populations had fewer healthy food options at food stores, fewer supermarkets
Hayes (2000)	NYC, NY	Urban	Income	Zip codes	Comparison of price of foods by neighborhood wealth using market basket surveys	N = 57 food stores with at least 4000 square feet of retail space within 28 zip codes	No differences in prices of food items surveyed by wealth of areas
Alwitt (1997)	Chicago, IL	Urban	Income	Zip codes	Comparison of the presence of grocery stores, restaurants, and other retailers by poor and nonpoor areas of Chicago	N = 53 zip codes	Poor areas have more small grocery stores and fewer supermarkets
Fisher (1999)	Seven New York counties, NY	Metropolitan; midsized-urban and rural	Income, race, and urbanization	Zip codes	Percent of low-fat milk on store shelves	N = 795 food stores from 53 zip codes (15 stores sampled from each zip code)	Percent of milk in stores that is low fat was positively associated with urbanization, higher income and greater than 50% non-Hispanic White zip codes

(Continued)

TABLE 4.1 (Continued)

Summary of Studies Aimed to Measure Disparities between Local Food Environments in the United States

First Author (Year)	Target Area(s)	Population Density	Neighborhood Characteristic	Geographic Unit	Target in LFE	N	Findings
Chung (1999)	Twin Cities, MN (Hennepin and Ramsey counties)	Urban and suburban	Income	Urban/ suburban	Store type availability and cost differences in Thrifty Food Plan market basket by neighborhood income level and store type	N = 526 stores in target areas; n = 55 stores surveyed	Chain supermarkets were disproportionately located in suburbs, chain supermarkets offer lower prices, price difference between urban and suburban areas were not observed although the availability of food types was lower in the inner city
Algert (2006)	Pomona, CA	Urban	Low-income food pantry (FP) clients	Network distances of FP clients to stores within walking distance, defined as 0.8 km (0.5 mile), to stores that sell produce	Stores classified as selling limited versus variety of produce. Verified by phone call	N = 84 store within 0.8-km buffer zone of Pomona city limits	83% of food pantry clients were within walking distance to small stores with limited or no produce
Block, D (2006)	Austin and Oak Park, IL	Urban and suburban	Race/ethnicity and Wealth	Neighborhood	Store type availability, price and quality differences in Thrifty Food Plan market basket by neighborhood income level and store type	N = 134 stores surveyed	Fewer supermarkets in predominately black neighborhood, prices within the same type of store were similar between areas, Supermarkets were the only type of food store that carried all items

Study	Location	Urban/Rural	Measures	Geographic unit	Objective	N stores	Findings
Zenk (2005)	Detroit, MI	Urban	African-American and poverty	Census tract, Manhattan block distance	Presence of supermarkets located in predominately African-American areas of Detroit compared to predominately white areas (accounting for poverty)	$N = 160$ stores identified from Michigan Department of Agriculture	Nearest supermarket was significantly further away in neighborhoods with high African-American population and most impoverished
Block, JP (2006)	New Orleans, LA	Urban	African-American and poverty	Census tract, 1-mile buffer zone	Presence of fast food restaurants located in predominately African-American areas compared to white areas, accounting for area wealth		For every 10% increase in fast-food restaurant density, neighborhood median household income decreased by 4.8% and percentage of black residents increased by 3.7
Starkey (2008)	Six rural counties, TX	Rural	Area deprivation and minority composition	Census block, block group and distance	Determine the distribution of distance from geographic center or centroid to nearest type of food store	$N = 213$ food store: 23 supermarket/grocery, 154 convenience, 20 discount, 3 beverage, and 13 specialty	Distance to supermarket was positively associated with area deprivation and minority status

urban centers (Sloane et al. 2003; Baker et al. 2006; Block and Kouba 2006; Jetter and Cassady 2006; Liese et al. 2007; Morland and Filomena 2007). Others have documented disparities in the availability of selected healthy food options independent of supermarket presence (Fisher and Strogatz 1999; Lewis et al. 2005; Horowitz et al. 2004; Algert et al. 2006; Hosler et al. 2006) and those differences have been associated with demographic and urbanization factors. Only one study documented lower prices of foods within supermarkets (Chung and Myers 1999), although other studies that have measured price difference (Hayes 2000; Block and Kouba 2006; Jetter and Cassady 2006; Cole et al. 2010) report price not being a significant factor between local food environments.

There is a remarkable consistency of findings across these studies. Most investigators have found disparities in access to healthy foods by racial and economic characteristics of areas, which supports earlier investigations. The consistency of findings has led to a report to Congress from the USDA called "Access to Affordable and Nutritious Foods: Measuring and Understanding Food Deserts and Their Consequences" (USDA 2009). The USDA reported that (1) 11.5 million low-income Americans live more than a mile away from a supermarket; (2) food costs are lower within supermarkets; and (3) low-income households are more likely to utilize supercenters, when possible, because of lower prices. These conclusions were drawn from the studies conducted by the ERS and from many of the studies summarized in Table 4.1. Findings between studies in Table 4.1 are rather consistent, even though investigators have utilized different methods. The size of the studies vary greatly, with some representing smaller geographic areas and others like Powell et al. (2007) measuring all areas of the United States. Variations between studies may be due to difference across the country, but can also be due to the selection of comparison groups, sampling and methods for determining food stores, food types to study, and measurement methods for the cost of foods.

Few studies have measured the changes in local food environments over time. This is an important component of understanding disparities between local food environments and how residents' exposure may be constant over time. One study measured the fluctuation of supermarket presence in Brooklyn from 2007 to 2011 and found that there was an increase in the number of supermarkets during that period; in fact, the greatest proportion of new supermarket locations was found in the lowest income areas. The higher wealth areas had the greatest supermarket stability, meaning the greatest proportion of stores remained open during the 5-year period of investigation (Filomena et al. 2013). A better understanding of the types of fluctuations within local food environments may aid in understanding chronic exposure and how motivations for behavior change are influenced by the stability of local food environments. For instance, within a community-based participatory project to address poor access to healthy foods, a community group opened a new community-owned and operated food store in East New York. Comments from store patrons as to why they were not using the new food store with any regularity reflected their familiarity with a volatile retail environment; stating they were hesitant to rely on a new food store because they expected it would shut down within a year or two. These comments were in spite of the recognition by the community that the store was needed and contained foods that were desired and served the community (Munoz-Plaza et al. 2007). Unfortunately, residents were correct and the store was not able to sustain itself more than two years (Rainlake Productions 2009; Morland 2010).

In summary, there is strong empirical evidence that some Americans currently live in areas with poor access to healthy foods and that these disparities appear to tract in communities with higher concentrations of people of color and low income. Some believe that these disparities are the result of a food system that has increasingly evolved toward factory farming and mass merchandising. Others blame a social class system predicated on the belief that people lacking resources should travel further or accept lesser to meet basic needs. Regardless, the end result is the same; as Bill Maher has said, *food racism* exists in the United States (2013). The extent to which public health researchers can measure any effect these disparities may have on food purchasing, eating, and subsequent disease will be described in Chapters 5–8.

REFERENCES

Acevedo-Garcia, D. and K. A. Lochner. 2003. Residential segregation and health. In *Neighborhoods and Health*, edited by I. Kawachi and L. F. Berkman. New York: Oxford University Press.

Akresh, I. R. 2007. Dietary assimilation and health among Hispanic immigrant to the United States. *J Health Soc Behav* 48:404–417.

Algert, S. J., A. Agrawal, and D. S. Lewis. 2006. Disparities in access to fresh produce in low income neighborhoods in Los Angeles. *Am J Prev Med* 30:365–370.

Alwitt, L. F. and T. D. Donley. 1997. Retail stores in poor urban neighborhoods. *J Cons Aff* 31:139–164.

Anderson, A. R. 1978. The Ghetto marketing life cycle: A case of the underachievement. *J Market Res* 15:20–28.

Baker, E. A., M. Schootman, E. Barnidge, and C. Kelly. 2006. The role of race and poverty in access to foods that enable individuals to adhere to dietary guidelines. *Prev Chronic Dis* 3:A76.

BBC History. 2013. http://www.bbc.co.uk/history/historic_figures/snow_john.shtml (Accessed August 4, 2013).

Bloch, M., S. Carter, and A. McLean. 2013. *The New York Times*. http://projects.nytimes.com /census/2010/explorer (Accessed August 4, 2013).

Block, D. and J. Kouba. 2006. A comparison of the availability and affordability of a market basket in two communities in the Chicago area. *Public Health Nutr* 9:837–845.

Block, J. P., R. A. Scribner, and K. B. DeSalvo. 2004. Fast food, race/ethnicity, and income: A geographic analysis. *Am J Prev Med* 27:211–217.

Bronfenbrenner, U. (Ed.) 1994. Ecological models of human development. In *International Encyclopedia of Education*, Vol 3, 2nd Ed. Oxford: Elsevier. Reprinted in *Readings on the Development of Children*, 2nd Ed., pp. 37–43. Edited by Gauvain M. and M. Cole. 1993. New York: WH Freeman.

Cassady, D., K. M. Jetter, and J. Culp. 2007. Is price a barrier to eating more fruits and vegetables for low-income families? *J Am Diet Assoc* 107:1909–1915.

Chung, C. and S. L. Myers. 1999. Do the poor pay more for food? An analysis of grocery store availability and food price disparities. *J Cons Aff* 33:276–296.

Cole, S., S. Filomena, and K. Morland. 2010. Analysis of fruit and vegetable cost and quality among racially segregated neighborhoods in Brooklyn, New York. *J Hun Env Nutr* 5:202–215.

Cooper, R. S., K. Wolf-Maier, A. Luke A, et al. 2005. An international comparative study of blood pressure in populations of European vs. African descent. *BMC Med* 3:2. http://www/pubmedcentral.nih.gov/articlerender.fcgi?artid = 545060 (Accessed February 21, 2013).

Cotterill, R. W. and A. W. Franklin. 1995. The Urban Grocery Store Gap. Food Marketing Policy Issue Paper, No. 8. Storrs, CT: Food Marketing Policy Center, University of Connecticut.

Davies, A. A., A. Basten, and C. Frattini. 2006. Migration: A Social Determinant of the Health of Migrants. International Organization of Migration (IOM). http://ec.europa.eu/ewsi/UDRW/images/items/docl_9914_392596992.pdf (Accessed August 5, 2013).

DeNavas-Walt, C., B.D. Proctor and J.C. Smith, U.S. Census Bureau, Current Population Reports, P60-239, Income, Poverty and Health Insurances Coverage in the United States: 2010, U.S. Government Printing Office, Washington DC 2011.

Drake, St. C. and H. R. Cayton. 1970. *Black Metropolis: A Study of Negro Life in a Northern City*. Chicago, IL: University of Chicago Press.

Filomena, S., K. Scanlin, and K. B. Morland. 2013. Brooklyn, New York foodscape 2007–2011: A five-year analysis of stability in food retail environments. *Int J Behav Nutr Phys Act* 10:46. http://www.ijbnpa.org/content/10/1/46.

Fisher, B. D. and D. S. Strogatz. 1999. Community measures of low-fat milk consumption: Comparing store shelves with households. *Am J Public Health* 89:235–237.

Galvez, M. P., K. Morland, C. Raines, et al. 2007. Race and food store availability in an inner-city neighborhood. *Public Health Nutr* 11:624–631.

Glanz, K., J. F. Sallis, B. E. Saelens, and L. D. Frank. 2007. Nutrition environment measures survey in stores (NEMS-S): Development and evaluation. *Am J Prev Med* 32:282–289.

Helper, R. 1969. *Racial Policies and Practices of Real Estate Brokers*. Minneapolis: University of Minnesota Press.

Hayes, L. R. 2000. Are prices higher for the poor in New York City? *J Cons Pol* 23:127–152.

Hays, R. A. 1985. *The Federal Government and Urban Housing: Ideology and Change in Public Policy*. Albany, NY: State University of New York Press.

Horowitz, C. R., K. A. Colson, P. L. Herbert, and K. Lancaster. 2004. Barriers to buying healthy foods for people with diabetes: Evidence of environmental disparities. *Am J Public Health* 94:1549–1554.

Hosler, A. S., D. Varadarajulu, A. E. Ronsani, B. L. Fredrick, and B. D. Fisher. 2006. Low-fat milk and high-fiber bread availability in food stores in urban and rural communities. *J Public Health Manag Pract* 12:556–562.

Jetter, K. M. and D. L. Cassady. 2006. The availability and cost of healthier food alternatives. *Am J Prev Med* 30:38–44.

Jonnalagadda, S. S. and S. Diwan. 2002. Nutrient intake of first generation Gujarati Asian Indian immigrants in the U.S. *J Am Coll Nutr* 21:372–380.

Jugo, R., T. Baranowski, and J. C. Baranowski. 2007. Fruit and vegetable availability: A micro environmental mediating variable? *Public Health Nutr* 10:681–689.

Kawachi, I. and L. F. Berkman. 2003. *Neighborhoods and Health*. New York: Oxford University Press.

Leise, A. D., K. E. Weiss, D. Pluto, E. Smith, A. Lawson. 2007. Food store type, availability, and cost of foods in a rural environment. *J Am Diet Assoc* 107:1916–1923.

Levy, B. S. and V. W. Sidel. 2006. The nature of social injustice and its impact on public health. In *Social Injustice and Public Health*, edited by B. S. Levy and V. W. Sidel. New York: Oxford University Press.

Lewis, L. B., D. C. Sloane, L. M. Nascimento et al. 2005. African Americans' access to healthy food options in south Los Angeles restaurants. *Am J Public Health* 95: 668–673.

Lieberson, S. 1963. *Ethnic Patterns in American Cities*. New York: Free Press of Glencoe.

Maher, B. 2013. Food Racism. http://www.real-time-with-bill-maher-blog.com/real-time-with-bill-maher-blog/2013/3/15/food-racism.html (Accessed March 17, 2013).

Marmot, M. and R. Bell. 2006. The socioeconomically disadvantaged. In *Social Injustice and Public Health*, edited by B. S. Levy and V. W. Sidel. New York: Oxford University Press.

Massey, D. S. and N. A. Denton. 1993. *American Apartheid: Segregation and the Making of the Underclass*. Cambridge, MA: Harvard University Press.

Moore, L. V. and A. V. Diez Roux. 2006. Associations of neighborhood characteristics with the location and type of food stores. *Am J Public Health* 96: 325–331.

Morland, K. B. 2010. An evaluation of a neighborhood-level intervention to a local food environment. *Am J Prev Med* 39:e31–e38.

Morland, K. and S. Filomena. 2007. Disparities in the availability of fruits and vegetables between racially segregated urban neighborhoods. *Public Health Nutr* 10:1481–1489.

Morland, K. and S. Filomena. 2008. The utilization of local food environments by urban seniors. *Prev Med* 47:289–293.

Morland, K., S. Wing, A. V. Diez Roux C. Poole. 2002. Neighborhood characteristics associated with the location of food stores and food service places. *Am J Prev Med* 22:23–29.

Munoz-Plaza, C. E., S. Filomena, and K. B. Morland. 2008. Disparities in food access: Inner-city residents describe their local food environment. *J Hun Environ Nutr* 2:51–64.

National Institutes of Health, National Heart Lung and Blood Institute. Stroke Belt Initiate. http://www.nhlbi.nih.gov/health/prof/heart/other/sb_spec.pdf (Accessed June 13, 2013).

National Institutes of Health, National Institute of Neurological Disorders and Stroke. 2009. Stroke: Challenges, Progress and Promise. NIH Publication No. 09-6451.

Pothukuchi, K. 2005. Attracting supermarkets to inner-city neighborhoods: Economic development outside the box. *Econ Dev Quart* 19:232–244.

Powell, L. M., S. Slater, D. Mirtcheva, Y. Bao, F. J. Chaloupka. 2007. Food store availability and neighborhood characteristics in the United States. *Prev Med* 44:189–195.

Rainlake Productions. 2009. *Building Food Justice in East New York*, edited by Kim Connell. New York: Rainlake Productions.

Rice, R. L. 1968. Residential segregation by Law, 1910–1917. *J South Hist* 34:179–199.

Sharkey, J. R. and S. Horel. 2008. Neighborhood socioeconomic deprivation and minority composition are associated with better potential spatial access to the ground-truthed food environment in a large rural area. *J Nutr* 138:620–627.

Sloane, D. C., A. Diamant, L. B. Lewis L. et al. 2003. Improving the nutritional resource environment for healthy living through community-based participatory research. *J Gen Intern Med* 18: 568–575.

Smedley, B., M. Jeffries, L. Adelman, J. Cheng. 2008. Race, Racial Inequalities and Health Inequities: Separating Myth from Fact. http://www.unnaturalcauses.org/assets/uploads/file/Race_Racial_Inequality_Health.pdf (Accessed February 15, 2013).

Troutt, D. D. 1993. *The Thin Red Line: How the Poor Still Pay More*. San Francisco, CA: West Coast Regional Office, Consumers Union of United States.

U.S. Administration on Aging. 2002. A profile of Older Americans: 2002. http://www.aoa.gov/AoAroot/Aging_Statistics/Profile/2002/13.aspx (Accessed August 5, 2013).

U.S. Bureau of the Census. 2013. http://www.census.gov/geo/reference (Accessed April 1, 2013).

U.S. Department of Agriculture (USDA). 2007. Thrifty Food Plan, 2006. CNPP-19. http://www.cnpp.usda.gov/Publications/FoodPlans/MiscPubs/TFP2006Report.pdf (Accessed April 12, 2013).

U.S. Department of Agriculture (USDA). 2009. Access to Affordable and Nutritious Food: Measuring and Understanding Food Deserts and Their Consequences: Report to Congress. http://www.ers.usda.gov/media/242675/ap036_1_pdf (Accessed April 22, 2013).

U.S. House of Representatives Select Committee on Hunger. 1992. Urban Grocery Gap. Washington, DC: U.S. Government Printing Office.

U.S. House of Representatives Select Committee on Hunger. 1987. Obtaining food: Shopping constraints on the poor. Washington, DC: U.S. Government Printing Office.

Wolf, P. A. 1994. Epidemiology of stroke. In *Primer in Preventive Cardiology*, edited by T. A. Pearson, M. H. Criqui, R. V. Luepker, A. Oberman, and M. Winston. New York: American Heart Association.

Zenk, S. N., A. J. Schulz, B. A. Israel, S. A. James, S. Bao, M. L. Wilson. 2005. Neighborhood racial composition, neighborhood poverty, and the spatial accessibility of supermarkets in metropolitan Detroit. *Am J Public Health* 95:660–667.

5 Local Food Environments and Dietary Intake

Barbara A. Laraia, Bethany Hendrickson, and Yun T. Zhang

Humans do not innately know how to select a nutritious diet; we survived in evolution because nutritious foods were readily available for us to hunt or gather.

Marion Nestle (2007)

The increase in prevalence of diet-related diseases and conditions like diabetes, heart disease, and obesity in the United States over the last 30 years is now well documented and has made its way as a topic of mainstream concern by individuals, the media, and policy makers. Within these data is the troubling trend that low-income and certain minority groups experience these diet-related diseases at disproportionately higher rates. Data from the 2009–2010 National Health and Nutrition Examination Survey (NHANES) indicated that the adult age-adjusted prevalence of obesity was 35.7%. The overall prevalence of obesity did not appear to increase between 2007/2008 and 2009/2010; however, significant increases from 2007/2008 and higher obesity rates were found among Mexican-American (44.9%) and African-American (58.5%) women aged 20 years and older (Ogden et al. 2012). The multibillion-dollar diet and weight loss industry is but one example of the individual focus abating these conditions has taken (Havrankova 2012). Yet, despite this investment, only limited success has occurred in this arena suggesting that these individually focused interventions inadequately address the complex factors associated with diet and physical activity. This over-emphasis on the role of individual behaviors in diet and health ignores the complex contexts in which many of these behaviors take place, one of which is the local food environment. A growing number of academics, public health practitioners, policy makers, and community groups believe that our environment shapes who we are, how we live, and what we eat; however, we have not identified what aspect of the local food environment is most influential and to what extent our environment determines dietary intake and risk of chronic conditions.

Early work by Cheadle et al. (1991) suggested that the type of food available in the local food environment was associated with dietary intake of those foods, and work by Morland et al. (2002) suggested that there are geographic disparities in fruit and vegetable intake by the ethnic/racial distribution of people residing in a neighborhood. This chapter focuses on the extent that food venues and our ability to access and interact with these resources determine what we purchase and consume. Previous chapters in this book have described the food environment, the food system and the distribution of the food supply, and assessment issues. This chapter focuses on the relationship between the food environment and dietary intake. There are two inherent challenges with attempting to assess this relationship. One challenge is in conceptualizing and measuring the diet—dietary intake is a complex and multidimensional construct. Thus, before confronting the logistical challenge of assessment, one must confront the conceptual challenge of identifying the specific aspect of diet that is theorized to "matter" for the health outcome of interest answering such questions as: what aspect of the diet will represent one's risk or benefit profile for some health outcome? For example, is underconsuming fresh, whole foods that are rich in nutrients (e.g., fruits, vegetables, whole grains, and lean meats), or overconsuming energy-dense foods (e.g., sugar-sweetened beverages, snacks, and fast foods), or a ratio of nutrient-dense to energy-dense foods, or the overall meal pattern, the important aspect of the diet? An additional challenge is to identify the instrument with which to measure the diet. Deciding on which aspect of the diet is the focus of measurement will guide what dietary assessment method to use. The other challenge relates to the difficulty in modeling or estimating the extent the environment shapes or determines dietary behaviors. The local food environment may be measured by type of food venue—supermarkets, grocery stores, small corner markets, convenience stores, fast-food, and other types of restaurants. These may be measured separately as the proximity (distance to the closest outlet), or the density (a count within a specified geographical unit), or a summary of these can be quantified. For example, the simple presence or absence of a food store may be associated with the dietary intake of an individual, but the person's age, ethnicity, gender, or income might explain this finding. In addition to the proximity and density, researchers have assessed price of food, availability, and quality of food within stores using audit tools, and the perception of food availability, cost, and quality. This chapter will attempt to provide a framework for answering these questions, review the burgeoning literature over the past two decades that focuses on these issues, and identify ways to measure dietary intake and the food environment.

As explained at the outset, one intention of this book is to explore the role, if any, of the local food environment in contributing to the wide disparities in health in the United States. Rates of noncommunicable diseases are seen in disproportionate numbers in low-income and minority populations. Many of these diseases have a strong dietary or weight component, meaning a poor diet is a contributing factor in the onset of some of these diseases, whereas a healthy diet can delay or prevent disease. Observational studies of the food environment have found that dietary patterns and obesity rates differ between neighborhoods with those in low-income or more deprived areas independently associated with a poor diet (Stimpson et al. 2007; Diez-Roux et al. 1999) and prevalence of obesity (Chang 2006; Nelson et al. 2006; Lopez 2007; Rundle et al. 2007). In addition, there is evidence that low-income and communities of color experience different access to different types of food outlets where fewer supermarkets (Morland et al. 2002) and, in turn, more liquor, fast food, and convenience stores are commonly found when compared with high-income neighborhoods (Moore and Diez Roux 2006). These observations provide a starting point for further exploration if these characteristics of neighborhood, retail food outlets, and diet are related.

When assessing the local food environment and diet relationship, one would like to capture a person's "usual" dietary intake, one that reflects dietary intake over some period. This is important because dietary intake is highly variable for each person.

Dietary intake is a unique health behavior because, unlike other behaviors, we must eat every day and usually at least three times per day. There are very few mandatory behaviors that we must engage in on a daily basis. The average individual makes 200 food-related decisions each day (Wansink and Sobal 2007); therefore, personal choice greatly factors into food purchases. No other mandatory behavior has a similar number of decisions that are made throughout each day, and the number of daily food-related thoughts and decisions may increase the risk of deciding to choose a less nutritious option under certain conditions. The number of food-related thoughts coupled with other cognitive and neurological interactions, such as poor executive function, cognitive load, stress, and depression, all have a role in our food-related choices, and when these systems are taxed we often make poor choices with regard to food (Adam and Epel 2007; Epel et al. 2012). Another issue pertaining to assessing the association between the local food environment and diet is identifying what aspect of the diet needs to be measured—nutrients, individual foods or beverages, meal patterns, or food preferences of individuals—to capture health risk. In addition, when and how often does dietary intake need to be measured when estimating the extent to which the food environment may influence food choice? What other important aspects of food choice do we need to measure, such as cost, quality, preference, and time? This chapter raises a number of measurement issues and conceptual considerations when assessing the diet.

The structure of this chapter is as follows: first, we will review diet–disease relationships that have been discovered in the last century, and review diet assessment methods and tools. Second, we will review tools and measures used to assess the local food environment. Third, we will review the literature that focuses on retail food venues, sometimes referred to as the built environment—convenience stores, corner stores, grocery stores, supermarkets, farmers' markets, fast-food establishments, and other restaurants—and food purchase and dietary intake. Fourth, we will present the trends in purchases of foods away from home and measurement issues related to how restaurants and takeaway foods influence dietary intake. Fifth, we will touch on initiatives that focus on the school food environment and food stores that surround schools.

Figure 5.1 is a simplistic representation of factors that may be involved and interact with the local food environment during food purchase decisions and eating events. A person's age, food preference, time/convenience, and mode of transportation will directly influence food purchases. Many of the characteristics that determine food purchases (e.g., age, food preference, and time/convenience) also influence what is eaten during an eating event. In addition, the household size and membership, sex, time of day (meal/snack), and time of month are depicted as arrows between food purchase and dietary intake.

DIET AND HEALTH

The role of nutrition in health is inextricable; however, we know mostly about nutrition through the extremes of malnutrition and nutrient deficiencies identified in the twentieth century. We are beginning to understand more about over-nutrition and disease of modern societies but we know very little about optimal nutrition and longevity. We often hear that all foods, if eaten in moderation, can fit into a healthy diet. Yet, dietary trends in the United States suggest that too few people meet the Dietary Guidelines for Americans (DGA) (Kirkpatrick et al. 2012) and too many people are eating in

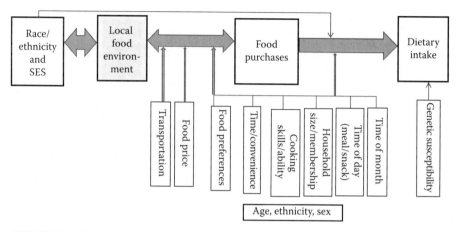

FIGURE 5.1   Hypothesized relationships between local food environments and diet for adults.

great excess of the suggested limits to *discretionary* calories, which are defined by the United States Department of Agriculture (USDA), as the number of calories available to an individual after they meet all of the dietary guidelines (http://www.health.gov /dietaryguidelines/dga2005/report/HTML/D3_Disccalories.htm). Using NHANES 2001–2004 data, Kirkpatrick et al. (2012) found that a small percent of children met dietary guidelines for nutritious plant-based foods. On average, only 0.5% met guidelines for whole grains, 1.0% for dark leafy green vegetables, 4.2% for orange vegetables, 5.1% for dry beans, 6.6% for total vegetable, and 28.7% for total fruit, while 37.1% met guidelines for milk, 42% for starchy vegetables, 43.8% for meat/dry beans, and 80.7% for total grains. Strikingly, the percent of low-income children that met guidelines was either roughly equivalent or higher to their upper-income peers.

This section will provide a short review of nutrient and related disease discoveries of the twentieth century, present the motivation of the public health sector in identifying ways to intervene on chronic disease risk, and review dietary assessment tools. Nutritional science is a relatively young science that began in the late nineteenth century with the discovery of essential micronutrients. These micronutrients are defined as essential because they must be consumed, as they cannot be produced by the body and are necessary to avoid diseases caused by their deficiency. There is causal evidence linking nutrient deficiencies with disease—niacin and pellagra, vitamin C and scurvy, thiamine and beriberi, vitamin D and rickets, iodine and goiter, and iron and anemia, to name just a few. These nutrient–disease relationships were all discovered in the late nineteenth and early twentieth century. For example, sailors on long voyages often contracted a rare disease characterized by extreme fatigue and malaise and eventually spotted or mottled skin, and spongy, sore red gums. If prolonged, the condition worsens with a loss of teeth, jaundice, fever, neuropathy, and death, but eventually, a simple treatment was identified. By providing fresh food, and specifically citrus foods (e.g., limes), sailors were safe from the disease. Not until 1932, with the discovery of vitamin C, was the cause-and-effect mechanism of scurvy identified. During the early twentieth century, there were several similar discoveries. For instance, niacin (vitamin B3), which is needed for metabolism of carbohydrates and creation of energy, causes pellagra when deficient in the diet. Niacin deficiency is largely due to poverty and results in the slowing of the metabolism and the three Ds— diarrhea, dermatitis, and dementia. Although niacin was first characterized in the late 1800s, it was not understood as a pellagra-preventing factor until 1937, when the biochemist Conrad Elvehjem made the connection. Along with vitamin C and niacin, thiamin (vitamin B1) deficiency (beriberi), vitamin D deficiency (rickets), vitamin A deficiency (night blindness and other symptoms) were all discovered during this same period. In 1897, Dr. Christiaan Eijkman, a Dutch physician and pathologist, demonstrated that beriberi is caused by poor diet, and discovered that feeding unpolished rice helped prevent beriberi in chickens. More recently, folate and supplementation of folic acid (the synthetic form of folate) in the diet was identified as playing a major role in decreasing neural tube defects (e.g., spina bifida) and heart disease among adults caused by elevated homocysteine levels that may be due to folate deficiency. Mineral deficiencies, such as iodine deficiency that caused goiter, were largely eradicated in the United States in the 1950s.

Although many of these curable vitamin and mineral deficiency-related diseases still exist in parts of the world, they were largely eradicated in the United States by the 1960s. With the exception of vitamins A and C, most of these identified micronutrient deficiencies have been treated by intervention in the food supply through fortification and enrichment. Today, most of our grains are fortified with niacin, thiamine, riboflavin, folic acid, and iron; our milk with vitamin D; and our salt with iodine. Major shifts in diet have occurred since the 1960s and the focus has turned to chronic disease, diet-related cancers, over-nutrition and the obesity epidemic. In 2008, it was estimated that, of all the deaths that occurred in the world, 63% were due to noncommunicable diseases (Alwan et al. 2010). Due to the rising prevalence of cardiovascular disease (CVD), some cancers, and diabetes, nutrition-related chronic disease will account for three quarters of deaths by 2020 (Alwan et al. 2010; Alwan and World Health Organization 2011). According to the reviews of the literature by World Health Organization, convincing evidence exists regarding the role that a handful of foods and nutrients play in preventing or promoting chronic diseases. Trends in food availability and consumption patterns suggest that there are more calories available per capita, more calories from fat and refined carbohydrates, and more processed food products in the market place (e.g., 24,000 new products each year), thus making "healthy" food choices difficult for individuals to navigate in the current food environment (Wells and Buzby 2008). When it comes to CVD, we know that certain fats, such as trans and saturated fatty acids, and sodium increase risk, whereas polyunsaturated fats, fruits, and vegetables are seen to be protective (Srinath and Katan 2004). In diabetes, high intake of saturated fat is a risk factor but intake of high-fiber complex carbohydrates is protective (Steyn et al. 2004). There is also evidence that energy-dense foods (those with high calories relative to size or weight of the food) and sugar-sweetened beverages may contribute to weight gain (Swinburn et al. 2004). This information is helpful to an extent but most humans do not eat single nutrients; rather, we eat a range of foods made up of varying levels of nutrients, with many of those that are listed as *protective* or *promoting* of disease appearing in the same food. Although we have a sense of the nutrients that are associated with disease, measures of diet that take a more holistic approach—those that account for quality, quantity, safety, and meal pattern—may have more relevance. However, a validated and standardized measure of the overall diet is not yet available.

Chronic disease, diet-related cancers, and the obesity epidemic have created a strong focus on the quality and quantity of macronutrient—protein, fat, and carbohydrate—intake. Scientific evidence of an optimal diet that minimizes morbidities, reduces obesity, reverses chronic disease, and increases longevity is emerging. Diets such as the successful DASH (Dietary Approaches to Stop Hypertension) diet focusing on foods such as fruits, vegetables, whole grains, nuts, lean cuts of meat, and low-fat dairy (thus maximizing calcium, potassium, magnesium, and fiber intake) was found to reduce hypertension (Sacks et al. 2001). In addition, low-fat vegetarian diets (Ornish 1998; 2008); and Mediterranean diets characterized by increased intake of fruits, root vegetables, green vegetables, fish, olive oil instead of butter, and less red meat (de Lorgeril et al. 1994) have consistently shown reduction of risk factors among adults with chronic conditions (de Koning et al. 2011). These diets are similar in that they are comprehensive approaches to an overall diet and serve to minimize the consumption of highly processed and refined grains, added sugar, red meat and saturated fats, and sugar-sweetened beverages. What is emphasized in an approach that assesses the overall diet is the habitual dietary pattern that reduces disease risk and, therefore, prevents the onset of chronic disease at some later date. Nutrition studies are needed that will help determine both an optimal diet and a sufficient food supply that will assist humans with living long and healthy lives relatively free of disease.

In the United States, with the exception of the National Cancer Institute's (NCI) 5-A-Day campaign that promotes daily consumption of at least five servings of fruits and vegetables daily (Heimendinger et al. 1996), there have been few whole foods campaigns that promote maximizing nutritional quality of foods and dietary intake of essential micronutrients. As a federal nutrition policy, the DGA is a scientifically-based assessment of necessary foods and food components needed for an optimal diet. This policy is the underpinning of most federal nutrition programs. Reviewed every 5 years, the 2010 DGA is the most recent set of guidelines and is the most comprehensive assessment to date. Specifically, the DGA offers one general set of guidelines, but they are not all quantifiable. The most recent 2010 DGA consists of 23 recommendations that fall into four categories: (1) Balancing Calories to Manage Weight; (2) Foods and Food Components to Reduce; (3) Foods and Nutrients to Increase; and (4) Building Health Eating Patterns (USDA 2010).

There are additional recommendations for vulnerable populations, such as pregnant women and the elderly. Based on the DGA, the UDSA created a diet quality index called the Healthy Eating Index (HEI), which is used to measure the overall diet quality of an individual and how well they are meeting the recommendations. Because not all 23 recommendations are quantifiable, the HEI has traditionally measured 10 or 12 items including fruits, vegetables, grain, dairy, meat, fats, sodium, and empty calories. The most recent version of the HEI, the HEI-2010, focuses on the following foods and nutrients: whole fruit, total fruit, total vegetables, greens and beans, whole grains, refined grains, dairy, total protein foods, sea and plant protein, fatty acids, sodium, and empty calories (Guenther et al. 2013) (Figure 5.2).

⋀⋁ Healthy Eating Index HEI-2010 Components and Scoring System

HEI-2010[1] Component	Maximum	Standard for Maximum Score	Standard for Minimum Score of Zero
▲ Adequacy *(Higher Score Indicates Higher Consumption)*			
Total fruit[2]	5	≥ 0.8 cup equiv./1,000 kcal[10]	No fruit
Whole fruit[3]	5	≥ 0.4 cup equiv./1,000 kcal	No whole fruit
Total vegetables[4]	5	≥ 1.1 cup equiv./1,000 kcal	No vegetables
Greens and beans[4]	5	≥ 0.2 cup equiv./1,000 kcal	No dark-green vegetables, beans, or peas
Whole grains	10	≥ 1.5 ounce equiv./1,000 kcal	No whole grains
Dairy[5]	10	≥ 1.3 cup equiv./1,000 kcal	No dairy
Total protein foods[6]	5	≥ 2.5 ounce equiv./1,000 kcal	No protein foods
Seafood and plant proteins[6,7]	5	≥ 0.8 ounce equiv./1,000 kcal	No seafood or plant proteins
Fatty acids[8]	10	(PUFAs + MUFAs)/SFAs ≥ 2.5	(PUFAs + MUFAs)/SFAs ≤ 1.2
▼ Moderation *(Higher Score Indicates Lower Consumption)*			
Refined grains	10	≤ 1.8 ounce equiv./1,000 kcal	≥ 4.3 ounce equiv./1,000 kcal
Sodium	10	≤ 1.1 gram/1,000 kcal	≥ 2.0 gram/1,000 kcal
Empty calories[9]	20	≤ 19% of energy	≥ 50% of energy

FIGURE 5.2 Healthy Eating Index—2010 scoring (http://www.cnpp.usda.gov /healthyeatingindex.htm. Accessed June 6, 2013). [1]Intakes between the minimum and maximum standards are scored proportionately. [2]Includes 100% fruit juice. [3]Includes all forms except juice. [4]Includes any beans and peas not counted as Total Protein Foods. [5]Includes all milk products, such as fluid milk, yogurt, and cheese, and fortified soy beverages. [6]Beans and peas are included here (and not with vegetables) when the Total Protein Foods standard is otherwise not met. [7]Includes seafood, nuts, seeds, soy products (other than beverages) as well as beans and peas counted as Total Protein Foods. [8]Ratio of poly-monounsaturated fatty acids (PUFAs and MUFAs) to saturated fatty acids (SFAs). [9]Calories from solid fats, alcohol, and added sugars; threshold for counting alcohol is >13 g/1000 kcal. [10]Equiv, equivalent; kcal, kilocalorie.

Dietary intake scores based on the HEI indicate that, on average, Americans are not eating well. The diets of American children aged 2–17, like those of adults, are on average very poor as evidenced by a 55.9 mean score of a possible 100 using the HEI-2005, a measure that assesses overall compliance with 2005 DGA (Fungwe et al. 2009). Among low-income children, the mean HEI-2005 score was about the same: 56.4 (Guenther et al. 2007).

MEASURING DIET FOR LOCAL FOOD ENVIRONMENT RESEARCH

Understanding the elements of the diet that promote or prevent disease is important in local food environment research for a multitude of reasons; namely, it provides a benchmark from which to compare the nutrition status and behaviors of individuals or groups. In local food environment research, sources of diet data come either from primary data collection or from existing databases representing nutritional status of certain populations. For example, at the national level the NHANES and National Health Interview Survey (NHIS) are annual surveys conducted on a representative sample of the U.S. population. The Behavioral Risk Factor Surveillance Study (BRFSS) and California Health Interview Survey (CHIS) are annual surveys conducted at the state level. All of these surveys are publicly available datasets that have dietary data and can be geocoded to residential neighborhood and can be used to assess the relationship between the local food environment and dietary intake for a given year.

There are a number of tools that are used to collect dietary intake data. Depending on time, resources, and the research question, diet data is collected using one of a few different methods. Three general types of dietary assessment tools are described in the following subsections. A full tutorial in dietary assessment is available in Thompson and Subar (2013).

24-Hour Recall

The 24-hour recall is often considered the *gold standard* for measuring actual diet intake in an individual or population because it provides the highest validity, least biased dietary information relative to other methods of diet data collection. In the 24-hour recall, the respondent is asked to report everything eaten and drunk during the previous 24 hours and to provide details regarding every item consumed (when, where, how, how much, with what). It is often conducted in person or over the phone by trained administrators who are taught to probe for all food details and usually takes 20 minutes to administer. It is recommended that two or more recalls are collected from individuals with both weekday and weekend intake represented to approximate one's usual intake. Collecting dietary data using the 24-hour recall approach necessitates dietary software that contains an extensive food and nutrient database. A number of software products are available and range in price depending on the extensiveness of the food/nutrient database and intricacy of the software interface (Pennington et al. 2007). The NCI has developed a computer-assisted self-report recall system, called the Automated Self-Administered 24-hour recall (ASA24), which is free to use (http://riskfactor.cancer.gov/tools/instruments/asa24/. Accessed August 15, 2013) (Table 5.1).

The benefit of the 24-hour recall is that it does not require a high level of literacy (if being administered by an interviewer) and because of the immediacy of the recall period, respondents are generally able to remember their intake. Further, it is the most accurate tool to determine usual intake distributions in a population, if two or more 24-hour recalls are collected. However, average dietary intakes of a population can be determined with just one 24-hour recall collection. The downsides of this method of data collection are that it tends to be impractical for large-scale research due to its expense and reliance on trained interviewers, and multiple days are needed to estimate the usual intakes of individuals. Estimating the *usual intake*, is important because dietary recommendations are intended to be met over time and diet-health hypotheses are based on dietary intakes over the long term. Unless multiple 24-hour recalls are assessed over a long period, there is a concern that seasonality is not captured. Despite this and other limitations, the 24-hour recall approach is the most accurate and

TABLE 5.1

Dietary Intake Software to Be Used with 24-h Dietary Recall Data Collection

Name	Uniform Resource Locator	Cost	Database	
ASA24	http://riskfactor.cancer.gov /tools/instruments/asa24/	FREE		NIH/NCI
USDA Food and Nutrient Database for Dietary Studies (FNDDS)	http://www.ars.usda.gov /Services/docs. htm?docid=12089	FREE	• Database of foods, their nutrient values, and weights for typical food portions • Includes 10 data files, plus comprehensive documentation and user's guide for ease of use • Used to analyze data from the survey *What We Eat in America*, the dietary intake component of the National Health and Nutrition Examination Survey (NHANES) • Underlying food composition data are from the USDA National Nutrient Database for Standard Reference	USDA
Nutrition Analyst 2.0	http://www.myfoodrecord .com/	FREE	The database used by Nutrition Analyst Tool (NAT) is composed of the USDA Standard Reference (SR) and information from food companies. The data should not be taken as an exact representation of the nutrient content of your diet. The numbers used for analysis are averages and there is great variance in nutrient content for each food item in the database. The nutrient data may not be complete for every food listed in NAT as there are still gaps in our knowledge of food composition	University of Illinois, Department of Food Science and Human Nutrition
Nutrition Data System for Research	http://www.ncc.umn.edu /products/ndsr.html	$5500	The Nutrition Coordinating Center Food and Nutrient Database serves as the source of food composition information in the program. This database includes over 18,000 foods including 7,000 brand name products. Ingredient choices and preparation methods provide more than 160,000 food variants. Values for 163 nutrient, nutrient ratios, and other food components are generated from the database. Also, food group assignments are provided. The database is updated annually to reflect marketplace changes and new analytic data	University of Minnesota

(Continued)

TABLE 5.1 (*Continued*)
Dietary Intake Software to Be Used with 24-h Dietary Recall Data Collection

Name	Uniform Resource Locator	Cost	Database	
Food Processor	http://www.esha.com /product/food-processor	$699	ESHA master database is composed of 50,000 + food items, with data from over 1,700 reputable sources. The data sources include the latest USDA Standard Reference database, manufacturer's data, restaurant data, and data from literature sources. Each of our 163 nutritional components is individually sourced. In addition, we provide several calculated fields, such as the percent calories from fat and niacin equivalents	ESHA Research 4747 Skyline Rd. S, Suite100 Salem, OR 97306
Nutritionist Pro Diet Analyst	http://www.nutritionistpro .com/	$595	Extensive Database—Accurate, up-to-date food and nutrient data for complete analysis on over 51,000 foods and ingredients, including brand-name, fast foods, ethnic foods, and enteral products. The Knowledge Database also includes over 500 brands from over 700 food manufacturers. Plus you can add an unlimited number of your own foods and recipes	Axxya Systems, 4800 Sugar Grove Blvd Suite 602 Stafford, TX 77477
Food Works 15	http://nutritionco.com/	$199.95	The FoodWorks Database consists of more than 39,000 food references. These foods are derived from the following sources: 1. The USDA National Nutrient Database for SR 2. The FNDDS 3. The Canadian Nutrient File 4. The pre-FNDDS Survey Data 5. Historic Data and Other Data Sources 6. The Fast Food Data Supplement: This data is obtained directly from selected fast-food restaurants (McDonald's, Burger King, Starbucks, Kentucky Fried Chicken, Sonic, Taco Bell, and Tim Horton's). Data includes current menu listings. Expanded nutrient data for selected items from these and other restaurants are also included in the SR and FNDDS databases	The Nutrition Company, P.O. Box 477, Long Valley, NJ 07853 USA

TABLE 5.1 (*Continued*)
Dietary Intake Software to Be Used with 24-h Dietary Recall Data Collection

Name	Uniform Resource Locator	Cost	Database	
Nutrition Software Solutions	http://www .nutritionsoftwaresolutions .com/	$179	Provides the most extensive collection of nutrition assessment tools, in electronic format, to help health-care professionals assess adult and pediatric nutritional needs, perform enteral/parenteral calculations, reference laboratory values, design diabetic and renal meal plans, and offers a host of other unique and useful tools	Nutrition Software Solutions, Inc. 13677 Samhill Drive Mount Airy, MD 21771-3918
Technology Assisted Dietary Assessment	http://www.tadaproject.org/	$179	Provides the most extensive collection of nutrition assessment tools, in electronic format, to help health-care professionals assess adult and pediatric nutritional needs, perform enteral/parenteral calculations, reference laboratory values, design diabetic and renal meal plans, and offers a host of other unique and useful tools	Purdue University, Video and Image Processing Laboratory

comprehensive and, if used to capture a group mean intake, it is the best approach. In addition, it is the only way to capture total caloric intake.

FOOD FREQUENCY QUESTIONNAIRES

The Food Frequency Questionnaires (FFQ) asks respondents to report the frequency of consumption of particular foods over a specified period. The FFQ is most often used to obtain a crude estimate of total diet intake over a specified time, such as the past month, 6 months or, year. A list of foods is provided to the respondent and details on frequency of consumption are asked. Some FFQs will incorporate questions on portion sizes but little detail regarding other food characteristics (such as method of cooking) is collected. For example, FFQs often group similar items into a single question (e.g., pork, beef, lamb), which could be considered cognitively challenging to someone who frequently eats beef, but only occasionally eats pork, lamb, or other similar meats. The challenge with an FFQ is creating an appropriate list of foods that captures as closely as possible the breadth of an individual's diet, is culturally appropriate, and is the least cognitively challenging. Compared to the 24-hour recall, the FFQ is less expensive as it is often self-administered. However, measurement error, especially underreporting of caloric intake, is common due to many details of diet intake not being measured and inaccuracies due to incomplete listings of foods. Research has suggested that longer FFQ lists may overestimate intake of fruits and vegetables, whereas shorter lists may underestimate intake (Krebs-Smith et al. 1994). The information from the FFQ is entered into a food and nutrient database to generate diet variables. There are many versions of the FFQ, which attests to its easy adaptability for specific populations and purposes. Most FFQ have between 120 and 160 food items or groups and take 45 minutes to an hour to complete. A few of the most common versions that have been evaluated include the Block Questionnaire (https://www.nutritionquest.com/assessment/list-of-questionnaires-and-screeners), the Fred Hutchinson Cancer Research Center FFQ (http://sharedresources.fhcrc.org /services/food-frequency-questionnaires-ffq), the Harvard University FFQ, or Willett Questionnaires (https://regepi.bwh.harvard.edu/health), and the NCI's Diet History Questionnaire (http://riskfactor.cancer.gov/dhq2/).

BRIEF DIETARY SCREENERS

Short dietary assessment instruments, often called screeners, can be useful in situations that do not require assessment of total caloric intake, the total diet, or quantitative accuracy in dietary estimates. Although estimates of intake from short dietary assessment instruments are not as accurate as those from more detailed methods, such as 24-hour dietary recalls, screeners are often used to characterize a population's median intakes, distinguishing between individuals or populations with regard to higher versus lower intakes, examining interrelationships between diet and other variables, and comparing findings from a smaller study to a larger population study. It is common for screeners to be developed if a specific component of diet is of interest, as is the case with fruit and vegetable screeners used in the BRFSS and the CHIS. Numerous screeners have been developed and evaluated against 24-hour recalls and full FFQ and can be found at the NCI website (http://riskfactor.cancer.gov/diet/screeners/) (Table 5.2).

The obvious advantage to using a short screener to assess intake is the time and fewer resources required to administer. For example, instead of relying on an extensive food and nutrient database, a score based on the frequency with which the foods are consumed can be tallied. However, despite this advantage, short screeners do have some limitations. First, they do not capture information about the entire diet and measurements are often not quantitatively meaningful (which prohibits the development of estimates of diet intake for a population).

FOOD ENVIRONMENT MEASURES AND METHODS

This section includes a review of the literature that assesses the association between the retail food environment and dietary intake. We first review the definitions and measurement of the retail food environment. This information is covered in more detail in Chapter 4; however, we highlight the definitions and measurements most commonly used in research studies that focus on the relationship between food retail and dietary intake.

The majority of research studies assessing the relationship between the local food environment and dietary intake use geographic information systems (GIS) to measure and define the local food environment. In addition to using GIS methodologies, a

TABLE 5.2
Selected Dietary Screeners to Collect Individual-Level Diet Information

	Screener Name	Number of Questions	Nutrients Measured						Validation Study
			Fruit and Veg.	Fiber or Whole Grains	Fat	Meat or Dairy	Sugar Foods or Bev.	Other	
ADULT	DASH Online Questionnaire	74	X	X	X	X	X	X	Apovian et al. (2010)
	Five-Factor Screener in the 2005 NHIS Cancer Control Supplement (CCS)	18	X	X			X	X	
	Dietary Screener Questionnaire in the NHANES 2009–10 and 2010 NHIS CCS	26	X	X		X	X	X	
	Dietary Screener in the 2009 CHIS	9	X				X		Hattori et al. (2013)
	NCI Multifactor Screener	17	X	X	X				Thompson et al. (2004)
	NCI 2-Factor Screener	11	X				X		Colón-Ramos et al. 2009
	NCI Fat Screener	16			X				Thompson et al. (2007)
	Block Rapid Screener	22	X		X				Block et al. (2000)
	Two-item Fruit and Vegetable Screener	2	X						Yaroch et al. (2012)
CHILDREN	Beverage and Snack Questionnaire	19	X			X	X	X	Neuhouser et al. (2009)
	Youth Risk Behavior Surveillance System questionnaire	4	X						Field et al. (1998)
	Fruit and Vegetable Brief	2	X						Prochaska and Sallis (2004)
	Child Dietary Fat Questionnaire	17			X				Dennison et al. (2000)
	Qualitative Dietary Fat Index Questionnaire	18			X				Yaroch et al. (2000)

Note: For further information please visit the National Cancer Institute site on Dietary Assessment: http://riskfactor.cancer.gov/diet/screeners/.

number of studies use audit tools to assess the local food environment and food availability, quality, and price within food stores. For an extensive presentation of methods used to measure these environments, including survey instruments (self-reported and observed) and methodologies, such as GIS, please see the National Institutes of Health National Cancer Institute website on Measures of the Food Environment: Defining Measures (Instruments and Methodologies) (https://riskfactor.cancer.gov /mfe/defining-measures-instruments-and-methodologies).

Common objective measures of the availability of outlets in the community food environment include the following: (1) count of outlets by type, (2) density of outlets by type (adjusting for population or area), (3) kernel density of outlets by type, (4) presence of outlets by type within buffer, or (5) opening of new store. Common objective measures of availability of food types in the consumer food environment include (1) presence/absence of select products within stores, (2) variety of select product types within stores, or (3) index or store summary score of food availability by store.

In addition to objective measurement of food availability, subjective measures of the availability are derived from survey questions that ask general questions regarding the availability or variety of foods within one's neighborhood, thus blurring the distinction between the community and consumer food environment. Past measures include (1) self-reported perceived availability of food types within one's *neighborhood*, (2) self-reported variety of products within food types in one's neighborhood, or (3) subjective reports from third parties such as neighbors (Moore et al. 2008; Zenk et al. 2005b, 2009).

Research studies have generally converged on a select number of diet-related constructs, but studies still vary widely in how those constructs are measured. The most common dietary outcome measure is fruit and vegetable intake. However, although validated diet instruments are available, they are not always used. Customized diet screeners are also common. Other measures include caloric intake, fat and sugar intake, the USDA Healthy Eating Index, dietary patterns, and fast-food consumption.

Two seminal ecological studies in the 1990s found that area-average product availability within stores was associated with area-average consumption of those food products (Cheadle et al. 1991; Fisher and Strogatz 1999). Cheadle et al. (1991) measured the proportion of shelf space dedicated to three specialty food products—non-white bread as a share of all bread shelf space, reduced-fat milk as a share of all milk shelf space, and red meat as a share of total meat shelf space within a county or zip code area—and investigated the relationship with the average consumption of those products. They found a significant positive correlation between the availability of healthful products in stores and the reported healthfulness of participants' diets. Fisher and Strogatz (1999) found that average availability of low-fat milk in a sample of 15–20 stores in the same zip code was associated with the proportion of zip code households that consumed low-fat milk. These observational studies were hypothesis generating, and the results—that the availability of nutritious foods and calorie-dense foods was positively correlated with consumption of those items—led to a number of studies over the next two decades.

We reviewed 34 studies that were based in the United States between 1990 and 2013. Tables 5.3 and 5.4 summarize the findings from the literature that look at associations between the food environment and diet. A number of studies examined multiple diet outcomes in their analyses, whereas others focused on one or two foods or behaviors, such as fruit and vegetable intake or fast-food consumption. The ability to measure various diet outcomes is largely dependent on the tool used. For example, 24-hour recalls, FFQs, and some screeners allow researchers to analyze multiple components of diet, whereas certain screeners only focus on one or two foods.

Table 5.3 focuses on findings from studies that have included fruits and vegetables measured separately and fruits and vegetables measured together as outcomes. There is now considerable evidence linking various health benefits to fruit and vegetable consumption, which is fueling increased focus from the scientific and policy communities on factors related to intake. The DGA have emphasized fruits and vegetables as separate food groups since the 1980s and continues to recommend a plant-based diet high in fruits and vegetables to reduce the risk of chronic disease and maintain a healthy weight (USDA 2010). Healthy People 2020, the report of health goals for the nation that is reviewed every 10 years, also outlines targets for increases in fruit and vegetable consumption for all populations over 2 years of age. Despite the array of health evidence underlying the promotion of fruits and vegetables, and advice from the scientific community, it is estimated that fewer than 20% of adults in the United States consume the recommended five daily servings (Blanck et al. 2008). In low-income populations, the consumption patterns appear to be worse, with even fewer servings of fruits and vegetables consumed (Kirkpatrick et al. 2012). Identifying the range of factors that may contribute to fruit and vegetable intake is one step that may lead to improvements in intake and reductions in risk of chronic disease.

A number of studies have looked at associations between the local food environment and intake of fruits and vegetables. A main premise driving much of this work is that a wide variety of reasonably priced fruits and vegetables of good quality found in one's neighborhood may promote fruit and vegetable intake. Often these qualities are found in larger supermarkets or grocery stores and sometimes even in well-stocked corner stores and markets. As Zenk et al. (2009) point out, researchers posit that larger, well-stocked stores can influence fruit and vegetable intake diet by "facilitating their purchase during major shopping trips or in between major shopping excursions as home stocks run low, or by serving as visual cues that prompt their purchase." Conversely, if a neighborhood food supply is made up of stores selling energy-dense items, such as convenience and liquor stores, fruit and vegetable intake may be negatively affected. This may be working through "disproportionate promotion of unhealthy foods, lower food costs per kilocalorie, shifts in social norms around food, or changes in food preferences (Zenk et al. 2009)." Yet, despite these reasonable theories, there is not yet a clear picture on what in the local food environment, if anything, might be influencing fruit and vegetable consumption.

Table 5.3 reviews the 24 studies that had at least one fruit and/or vegetable outcome. Of the eight studies that assessed fruit intake, four studies found no association and ran multiple tests to identify if a significant relationship could be found (e.g., between 7 and 30 tests) (Bodor et al. 2008 Powell and Han 2011; An and Sturm 2012;

TABLE 5.3

Studies Examining Relationships between the Local Food Environment and Fruit and Vegetable Intake

Author, Year[a]	Outcome[a]	Design[b]	Sample		Setting[e]	Potential or Realized Access[f]	Food Environment Measurement			Objective or Self-Report[j]	Results		
			Age[c]	Minority or Low-Income[d]			Food Environment Measure[g]	Geographic Unit[h]	Assessed Outlets[i]		Positive Diet Association[k]	Negative Diet Association[l]	No Significant Association[m]
Specific Foods													
Fruit													
Gustafson et al. (2013)	Fruit (24-h recall)	C (2010)	Adult (147)	Low (SNAP)	Res	P	Count	Buff (0.5, 1 mi.)	Super, Groc, Conv, FM, Gas	Ob	Conv (1)	0	5
Hattori et al. (2013)	Fruit (CHIS)	C (2007 and 2009)	Adult (97,678)	NA	Res	P	Count	Buff (0.25, 0.5, 1.0, 1.5, 3 mi., E)	SupGr, Groc, Super, Conv, FullR, FFR	Ob	0	FFR (2)	16
An and Sturm (2012)	Fruit (CHIS)	C (2005 and 2007)	Teen (7,574) Adult (11,851)	N/A	Res, Sch	P	Count	Buff (0.1, 0.5, 1.0, 1.5 mi.)	Super, Groc, SMGr, Conv, FFR	Ob	0	0	30
An and Sturm (2012)	100% Juice (CHIS)	C (2005 and 2007)	Teen (7,574) Child (11,851)	N/A	Res, Sch	P	Count	Buff (0.1, 0.5, 1.0, 1.5 mi.)	Super, Groc, SMGr, Conv, FFR	Ob	0	Teen: Conv, (1)	29
Powell and Han (2011)	Fruit (BrScr)	C (1997, 2002–2003)	Teen (O: 1,134, L: 342, H: 792)	Inc strata	Res	P	Dens, Price	Zip, City	Super, Groc, Conv, FFR, FFP, FHP, FullR	Ob	0	0	21

(Continued)

					P, R		CBG		Ob, SR	Variety	Prox N	
Sharkey et al. (2010)	Fruit (BrScr)	C (2006–2007)	Older Adult (582)	N/A	Res		Prox N, Avail, Variety	CBG	Super, Groc, OthS	Ob, SR	Variety (3)	Prox N (2)	4
Bodor et al. (2008)	Fruit (24 h)	C (2001)	Adults (102)	Min, Low	Res	P	Count, Avail, Prox N	Buff (100 m, 1,000 m)	Super, OthS	Ob	0	0	7
Jago et al. (2007)	Fruit (Cullen FFQ)	C (2003)	Boys/Teens (204)	N/A	Res	P	Prox N, Dens	Buff (1 mi., E)	LgGroc, OthS, FFR	Ob	OthS (Prox N)	FFR (Prox N)	4
Rose and Richards (2004)	Fruit (Other)	C (1996–1997)	Adults (963)	Min, Low	Res	R	Prox N, Travel Time, Access	N/A	Super, PrimS	SR	Access, Prox N	0	3
Vegetables												
Gustafson et al. (2013)	Veg (24-h recall)	C (2010)	Adult (147)	Low (SNAP)	Res	P	Count	Buff (0.5, 1 mi.)	Super, Groc, Conv, FM, Gas	Ob	Conv, FM, Super (5)	0	1
Hattori et al. (2013)	Veg (CHIS)	C (2007 and 2009)	Adult (97,678)	N/A	Res	P	Count	Buff (0.25, 0.5, 1.0, 1.5, 3 mi., E)	SupGr, Groc, Super, Conv, FullR, FF	Ob	0	FFR	29
An and Sturm (2012)	Veg (CHIS)	C (2005 and 2007)	Child (11,851) Teen (7,574)	N/A	Res, Sch	P	Count	Buff (0.1, 0.5, 1.0, 1.5)	Super, Groc, SMGr, Conv, FFR	Ob	Teen: FFR (2)	0	28
Powell and Han (2011)	Veg (BrScr)	C (1997, 2002–2003)	Teen (O: 1,134, L: 342, H: 792)	Inc strata	Res	P	Dens, Price	Zip, City	Super, Groc, Conv, FFR, FFP, FHP, FullR	Ob	L: Super, Groc	0	20

TABLE 5.3 (Continued)
Studies Examining Relationships between the Local Food Environment and Fruit and Vegetable Intake

Author, Year	Outcome[a]	Design[b]	Sample: Age[c]	Minority or Low-Income[d]	Setting[e]	Potential or Realized Access[f]	Food Environment Measures[g]	Geographic Unit[h]	Assessed Outlets[i]	Objective or Self-Report[j]	Positive Diet Association[k]	Negative Diet Association[l]	No Significant Association[m]
Izumi et al. (2011)	Select Veg (Mod Block FFQ)	C (2002–2003)	Adults (919)	Min, Low	Res	P	Count	Buff (0.5, E)	VegS	Ob	VegS	0	0
Laska et al. (2010)	Veg (24-h)	C	Teen (349)	N/A	Res, Sch	P	Dist Dens	Dist. to nearest facility, 800 m, 1,600 m, 3,000 m	Groc, Conv, OthS, FFR, OthR	Ob	0	0	19
Sharkey et al. (2010)	Veg (BrScr)	C (2006–2007)	Older Adult (582)	N/A	Res	P, R	Prox N, Avail, Variety	CBG	Super, Groc, OthS	Ob, SR	Avail (3)	Prox N (2)	4
Bodor et al. (2008)	Veg (24-h)	C (2001)	Adults (102)	Min, Low	Res	P	Count, Avail, Prox N	Buff (100 m, 1,000 m)	OthS, Super	Ob	Avail	0	6
Rose and Richards (2004)	Veg (Other)	C (1996–1997)	Adults (963)	Min, Low	Res	R	Prox N, Travel Time, Access	N/A	Super, PrimS	SR	0	0	5
Jago et al (2007)	Low-fat Veg (Cullen FFQ)	C (2003)	Boys/Teens (204)	N/A	Res	P	Prox N, Dens	Buff (1 mi., E)	LgGr, OthS, FFR	Ob	0	0	6

Study	Diet measure		Population					Buff	Store types		OthS (Prox N)	FFR (Prox N)	
Jago et al. (2007)	High-fat Veg (Cullen FFQ)	C (2003)	Boys/Teens (204)	N/A	Res	P	Prox N, Dens	Buff (1 mi, E)	LgGr, OthS, FFR	Ob		0	4
Fruit and Vegetables													
Ollberding et al. (2012)	Fruit and Veg (NCI FV All-Day Scr)	C (2006)	Adult (384)	Min	Res	P	Count	Buff (.5, 1, 1.5, 2, 2.5, 3, 3.5 km, E)	TotS, HlthO, UnHlthO	Ob	TotS, HlthO	0	21
Fuller et al. (2013)	Fruit and Veg (Block FFQ)	C (2006)	Adult (1,266)	Min	Res	P	Prox N	N/A	PrimS	Ob	0	0	1
Christian (2012)	Fruit and Veg (25-item NHANES Scr)	C (2011)	Adult (121)	N/A	Res	P	UH/H Ratio	Activ	RatioO	Ob	0	0	1
Caspi et al. (2012)	Fruit and Veg (6-item Prime Screen)	C (2007–2009)	Adult (743)	Min, Low	Res	P, R	Prox N	Drive, Walk	Super	Ob, SR	Walk	0	2
Boone-Heinonen et al. (2011)	Fruit and Veg (Diet History, DQI)	L (1985–1986; 1987–1988; 1990–1991; 1992–1993; 1995–1996; 2000–2001)	Adult (5,115)	N/A	Res	P	Count, Dens, Prox	Buff (1, 3, 5, 8.05 km, E)	Super, SMGr	Ob	Super (1)	0	15
Gustafson et al. (2011)	Fruit and Veg (Block Rapid Screener)	C (2005)	Older Wom 40–64 (186)	Low	Res	P, R	Travel Time, Avail, Count, Prox N	N/A	PrimS, Super, Conv, OthS.	Ob, SR	0	0	11

(Continued)

TABLE 5.3 (Continued)
Studies Examining Relationships between the Local Food Environment and Fruit and Vegetable Intake

Author, Year	Outcome[a]	Design[b]	Sample		Food Environment Measurement					Objective or Self-Report[j]	Results		
			Age[c]	Minority or Low-Income[d]	Setting[e]	Potential or Realized Access[f]	Food Environment Measures[g]	Geographic Unit[h]	Assessed Outlets[i]		Positive Diet Association[k]	Negative Diet Association[l]	No Significant Association[m]
Beydoun et al. (2011)	Fruit and Veg (24-h)	C (1994–1996)	Child (O: 6,759, L: 3,186, H: 3,573) Teen (O: 1,679, L: 685, H: 994)	Inc strata	Res	P	Price	County	FFP, FVP	Ob	Child – O,H: FFP	0	10
Laska et al. (2010)	Fruit and Veg (24 h)	C	Teen (349)	N/A	Res, Sch	P	Dist, Dens	Dist. to nearest facility, 800 m, 1,600 m, 3,000 m	Groc, Conv, OthS, FFR, OthR	Ob	0	0	19
Sharkey et al. (2010)	Fruit and Veg (BrScr)	C (2006–2007)	Older Adults (582)	N/A	Res	P, R	Prox N; Avail, Variety	CBG	Super, Groc, OthS	Ob, SR	Avail (3), Variety (3)	Prox N (2)	1
Michimi and Wimberly (2010)	Fruit and Veg (BRFSS FFQ)	C (2006)	Adults (Metro: 568,584; Nonmetro: 267,697)	N/A	Res	P	Prox N	County	Super, SuperC	Ob	0	Prox N (2)	4

	Outcome (assessment method)										LgGr	Afford	
Zenk et al. (2009)	Fruit and Veg (Mod Block FFQ)	C (2002–2003)	Adults (919)	Min, Low	Res	P	Count, Prox N, Avail, Variety, Qual, Afford	Buff (0.5 mi., E)	Super, LgGr, OthS, Conv, SMGr, Produce	Ob, SR		Afford	12
Powell et al. (2009)	Fruit and Veg (BrSc)	C (2002)	Y. Adults 18–23 (3,739)	N/A	Res	P	Price	County	FFP, FVP, OthP	Ob	0	Price	6
Caldwell et al. (2009)	Fruit and Veg (YRBS Scr)	C (2002–2005)	Teens, Adults (130)	N/A	Res	P, R	Count, Access, Avail, Variety, Qual, Price	Oth	Groc	Ob, SR	Prod Avail (3), Variety, Qual, Count, Price (3)	0	9
Beydoun et al. (2008)	Fruit and Veg (24 h)	C (1994–1996)	Adults (O: 7,331, L: 1,616, M: 2,713, H: 3,002)	Inc strata	Res	P	Price	County	FFP, FVP	Ob	0	0	8
Zenk et al. (2005b)	Fruit and Veg (BRFSS Scr)	C (2001)	Women (266)	Min	Res	R	Afford, Variety, Qual, CommO	N/A	PrimS, OthS	SR	OthS, Variety, Qual	0	3
Morland et al. (2002)	Fruit and Veg (FFQ)	C (1993–1995)	Adults (W: 8,231, B: 2,392)	Race strata	Res	P	Count	CT	Super, Groc, FullR, FFR	Ob	B: Super	0	7

a Outcome (assessment method): Indices: HEI, Healthy Eating Index; AHEI, Alternate Healthy Eating Index; FPM, Fats and Processed Meat Pattern; WGF, Whole Grains and Fruit Pattern; AMED, Alternate Mediterranean Diet Score. Assessment Methods: BrSc, Brief Screener; FFQ, Food Frequency Questionnaire; 24 h, 24-hour recall; Mod Block FFQ, Modified Block Food Frequency Questionnaire.

TABLE 5.3 (Continued)

Studies Examining Relationships between the Local Food Environment and Fruit and Vegetable Intake

[b] Design (year of data collection): C, cross-sectional; L, longitudinal.

[c] Sample (sample size): Older adult, Ages 50+ only; Adult, Ages 18–49 only or 18+; Teen, Ages 12–17 or middle/high school; Child, Ages <12 or elementary school. Strata-specific samples: O, Overall sample; L, Low-income; M, middle-income; H, high-income; W, non-Hispanic White; B, non-Hispanic Black.

[d] Minority or low income: Min, >50% Black or African-American, Hispanic, American Indian, or Asian; Low, Author identified as low-income or low SES sample (includes WIC only, SNAP/food stamp recipients only, and public housing residents). Income or race strata-specific analyses presented if applicable.

[e] Setting: Res, residential; Sch, school; Work, workplace; Activ, activity space; NA, not applicable.

[f] Potential or realized access: P, potential spatial access measure; R, realized access or utilization measure.

[g] Food environment measure: Count, count (unadjusted) of outlets (including presence or absence); Dens, density of outlets (adjusted for land area, population, street network length); Prox, proximity of outlets (N, street network distance; E, euclidean distance); Ratio, ratio of outlets (e.g., healthy to unhealthy); CommO, other community food environment measure; Avail, food availability, including shelf space; Price, food prices; Variety, food variety or selection; Qual, perceived food quality; Afford = Perceived affordability; ConsO, other consumer food environment measure.

[h] Geographic unit: CBG, census block group; CT, census tract; ZIP, ZIP code; Buff, geographic buffer (buffer size; N, street network distance; E, euclidean distance); Walk, walking distance; Drive, driving distance; Oth, other; NA, not applicable or not specified.

[i] Assessed outlets: Super, supermarket; SupGr, supermarket or grocery store; LgGr, large grocery store; SMGr, small or medium grocery store; Groc, grocery store, all or size not specified; Conv, convenience store; OthS, other food store; TotS, total food stores; FFR, fast-food or limited service restaurant; FullR, full service or sit-down restaurant; OthR, other restaurant (not fast-food or full service or not specified); TotR, total restaurants; HlthO, *healthy* outlets; UnHlthO, *unhealthy* outlets; RatioO, ratio of one outlet type to another; VegS, Store with 5 + vegetables; PrimS, reported primary food store; NA, not applicable or not specified; FM, farmers market; Gas, gas station with food.

[j] Objective or self-report: Ob, objectively measured or observed food environment measure; SR, self-reported or perceived food environment measure.

[k] Positive health outcome (number of findings if >1): Food environment measure has positive association with diet outcome. Codes shown under Food Environment Measure and Assessed Outlets. Subsample specific results presented when applicable—subsample codes under Sample.

[l] Negative health outcome (number of findings if >1): Food environment measure has negative association with diet outcome. Codes shown under Food Environment Measure and Assessed Outlets. Subsample-specific results presented when applicable—subsample codes under Sample.

[m] No significant association: Number of nonsignificant results out of all comparisons tested.

TABLE 5.4

Studies Examining Relationships between Unhealthy Food Exposure (Fast-Food Outlets, Convenience Stores, Fast-Food Price) and Unhealthy Food Purchase or Consumption (Fast Food, High Sugar Food, and Fried Food)

			Sample			Food Environment Measurement					Results		
Author, Year	Outcome[a]	Design[b]	Age[c]	Minority or Low-Income[d]	Setting[e]	Potential or Realized Access[f]	Food Environment Measure[g]	Geographic Unit[h]	Assessed Outlets[i]	Objective or Self-Report[j]	Positive Diet Association[k]	Negative Diet Association[l]	No Significant Association[m]
Jeffrey (2006)	Fast-Food Purchase (BrSc)	C (NR)	Adults (913)	N/A	Res, Work	P	Count	Buff (2 mi., E)	FFR	Ob	FFR	0	1
	Full Service Restaurant Freq (BrSc)								TotR, FullR	—	0	0	4
Jago et al (2007)	Fruit and 100% Juice (FFQ)	C (2003)	Boys (10–14)	N/A	Res	P	Prox, Dens	Buff (1 mi., E)	FFR, LgGr, SMGr	Ob	SMGr	FFR	4
	Low Fat Veg									—	0	0	6
	High-Fat Veg									—	SMGr	FFR	4
Beydoun et al. (2008)	Fast Food (24 h)	C (1994–1996)	Adults (O: 7,331, L: 1,616, M: 2,713, H: 3,002)	Inc strata	Res	P	Price	County	FFP, FVP	Ob	0	L: FVP	15
Beydoun et al. (2008)	Sugar (24 h)	—	—							—	0	0	8
Moore et al. (2009)	Fast Food (FFQ)	C (2000–2002)	Adults (5,633)	Min	Res	R	Prod Avail, Access, Dens	Buff (1 mi.)	FFR	SR, CR	FF (2)	0	1
Boone-Heinonen et al. (2011)	Fast Food (FFQ)	L (1992–1993, 1995–1996, 2000–2001)	Adult (5,115)	N/A	Res	P	Count, Dens, Prox	Buff (1, 3, 5, 8.05 km, E)	FFR	Ob	FFR (4)	FFR (2)	18

(Continued)

TABLE 5.4 (Continued)

Studies Examining Relationships between Unhealthy Food Exposure (Fast-Food Outlets, Convenience Stores, Fast-Food Price) and Unhealthy Food Purchase or Consumption (Fast Food, High Sugar Food, and Fried Food)

Author, Year	Outcome[a]	Design[b]	Age[c]	Minority or Low-Income[d]	Setting[e]	Potential or Realized Access[f]	Food Environment Measure[g]	Geographic Unit[h]	Assessed Outlets[i]	Objective or Self-Report[j]	Positive Diet Association[k]	Negative Diet Association[l]	No Significant Association[m]
							Food Environment Measurement					**Results**	
				Sample									
Beydoun et al. (2011)	Fast Food (24 h)	C (1994–1996)	Child (O: 6,759, L: 3,186, H: 3,573; Teen (O: 1,679, L: 685, H: 994)	Inc strata	Res	P	Price	County	FFP, FVP	Ob	0	Child—O,L: FF; L: FVP; Teen—L: FVP	8
	Sugar (24 h)	—	—	—	—	—	—	—	—	—	0	Child—O,H: FVP; Teen—O,H: FVP	8
Powell et al. (2011)	Sweets (BrScr)	C (1997, 2002–2003)	Teen (O: 1,134, L: 342, H: 792)	Inc strata	Res	P	Dens, Price	Zip, City	Super, Groc, Conv, FFR, FFP, FHP, FullR	Ob	0	0	21
An and Sturm (2012)	Fast Food (CHIS)	C (2005 and 2007)	Child (11,851) Teen (7,574)	N/A	Res, Sch	P	Count	Buff (0.1, 0.5, 1.0, 1.5)	Super, Groc, Smgr, Conv, FFR	Ob	0	Teen: Super, Groc, SMGr Conv, (4)	26
	Soda (CHIS)	—	—	—	—	—	—	—	—	—	0	Child: Super (1) Teen: Groc, Conv, (3)	26

Study	Dietary outcome	Design	Population (N)										
Christian (2012)	High sugar food (CHIS)	—	—	—	—	—	—	—	—	—	0	0	30
Christian (2012)	Fast-Food Purchase (BrScr)	C (2011)	Adult (121)	N/A	Res	P	Dens, Prop	Activ	RatioO	Ob	0	0	2
Christian (2012)	Fried Potatoes (25-item NHANES Scr)	—	—	—	—	—	—	—	—	—	0	0	1
Christian (2012)	Added Sugar (25-item NHANES Scr)	—	—	—	—	—	—	—	—	—	0	0	1
Hattori et al. (2013)	Fast Food (CHIS Scr)	C (2007 and 2009)	Adult (97,678)	NA	Res	P	Count	Buff (0.25, 0.5, 1.0, 1.5, 3 mi., E)	SupGr, Groc, Super, Conv, FullR, FFR	Ob	FFR (3)	0	27
	Fried Potatoes (CHIS)	—	—	—	—	—	—	—	—	—	FFR	0	29
	Sugary Soft Drink (CHIS Scr)	—	—	—	—	—	—	—	—	—	FFR	Super (2)	27
Zenk et al. (2013)	Eating Out (Block FFQ)	C (2008)	Adult >25 (460)	Min, Low	Res	P	Count, Prop	Buff (0.5 mi., E)	LgGr, SupGr, Conv, FFR	Ob	0	0	4
	Snack Food (Block FFQ)	—	—	—	—	—	—	—	—	—	Conv	LgGr	2

(Continued)

TABLE 5.4 (*Continued*)

Studies Examining Relationships between Unhealthy Food Exposure (Fast-Food Outlets, Convenience Stores, Fast-Food Price) and Unhealthy Food Purchase or Consumption (Fast Food, High Sugar Food, and Fried Food)

a Outcome (assessment method): Indices: HEI, Healthy Eating Index; AHEI, Alternate Healthy Eating Index; FPM, Fats and Processed Meat Pattern; WGF, Whole Grains and Fruit Pattern; AMED, Alternate Mediterranean Diet Score. Assessment Methods: BrSc, Brief Screener; FFQ, Food Frequency Questionnaire; 24 h, 24 hour recall; Mod Block FFQ, Modified Block Food Frequency Questionnaire.

b Design (year of data collection): C, cross-sectional; L, longitudinal.

c Sample (sample size): Older adult, Ages 50+ only; Adult, Ages 18–49 only or 18+; Teen, Ages 12–17 or middle/high school; Child, Ages <12 or elementary school. Strata-specific samples: O, Overall sample; L, Low-income; M, middle-income; H, high-income; W, non-Hispanic White; B, non-Hispanic Black.

d Minority or low income: Min, >50% Black or African–American, Hispanic, American Indian, or Asian; Low, Author identified as low-income or low SES sample (includes WIC only, SNAP/food stamp recipients only, and public housing residents). Income or race strata-specific analyses presented if applicable.

e Setting: Res, residential; Sch, school; Work, workplace; Activ, activity space; NA, not applicable.

f Potential or realized access: P, potential spatial access measure; R, realized access or utilization measure.

g Food environment measure: Count, count (unadjusted) of outlets (including presence or absence); Dens, density of outlets (adjusted for land area, population, street network length); Prox, proximity of outlets (N, street network distance; E, euclidean distance); Ratio, ratio of outlets (e.g., healthy to unhealthy); CommO, other community food environment measure; Avail, food availability, including shelf space; Price, food prices; Variety, food variety or selection; Qual, perceived food quality; Afford = Perceived affordability; ConsO, other consumer food environment measure.

h Geographic unit: CBG, census block group; CT, census tract; ZIP, ZIP code; Buff, geographic buffer (buffer size; N, street network distance; E, euclidean distance); Walk, walking distance; Drive, driving distance; Oth, other; NA, not applicable or not specified.

i Assessed outlets: Super, supermarket; SupGr, supermarket or grocery store; LgGr, large grocery store; SMGr, small or medium grocery store; Groc, grocery store, all or size not specified; Conv, convenience store; OthS, other food store; TotS, total food stores; FFR, fast-food or limited service restaurant; FullR, full service or sit-down restaurant; OthR, other restaurant (not fast-food or full service or not specified); TotR, total restaurants; HlthO, *healthy* outlets; UnHlthO, *unhealthy* outlets; RatioO, ratio of one outlet type to another; VegS, Store with 5 + vegetables; PrimS, reported primary food store; NA, not applicable or not specified; FM, farmers market; Gas, gas station with food.

j Objective or self-report: Ob, objectively measured or observed food environment measure; SR, self-reported or perceived food environment measure.

k Positive health outcome (number of findings if >1): Food environment measure has positive association with diet outcome. Codes shown under Food Environment Measure and Assessed Outlets. Subsample specific results presented when applicable—subsample codes under Sample.

l Negative health outcome (number of findings if >1): Food environment measure has negative association with diet outcome. Codes shown under Food Environment Measure and Assessed Outlets. Subsample-specific results presented when applicable—subsample codes under Sample.

m No significant association: Number of nonsignificant results out of all comparisons tested.

Hattori et al 2013). Four other studies found at least one relationship between the local food environment and fruit intake (Rose and Richards 2004; Jago et al. 2007; Sharkey et al. 2010; Gustafson et al. 2013). Both Sharkey et al. (2010) and Rose and Richards (2004) found an inverse association between distance and access to a supermarket and fruit intake—meaning that as distance to the nearest supermarket increased, fruit intake decreased. Sharkey et al. (2010) looked at an older, rural population and assessed both distance to supermarket and variety of foods offered in a supermarket and differences in fruit intake as assessed by a brief screener. Rose used a low-income population that received food stamps to look at various measures of access, which was determined by car availability, distance, and travel time to preferred supermarket. Although these two populations came from rural and urban areas, both found that an increased distance to supermarkets resulted in lower intake of both fruits and vegetables in the study of Sharkey and fruit but not vegetables in that of Rose. Using an FFQ to assess diet and a 1-mile buffer around the study population's home, Jago et al. (2007) found that living further away from small food stores, such as convenience and drug stores, resulted in an unexpected direction of higher intakes of fruit and juice in a small sample of teen boys. Gustafson et al. (2013) also found a small, unexpected association of increased fruit intake of a small sample of adults in Kentucky living near a convenience store. Although only half of the studies found an association between the local food environment and fruit intake, those that did found associations in both directions, casts doubt on our understanding of the true relationship between the local food environment and fruit intake.

Nine studies assessed vegetable intake. Again, many of the studies conducted multiple statistical tests using several operational definitions of food environment exposure and/or several diet outcomes. Two studies found no significant relationship between the local food environment measures and vegetable intake (Rose and Richards 2004; Jago et al. 2007); however, six studies found at least one association (Bodor et al. 2008; Sharkey et al. 2010; Izumi et al. 2011; An and Sturm 2012; Gustafson et al. 2013; Hattori et al. 2013). As the authors theorized, being closer to a supermarket, grocery store, or market with five or more vegetables was associated with increased vegetable intake in a small sample of Supplemental Nutrition Assistance Program (SNAP) participants (Gustafson et al. 2013) and low-income adults (Izumi et al. 2011) and a smaller, but significant association was seen in a large sample of teens (Powell and Han 2011). Vegetable availability, identified by in-store assessments, was positively associated with vegetable intake in a rural population of older adults (Sharkey et al. 2010), as well as in a small sample of low-income adults (Bodor et al. 2008). Studies looking at the local food environment and vegetable intake are showing small but significant associations in the expected direction, which may indicate a true relationship.

Fifteen studies combined fruit and vegetable consumption as an outcome. Five studies used a nationally representative dataset or based the analysis on a large population study and found no associations between supermarkets and fruit and vegetable intake (Michimi and Wimberly 2010; Powell and Han 2011; An and Sturm 2012; Gustafson et al. 2013; Hattori et al. 2013). Four studies that used data from a smaller geographic location also found no association between the food environment and fruit and vegetable intake (Beydoun et al. 2008; Gustafson et al. 2011; Christian 2012; Fuller et al.

2013). Three studies found that stores with more variety or availability of fruits and vegetables were positively associated with their intake (Zenk et al. 2005b; Caldwell et al. 2009; Sharkey et al. 2010).

Three studies found that proximity to a supermarket or large grocery store was positively associated, at varying degrees of magnitude, with fruit and vegetable intake (Morland et al. 2002; Zenk et al. 2009; Boone-Heinonen et al. 2011). In one of the few longitudinal studies looking at food environment and diet in the United States, few strong associations were seen. Boone-Heinonen and colleagues used data collected at six different points over 15 years through the Coronary Artery Risk Development in Young Adults (CARDIA) study, a cohort of U.S. young adults ($n = 5115$, 18–30 years at baseline) from four different cities. Diet was collected using a quantitative diet history to capture fast-food consumption, diet quality, and meeting fruit and vegetable recommendations. Availability of fast-food chains, supermarkets, or grocery stores was assessed using counts per population within 1 km, 1–2.9 km, 3–4.9 km, and 5–8 km of respondents' homes. Models were sex-stratified, controlled for individual socio-demographics and neighborhood poverty, and tested for interaction by individual-level income. They found that neighborhood supermarket and grocery store availability were generally unrelated to diet quality and meeting fruit and vegetable recommendations with a small association seen in men (Boone-Heinonen et al. 2011). Efforts should be made to fund and carry out more longitudinal studies to confirm or refute this lack of relationship.

Table 5.4 presents studies that examine relationships between unhealthy food exposure and unhealthy food purchase or consumption. Fast food has become a focus of public health nutrition due to its poor nutritional content and ubiquity in the United States. Americans now work more hours and fast-food restaurants are more pervasive than in past decades. Not surprisingly, food consumption away from home is on the rise. Between 1970 and 2006 foods purchased and eaten away from home have increased from 26.1% to 41.7% (McGuire et al. 2011). Specifically, 37.4% of sales of meals and snacks outside of the home are at limited service eating establishments like fast-food restaurants. Fast food accounts for 15% of daily energy intake, and in children the percent of energy consumed at these locations now surpasses the amount consumed in schools (Poti and Popkin 2011). This trend is alarming due to the associations with fast-food consumption and diet quality (Bowman et al. 2004; Bowman and Vinyard 2004; Sebastian et al. 2009), diet-mediated outcomes such as BMI (Duffey et al. 2007; Duffey et al. 2009; French et al. 2000), and poor metabolic outcomes such as insulin resistance (Duffey et al. 2009) and metabolic syndrome in adults (Pereira et al. 2005).

Although fewer studies have focused on fast-food intake as a diet outcome in food environment research, it remains an important focus of attention as it can act as a proxy for poorer dietary intake. Four cross-sectional studies and one longitudinal study examined the relationship between the fast-food outlet availability and fast-food purchasing or consumption. Three found evidence that greater fast-food availability is associated with greater fast-food consumption, and two studies found mixed or null results. Although most studies created GIS measures of food outlet availability from commercial store lists (i.e., InfoUSA or Dunn & Bradstreet), a few studies also examined alternate measures of food exposure, including fast-food price and perception of fast-food availability. As mentioned early, Boone-Heinonen et al. (2011) conducted one of the most methodologically rigorous studies relating the retail food environment with food consumption using data from the longitudinal CARDIA study. Although results were mixed, their findings suggest that the magnitude and direction of the relationship between the retail food environment and fast-food consumption may vary by income level and gender. Although a higher number of fast-food outlets close to respondents' homes (<1 km compared with 1–2.99 km) predicted greater fast-food consumption among low-income men, among women and men in higher income groups, over the 15 years the associations between fast-food exposure and fast-food consumption were not significant or were counterintuitive. Hattori et al. (2013) conducted another notable recent study using data from 97,678 respondents of the CHIS. They found that the number of fast-food restaurants within a 3-mile buffer of participant's homes was positively associated with increased intake of fast food along with other foods of low nutritional quality, such as sugar-sweetened soft drinks and fried potatoes (2013). However, in a youth sample of the CHIS, An and Sturm (2012) found no significant robust association in either direction between the geographic count of food outlets by type around youths' home or school and fast-food consumption.

One study by Moore et al. (2009), compared results obtained from GIS measures of fast-food exposure with subjective measures of fast-food availability. Perception-based measures were obtained from participant self-reported fast-food availability and informant-reported fast-food availability by neighbors. In fully adjusted models, greater perceived fast-food access as measured by self-report or informant report, was associated with greater odds of consuming fast food near home. In contrast, the *objective* GIS measure of fast-food outlet density near home was not associated with fast-food consumption. The authors also found that for every standard deviation increase in fast-food exposure, the odds of consuming fast food near home increased 11%–61% and the odds of a healthy diet decreased 3%–17%, depending on the model (2009).

The contrasting diet association with objective versus subjective measures of the food environment raises a number of questions. First, the different findings may indicate that our perception of the food environment, rather than the actual food landscape itself, matters for dietary behavior change. This conclusion, if true, has ramifications for community-level diet interventions that alter the built environment. The conflicting results obtained using subjective measures compared to GIS measures also calls into question the suitability of GIS measures for capturing the construct of healthy or unhealthy food availability. A number of studies have demonstrated that commercial databases (from which most GIS food availability measures are computed) are error-prone (Hoehner and Schootman 2010; Liese et al. 2010; Powell et al. 2011; Auchincloss et al. 2012). Store records may be omitted, miscategorized, or obsolete, resulting in considerable measurement error and often consequently, a bias toward null findings. Moreover, even in the unlikely scenario that the commercial databases on which studies rely were accurate, we must still consider whether these simple density, count, and proximity measures actually capture the multidimensional and complex constructs attributed to them, such as food accessibility and food availability. These constructs cannot be adequately measured by any one metric. Thus, future studies can improve on existing research by augmenting GIS metrics with other measures of access and availability, including in-store audits of food offerings, prices, and hours and subjective informant reports. A strong association between the food environment and a diet outcome should be robust to multiple metrics of the same overall exposure.

A very limited number of studies have examined the association between food prices (using a regional food price index) and fast-food consumption. The public health literature on the impact of food prices on fast-food consumption is in a nascent stage. No longitudinal studies have been conducted to date and results from the two existing cross-sectional studies are mixed. Both studies use data from the Continuing Survey of Food Intakes by Individuals (CSFII), a national diet survey with a youth supplement. Beydoun et al. (2011) found that higher average metropolitan fast-food price was associated with lower fast-food consumption among children; however, the result was not replicated in adolescents. An earlier 2008 study examining data from the adult respondents of the CSFII found no relationship between fast-food price and fast-food consumption.

In addition to fast-food consumption, fast-food outlet availability has been theorized to influence consumption of other food items—either because the food item is seen as a complement (i.e., soda, high-fat vegetables) or as a substitute (i.e., fruit and low-fat vegetables). Three out of five studies found no evidence that fast-food outlet availability affected the consumption of other food items. In the Hattori et al. (2013) study referenced above, fast-food outlet density was positively associated with fried potato consumption and soda consumption. Similarly, in a sample of Boy Scouts (10–14 years) from Houston, Texas, Jago et al. (2007), found that greater residential distance to the nearest fast-food restaurant predicted lower fruit and juice intake and lower high-fat vegetable intake. However, additional studies found no association between fast-food outlet availability and sweets (Powell and Han 2011); soda or high-sugar food (An and Sturm 2012); or snack foods (Zenk et al. 2013). The study by Zenk et al. (2013) was unique in that it assessed the interaction between stress and the food environment hypothesizing that indicators of high stress in a neighborhood would lead to greater consumption of high sugar and fat foods. They found a significant, positive direct association between snack food intake and convenience store availability, and snack food intake was negatively associated with large grocery store availability; however, chronic stress and major life events were generally not associated with dietary behavior. Latinos were less likely to eat out at high levels of major life events than African-Americans. Stress–neighborhood food environment interactions were not statistically significant. Important questions remain regarding the role of the neighborhood food environment in the stress–diet relationship that warrants further investigation (Zenk et al. 2013).

Additional studies have looked at specific food groups such as whole grains, meats, and dairy (Gustafson et al. 2013; Hattori et al. 2013; An and Sturm 2012; Christian 2012; Powell and Han 2011; Beydoun et al. 2008, 2011), diet quality (Laraia et al. 2004; Beydoun et al. 2008, 2011; Franco et al. 2009; Moore et al. 2008, 2009; Osypuk et al. 2009; Boone-Heinonen et al. 2011; Gustafson et al. 2013), or specific nutrients such as fat, cholesterol, sodium, calcium, or fiber (Beydoun et al. 2008, 2011). Studies that have used a diet quality index to assess the relationship between the local food environment and overall diet quality find mixed results as well. Franco et al. (2009) found no association between measures of the food environment and a healthy and an unhealthy diet pattern score. Carroll-Scott et al. (2013) found that the number of fast-food restaurants within a census tract were associated with unhealthy eating scores; however, living within 0.5 mile of a supermarket, while associated with lower BMI, was not associated with a healthy eating score (after controlling for a number of individual and neighborhood characteristics). Conversely, several studies found that living within close proximity of a supermarket was associated with a better diet quality score. Moore et al. (2008) found that participants with no supermarkets within a mile of their homes scored lower on the Alternative Healthy Eating Index than those with the most stores, after controlling for a number of individual characteristics. In a study in North Carolina, Laraia et al. (2004) found that pregnant women living greater than 4 miles from the nearest supermarket were at greater than twice the odds of falling into the lowest tertile of a comprehensive diet quality index that measured foods and nutrients needed for pregnancy compared to women who lived 2 miles or less to the nearest supermarket, after controlling for a number of socioeconomic and demographic variables as well as distance to the closest grocery store and convenience store.

A number of the research studies reviewed use large commercial databases to characterize the proximity and/or density of food venues and there are some large research efforts that assess the influence of food price on purchase and consumption patterns. However, these large-scale studies often lack detailed information on availability and quality of foods within the store. Because the food environment is multidimensional the assessment of it should strive to take into account the factors of proximity, density, as well as food availability, cost and quality (Rose et al. 2010). Local efforts can take advantage of systematically assessing the food environment. A burgeoning area of research focused on assessing healthy food availability, quality, and cost in small stores in low-income areas uses audit tools such as the Nutrition Environment Measurement System (Honeycutt et al. 2010) and the Communities of Excellence in California (Ghirardelli et al. 2010). These audit tools can be used in combination with GIS measures and shopping behaviors (Christian 2012). Researchers have also used intercept interviews with adults and children shopping in small stores in low-income areas. These studies have confirmed a lack of healthful and nutritious foods in small stores (Zenk, et al. 2005a; Gittelsohn and Sharma 2009; Laska et al. 2010). Improving food offerings in small ethnic or convenience stores was related to perceived and actual increases in sales of those foods (Song et al. 2009; Ayala 2013). Many of these studies use food store audit tools to collect data on availability, quality, diversity, and price of common foods that may be available in a small food store that can better inform interventions, programs, and policies.

ASSOCIATION BETWEEN DIET AND FOOD PRICES AND QUALITY

Food Prices

Current research on food prices has used price indices or price averages across large-scale geographic areas such as counties or states as exposure. There have been no studies looking at small-scale geographic variation in price and its association with small-scale variation in diet. Association between food prices and diet is inconsistent and not uncommonly the association is in the unexpected direction.

Seven studies tested the association between food prices and diet. Prices were defined as regional price indices for specific foods or the general food category or store-specific prices for specific foods were obtained from in-store audits. All studies examined the impact of prices on fruit and vegetable consumption, a few studies also examined alternate dietary outcomes including, fast-food consumption, summary diet indices, energy intake, and intake of specific nutrients. Four studies found no significant association between food price and fruit and vegetable consumption after adjustment for covariates (Beydoun et al. 2008, 2011; Powell and Han 2011). Powell et al. (2009) analyzed data from the nationally representative National Longitudinal Study of Youth and found that for each $1 increase in the regional price index for fruits and vegetables there was an associated 32% reduction in weekly consumption of fruits and vegetables. In contrast, Zenk et al. (2009) found that residents in three Detroit communities with stores present in upper quartile of affordability (i.e., had lower priced produce) had lower fruit and vegetable consumption compared to residents with stores not in upper quartile of affordability ($p = 0.052$). In addition, Caldwell et al. (2009) found that among participants of regional Colorado Healthy People 2010 Initiative programs to encourage physical activity or prevent diabetes, residents of neighborhoods with a greater minimum price for a six-item produce basket reported a greater increase in fruit and vegetable increase from program start to end.

In addition to studies that measured food prices, the perception of the cost of produce was studied. Two studies investigated the association between perceived affordability of fruit or produce and diet. However, perceived measures are subject to same source bias. Zenk et al. (2005b) found no significant association between perceived affordability of fresh produce at the store where women shopped and fruit and vegetable consumption.

Quality of Produce

Three studies investigated the association between produce quality/freshness and produce consumption (Zenk et al. 2005b, 2009; Caldwell et al. 2009). Two studies found a positive association between produce quality and produce consumption. Zenk et al. (2005b) found that respondents who reported greater satisfaction with the produce at their primary food store also reported greater fruit and vegetable consumption. Caldwell et al. (2009) audited two randomly selected neighborhood grocery stores in 24 communities in Colorado. They found that residents of communities with a greater proportion of produce that was fresh (not overripe or wilted) experienced a greater increase in fruit and vegetable intake over the period of a community health intervention.

SCHOOL ENVIRONMENT

The influence of the local food environment on children's dietary intake, eating patterns, and health cannot be assessed in the absence of the intervention and evaluation research being conducted on the school food environment. The concern over the rising rates of childhood obesity has been a main impetus for turning attention to the school food environment and its influence on diet. In 2007–08, the prevalence of obesity in children aged 6–11 had increased to five times what it was in 1971–74 (20% vs. 4%), (Fox et al. 2009). The majority of U.S. children are enrolled in public or private schools, with no other institution having as continuous and intensive contact. This leaves schools in a unique position to influence one aspect of children's food environment. School age children spend 50% or more of their day in sedentary activity (Matthews et al. 2008). Children spend on average 7 hours per weekday in school; therefore, the school setting has been the target of numerous studies aimed at understanding the role of school's internal environment on diet intake. Before the 1990s, studies looking at the school food environment largely focused on National School Lunch Program (NSLP) participation rates and found that elementary students are more likely than high school students to use the program, males more likely than females and students in schools with a closed campus policy being more likely to consume NSLP meals. During this time, the primary concern was to make sure that children from low-income households had access to this federal program. As the program expanded and participation rates increased, evaluation research focused on the quality of the NSLP in the context of the growing rate of obesity. In addition, various interventions and policies have targeted the school environment in hopes of decelerating the childhood obesity trend through improved diet. This area of research has now extended to the local food environment near schools in an effort to identify the influence of small stores and fast-food restaurants on children's dietary intake. Identifying and quantifying how the local food environment around schools may influence children is important because this information can inform school policies such as open campus policies in high school; municipal policies such as local zoning laws, and street vending regulation; and interventions such as farmer's markets on school grounds.

Researchers cite two main avenues through which schools influence diet, the first of which is the federally supported NSLP and School Breakfast program (SBP), which provides subsidized meals to children in school; and the second being *competitive foods*. Competitive foods are foods sold, served, or given to students in schools but so named because they are sold in competition to NSLP and SBP meals (e.g., food sold a la carte in the cafeteria, or food and beverages in vending machines, among other venues). Research has shown that competitive foods are low in nutritional quality and widely available to students. In addition, despite being required to meet dietary guidelines, meals provided in the NSLP are also generally low in nutritional value, making these two areas large targets of research and intervention with aims of exploring how the NSLP and competitive foods impact student diet intake. Students consuming school meals through the NLSP do tend to have healthier intakes of important micronutrients like vitamin A, vitamin B-12, riboflavin, calcium, phosphorus, potassium, and zinc. When compared to nonparticipants, lunches consumed by NLSP participants had higher dietary quality and were more nutrient-dense; however, NSLP participation was associated with increased prevalence of excessive sodium intakes among high school students (Clark and Fox 2009). However, offerings and consumption of healthier foods, such as fruits and vegetables, is low among all school-age children and efforts have been made through various programs and interventions to reverse this trend. Yet, studies that have examined the extent to which introducing more opportunities to consume healthier foods such as fruits and vegetables in school would result in better diets have found mixed results (Nagata et al. 2012; Davis et al. 2009; Coyle et al. 2009; Terry-McElrath et al. 2009). Studies have also identified that the SBP is reaching targeted levels; however, one study found that while 50% of students eat breakfast, 25% eat two or more breakfast meals (e.g., at home, on the way to school, and at school) and 25% do not eat any breakfast during the day, showing that overconsumption and underconsumption may still need to be addressed. When it comes to competitive foods, a number of studies have shown an association between availability and poor diet intake. Those with more opportunities to consume competitive foods were found to consume more fat and saturated fat and fewer fruits and vegetables than those with limited accessibility (Wordell et al. 2012). Although interventions to improve the school environment have been met with both success and failure, a new focus is on the greater food environment around schools.

In addition to the numerous intervention studies to improve dietary intake that occur in schools, recent efforts to intervene on what food is available to children include policies both inside and immediately outside of the school. In 2003, California passed the Childhood Obesity Prevention Act, prohibiting the sale of unhealthy beverages from vending machines or sources at all times for elementary school-age children and during the school day for middle school students. They followed up this Act in 2007 with Senate Bills 12 and 965, banning the sale of soda and sugar-sweetened beverages in all public schools and setting nutrition standards for competitive foods. Meanwhile, in 2004, the U.S. Congress required all schools participating in the NSLP to develop school wellness policies with goals for physical activity, nutrition education, and nutrition guidelines for all foods available on campus; however, the strength of these policies has been found to vary greatly. Six years later, in 2010, the Healthy Hunger Free Kids Act was passed, which included increasing funding to the NSLP to provide healthier meals and more funding for farm to school programs. The legislation also authorized the USDA to set nutrition standards for all foods sold in schools, including competitive foods. In February of 2013, the USDA released the proposed nutritional rules for competitive foods, which would require these foods and beverages to meet the dietary guidelines for Americans. It is still undetermined at this time when these changes will go into effect.

EXTERNAL SCHOOL ENVIRONMENT

Efforts within schools to improve the dietary intake of adolescents have shown mixed results, but certain policies and school attributes have been successful in improving diet. Although attention has appropriately focused on the internal school food environment, it is not the only setting where adolescents acquire food during the school day. Current research is focused on examining what influence, if any, the food environment surrounding schools has on the health and diet of attending adolescents. Arguably, this external environment has the potential to negate any efforts within schools working to improve health and diet, especially if the external offerings are in contrast.

The eating patterns of adolescents have changed, a trend in line with the consumption patterns of the entire U.S. population. Relying increasingly on foods away from home and school, 35% of adolescents' total daily calories are consumed outside the home with 19% coming from fast-food restaurants and 5% from foods purchased at a store and consumed outside the home (Guthrie et al. 2002; Nielsen et al. 2002). On a typical day, 39% of adolescents will consume foods from a fast-food establishment (Bowman et al. 2004). More research is now needed to determine whether or not these consumption patterns are influenced by what adolescents encounter around the place where they spend a large part of their day—primary and secondary schools.

According to Sturm (2008), about one-third of high schools have an open campus policy that allows students to leave the school during their lunch break. With an open campus policy, the probability that students will get lunch from a convenience store or fast-food restaurant triples (Neumark-Sztainer et al. 2005). In addition, 68% of adolescents take public transportation, walk, bike, or ride in a public vehicle to and from school (rather than ride a school bus). These modes of transport to school present opportunities to access nearby retail food outlets that differ from in-school food opportunities. Surrounding retail food outlets often offer a wider range of snack foods and sugar-sweetened beverages, have extended hours, and expose students to advertising on their way to and from school.

There is concern that these retail food outlets disproportionately cluster around schools. Zenk et al. (2008) assessed the retail food outlet availability within walking distance (0.5 mile) of U.S. schools and in the 20 most populous cities. The authors found that public secondary schools nationwide have at least 37% fast-food restaurants and 33% convenience stores within walking distance. Around the most populous cities, 68% had one or more fast-food restaurant and 56% had one or more convenience stores. One Chicago study found that 78% of all kindergarten, primary, and secondary schools had at least one fast-food restaurant within 800 m. Areas within 1.5 km of the schools studied had three to four times as many fast-food restaurants than would be expected if they were evenly distributed through the city (Austin et al. 2005). A study of four communities in the Atlanta region by Frank et al. (2007) found that fast-food restaurants were closer to middle schools than sit-down restaurants and that convenience stores were closer than grocery stores in three of the four communities. Additional studies show similar relationships with fast-food restaurants clustering near schools (Seliske et al. 2009). Whether this clustering is associated with actual health and diet outcomes in children and adolescents is not well understood.

Studies have examined the relationship between neighborhood environments and diet and external school environments and weight with mixed results. In eighth and tenth graders, Powell et al. (2007) found higher BMI and overweight was associated with convenience store access at the zip code level (though a second article found that the price of fast food was more important than location for determining eating and BMI). Borradaile et al. (2009) found among a sample of 833 students in grades 4 through 6 attending one of 10 elementary schools in Philadelphia, children spent an average of $1.07 and purchased two items averaging 356 calories: usually a sugar-sweetened beverage and a snack. The study was conducted using intercept interviews with children before and after school. This study suggests that among the children frequenting small food stores before and after school, they consume a large number of calories from high-energy-dense foods (Borradaile et al. 2009). A study by Davis and Carpenter (2009b) looked at the presence of fast-food outlets near schools and food consumption using data on 500,000 youth collected from the California Health Kids Survey. Food intake outcomes come from questions that asked about the student's reported intake of vegetables, fruit, juice, soda, and fried potatoes. Restaurants were located using Microsoft Streets and Trips database with latitude and longitude coordinates and a list of restaurant brands classified as "top limited-service restaurants" by Technomic. All restaurants within half a mile of California middle and high schools were identified. This is a distance one could walk in 10 minutes and is commonly used in other research. Over half of the sample attended schools within half a mile of a fast-food restaurant. For youths attending schools near a fast-food restaurant, they were less likely to report having consumed vegetables or juice and more likely to have consumed soda the previous day than did students who went to schools further from fast food. No difference was found in fried potato consumption. Although Davis and Carpenter found some association between food outlet proximity to school and diet, corresponding results were not seen in a study by An and Sturm (2012) on a similar population. Data from the 2005 and 2007 waves of the CHIS of children and adolescents was used that asked about one day of fast-food consumption. They compared consumption of a variety of foods, such as fruits, vegetables, 100% juice, milk, sweetened beverages, high-sugar foods, as well as fast-food consumption, with the number of food outlets including fast food, convenience stores, and small-, medium-, and large-size grocery stores within 0.1, 0.5, 1.0, and 1.5 miles from both home and schools. They found no evidence to support the theory that the food environment around schools or proximity to supermarkets, fast food, or convenience stores within walking distance of schools is related to diet intake in youth in California. A study in Minnesota found that although there was a median number of four fast-food restaurants within a mile from the schools studied, no relationship was found with these food outlets and diet (Forsyth et al. 2012). This study was also one of the few that looked at a school's open campus policy to see if the ability to go outside of school during the lunch hour was associated with diet. No relationship was seen in this study, but associations have previously been reported (Neumark-Sztainer et al. 2005).

The external school food environment differs according to grade and location of school. While at least one-third of all secondary schools nationwide and upward of two-thirds of secondary schools in the 20 most populous cities are within walking distance to fast-food or convenience stores, there is still no clear answer as to whether the presence of these food stores influences diet. Existing research on this topic carries limitations. First, measures of exposure differ with some assessing the presence or absence of just one type of food outlet, such as fast-food restaurants, whereas others use an expanded measure that includes all types of markets, restaurants, and convenience stores. Further, the quality of business listings used to classify food outlets varies. Powell advises caution when using databases like InfoUSA, finding only fair agreement between commercial data and actual field observations for supermarkets, grocery stores, convenience stores, and full-service markets and finding poor agreement for fast-food restaurants. It may also be inadequate to simply count the presence or absence of a food outlet as a predictor of diet without collecting more descriptive measures (e.g., store inventories or food quality). Unfortunately, gathering such data is very costly and time consuming and may never exist on a national scale. Measurements of dietary outcomes also differ across studies and few, if any, relied on multiple 24-hour diet recalls, which are considered the gold standard for collecting dietary intake information.

SUMMARY AND CONCLUSIONS

This chapter reviewed the measurement issues pertaining to the local food environment and dietary intake, summarized the state of the literature, and focused on local efforts that are trying to understand how best to measure both the local food environment and dietary intake or eating behaviors. Measuring the local food environment and dietary intake are both complex and multifaceted endeavors because there are a number of potential attributes that need to be measured, both are dynamic and ever changing, and both appear to be influenced by individuals' preferences, socioeconomic status, and demographic characteristics including age, sex, and race/ethnicity. Because of these complexities, answering the question "To what extent does the local food environment influence (i.e., cause) the quality of an individual's dietary intake?" is extremely challenging.

The local food environment in the articles reviewed within this chapter was mostly characterized using GIS that measured proximity/distance to the nearest food venue type and the density of food venue type. This was especially true of large-scale studies that covered a large geographic area; for the most part, these studies found no association between the local food environment and diet (Hattori et al. 2013; An and Sturm 2012; Boone-Heinonen et al. 2011; Franco et al. 2009). Small-scale studies benefited from using commercial data sources to characterize the local food environment, as well as to use food store audit tools and collect individual-level information on perceptions of the local environment and shopping behaviors (Gustafson et al. 2013; Zenk et al. 2013). These studies suggest that where people choose to shop is correlated with dietary intake.

Collecting dietary information and creating appropriate measures of the diet are inherently challenging. What seems to be essential is to capture some measure of overall diet quality and to know to what extent an individual is eating more nutritious and healthful foods compared to energy-dense, processed foods of low nutrient value.

Many of the studies reviewed use fruit and vegetable intake to simplify the data collection process. Although selecting fruit and vegetable intake is appropriate given the extensive literature linking these nutrient-dense foods to a number of nutrient deficiency and chronic diseases, we cannot know if an association between the food environment and fruit and vegetable intake is important for only fruit and vegetable intake or if fruit and vegetable intake is a proxy for some other aspect of the diet.

The research on food environment largely using distance and density of various types of food venues near a person's home and their dietary intake and eating pattern has largely been conducted using cross-sectional study designs. This means that the food environment was observed and data was collected on it at the same time that dietary intake was observed and collected. The majority of the studies, especially the large, representative samples, finds no association once they account for age, sex, income, education, and race/ethnicity. So it appears that these individual attributes are highly correlated with dietary intake and explain the relationship between the local food environment and diet. If the question to answer is "Does the local food environment causes certain types of dietary intake and eating patterns?", these studies do not support a causal relationship. The one study that used a longitudinal study design that started with a large sample of young adults and followed them over 15 years also did not find that the food environment was associated with dietary intake. However, as mentioned earlier, the measurement of various food environment exposures is prone to inaccuracies for a number of reasons, chief among them is the overreliance on commercial vendor databases that were not created for epidemiologic research purposes. Errors in the measurement of food environment exposures such as the miscategorization of store types, omitted and fabricated store locations, and delayed assessment of store closings and new store openings can all bias research results. The use of in-store audits and *groundtruthing* or field verification of store type and location can help improve the accuracy of commonly used food environment measures but such methods are more labor intensive and can be cost prohibitive if the study population is dispersed over a large region (Auchincloss et al. 2012).

However, if the research question is a social justice and food inequity question, then the focus is different. If we see disparate patterns of the price, quality, and type of food that is available to individuals based on their socioeconomic status (SES) or race/ethnicity quantifying these differences can inform policy and public health programs. If ethnic or low-SES communities have restricted access to the foods that are highlighted in federal food and nutrition policy, such as the DGA, then we must make strides to level the playing fields.

REFERENCES

Adam, T. C., and E. S. Epel. 2007. Stress, eating and the reward system. *Physiol Behav* 91 (4):449–58.
Alwan, A. and World Health Organization. 2011. *Global Status Report on Noncommunicable Diseases 2010*. Genevea, Switzerland: World Health Organization.
Alwan, A., D. R. MacLean, L. M. Riley, E. T. d'Espaignet, C. D. Mathers, G. A. Stevens, and D. Bettcher. 2010. Monitoring and surveillance of chronic non-communicable diseases: Progress and capacity in high-burden countries. *Lancet* 376 (9755):1861–8.

An, R., and R. Sturm. 2012. School and residential neighborhood food environment and diet among California youth. *Am J Prev Med* 42 (2):129–35.

Apovian, C. M., M. C. Murphy, D. Cullum-Dugan, P. H. Lin, K. M. Gilbert, G. Coffman, M. Jenkins, P. Bakun, K. L. Tucker, and T. J. Moore. 2010. Validation of a web-based dietary questionnaire designed for the DASH (dietary approaches to stop hypertension) diet: The DASH online questionnaire. Public Health Nutr 13 (5):615–22.Auchincloss, A, K. Moore, L. Moore, A. Diez Roux. 2012. Improving retrospective characterization of the food environment for a large region in the United States during a historic time period. *Health Place* 18:1341–7.

Austin, S. B., S. J. Melly, B. N. Sanchez, A. Patel, S. Buka, and S. L. Gortmaker. 2005. Clustering of fast-food restaurants around schools: A novel application of spatial statistics to the study of food environments. *Am J Public Health* 95 (9):1575–81.

Ayala, G.X., B. Baquero, B. A. Laraia, M. Ji, and L. Linnan. 2013. Efficacy of a store-based environmental change intervention compared with a delayed treatment control condition on store customers' intake of fruits and vegetables.

Beydoun, M. A., L. M. Powell, and Y. Wang. 2008. The association of fast food, fruit and vegetable prices with dietary intakes among US adults: Is there modification by family income? *Soc Sci Med* 66 (11):2218–29.

Beydoun, M. A., L. M. Powell, X. Chen, and Y. Wang. 2011. Food prices are associated with dietary quality, fast food consumption, and body mass index among U.S. children and adolescents. *J Nutr* 141 (2):304–11.

Blanck, H. M., C. Gillespie, J. E. Kimmons, J. E. Seymour, and M. K. Serdula. 2008. Trends in fruit and vegetable consumption among U.S. men and women, 1994–2005. *Prev Chronic Dis* 5 (2):A35.

Block, G., C. Gillespie, E. H. Rosenbaum, and C. Jenson. 2000. A rapid food screener to assess fat and fruit and vegetable intake. Am J Prev Med 18 (4):284–8.

Bodor, J. N., D. Rose, T. A. Farley, C. Swalm, and S. K. Scott. 2008. Neighbourhood fruit and vegetable availability and consumption: The role of small food stores in an urban environment. *Public Health Nutr* 11 (4):413–20.

Boone-Heinonen, J., P. Gordon-Larsen, C. I. Kiefe, J. M. Shikany, C. E. Lewis, and B. M. Popkin. 2011. Fast food restaurants and food stores: Longitudinal associations with diet in young to middle-aged adults: The CARDIA study. *Arch Intern Med* 171 (13):1162–70.

Borradaile, K. E., S. Sherman, S. S. Vander Veur, T. McCoy, B. Sandoval, J. Nachmani, A. Karpyn, and G. D. Foster. 2009. Snacking in children: The role of urban corner stores. *Pediatrics* 124 (5):1293–8.

Bowman, S. A. and B. T. Vinyard. 2004. Fast food consumption of U.S. adults: Impact on energy and nutrient intakes and overweight status. *J Am Coll Nutr* 23 (2):163–8.

Bowman, S. A., S. L. Gortmaker, C. B. Ebbeling, M. A. Pereira, and D. S. Ludwig. 2004. Effects of fast-food consumption on energy intake and diet quality among children in a national household survey. *Pediatrics* 113 (1 Pt 1):112–8.

Briefel, R. R., M. K. Crepinsek, C. Cabili, A. Wilson, and P. M. Gleason. 2009. School food environments and practices affect dietary behaviors of US public school children. *J Am Diet Assoc* 109 (2 Suppl):S91–107.

Caldwell, E. M., M. Miller Kobayashi, W. M. DuBow, and S. M. Wytinck. 2009. Perceived access to fruits and vegetables associated with increased consumption. *Public Health Nutr* 12 (10):1743–50.

Carroll-Scott, A., K. Gilstad-Hayden, L. Rosenthal, S. M. Peters, C. McCaslin, R. Joyce, and J. R. Ickovics. 2013. Disentangling neighborhood contextual associations with child body mass index, diet, and physical activity: The role of built, socioeconomic, and social environments. *Soc Sci Med* 95:106–114.

Caspi, C. E., I. Kawachi, S. V. Subramanian, G. Adamkiewicz, and G. Sorensen. 2012. The relationship between diet and perceived and objective access to supermarkets among low-income housing residents. *Soc Sci Med* 75 (7):1254–62.

Chang, V. W. 2006. Racial residential segregation and weight status among US adults. *Soc Sci Med* 63 (5):1289–303.

Cheadle, A., B. M. Psaty, S. Curry, E. Wagner, P. Diehr, T. Koepsell, and A. Kristal. 1991. Community-level comparisons between the grocery store environment and individual dietary practices. *Prev Med* 20:250–61.

Christian, W. J. 2012. Using geospatial technologies to explore activity-based retail food environments. *Spat Spatiotemporal Epidemiol* 3 (4):287–95.

Clark, M. A. and M. K. Fox. 2009. Nutritional quality of the diets of US public school children and the role of the school meal programs. *J Am Diet Assoc* 109 (2 Suppl):S44–56.

Colón-Ramos, U., F. E. Thompson, A. L. Yaroch, R. P. Moser, T. S. McNeel, K. W. Dodd, A. A. Atienza, S. B. Sugerman, and L. Nebeling. 2009. Differences in fruit and vegetable intake among Hispanic subgroups in California: Results from the 2005 California Health Interview Survey. *J Am Diet Assoc* 109 (11):1878–85.

Coyle, K. K., S. Potter, D. Schneider, G. May, L. E. Robin, J. Seymour, and K. Debrot. 2009. Distributing free fresh fruit and vegetables at school: Results of a pilot outcome evaluation. *Public Health Rep* 124 (5):660–9.

Davis, B. and C. Carpenter. 2009. Proximity of fast-food restaurants to schools and adolescent obesity. *Am J Public Health* 99 (3):505–510.

Davis, E. M., K. W. Cullen, K. B. Watson, M. Konarik, and J. Radcliffe. 2009. A Fresh Fruit and Vegetable Program improves high school students' consumption of fresh produce. *J Am Diet Assoc* 109 (7):1227–31.

de Koning, L., S. E. Chiuve, T. T. Fung, W. C. Willett, E. B. Rimm, and F. B. Hu. 2011. Diet-quality scores and the risk of type 2 diabetes in men. *Diabetes Care* 34 (5):1150–6.

de Lorgeril, M., S. Renaud, N. Mamelle, P. Salen, J. L. Martin, I. Monjaud, J. Guidollet, P. Touboul, and J. Delaye. 1994. Mediterranean alpha-linolenic acid-rich diet in secondary prevention of coronary heart disease. *Lancet* 343 (8911):1454–9.

Dennison, B. A., P. L. Jenkins, and H. L. Rockwell. 2000. Development and validation of an instrument to assess child dietary fat intake. *Prev Med* 31 (3):214–24.

Diez-Roux, A. V., F. J. Nieto, L. Caulfield, H. A. Tyroler, R. L. Watson, and M. Szklo. 1999. Neighbourhood differences in diet: The Atherosclerosis Risk in Communities (ARIC) Study. *J Epidemiol Community Health* 53 (1):55–63.

Drewnowski, A., N. Darmon, and A. Briend. 2004. Replacing fats and sweets with vegetables and fruits: A question of cost. *Am J Public Health* 94 (9):1555–9.

Duffey, K. J., P. Gordon-Larsen, D. R. Jacobs, O. D. Williams, and B. M. Popkin. 2007. Differential associations of fast food and restaurant food consumption with 3-y change in body mass index: The Coronary Artery Risk Development in Young Adults Study. *Am J Clin Nutr* 85 (1):201–8.

Duffey, K. J., P. Gordon-Larsen, L. M. Steffen, D. R. Jacobs, and B. M. Popkin. 2009. Regular consumption from fast food establishments relative to other restaurants is differentially associated with metabolic outcomes in young adults. *J Nutr* 139 (11):2113–8.

Epel, E.S., A.J. Tomiyama, and M.F. Dallman. 2012. Stress and reward: Neural networks, eating, and obesity. In *Food and Addiction: A Comprehensive Handbook*, edited by K. D. Brownell. and M. S. Gold. New York, NY: Oxford University Press.

Field, A. E., G. A. Colditz, M. K. Fox, T. Byers, M. Serdula, R. J. Bosch, and K. E. Peterson. 1998. Comparison of 4 questionnaires for assessment of fruit and vegetable intake. *Am J Public Health* 88 (8):1216–8.

Fisher, B. D. and D. S. Strogatz. 1999. Community measures of low-fat milk consumption: Comparing store shelves with households. *Am J Public Health* 89:235–7.

Forsyth, A., M. Wall, N. Larson, M. Story, and D. Neumark-Sztainer. 2012. Do adolescents who live or go to school near fast-food restaurants eat more frequently from fast-food restaurants? *Health Place* 18 (6):1261–9.

Fox, M. K., A. H. Dodd, A. Wilson, and P. M. Gleason. 2009. Association between school food environment and practices and body mass index of US public school children. *J Am Diet Assoc* 109 (2 Suppl):S108–17.

Franco, M., A. V. Diez-Roux, J. A. Nettleton, M. Lazo, F. Brancati, B. Caballero, T. Glass, and L. V. Moore. 2009. Availability of healthy foods and dietary patterns: The multi-ethnic study of atherosclerosis. *Am J Clin Nutr* 89 (3):897–904.

Frank, L. D., B. E. Saelens, K. E. Powell, and J. E. Chapman. 2007. Stepping towards causation: Do built environments or neighborhood and travel preferences explain physical activity, driving, and obesity? *Soc Sci Med* 65 (9):1898–914.

French, S. A., L. Harnack, and R. W. Jeffery. 2000. Fast food restaurant use among women in the Pound of Prevention study: Dietary, behavioral and demographic correlates. *Int J Obes Relat Metab Disord* 24 (10):1353–9.

Fuller, D., S. Cummins, and S. A. Matthews. 2013. Does transportation mode modify associations between distance to food store, fruit and vegetable consumption, and BMI in low-income neighborhoods? *Am J Clin Nutr* 97 (1):167–72.

Fungwe T, Guenther PM, Juan WY, Hiza HA, and Lino M. 2009. The quality of children's diets in 2003–04 as measured by the Healthy Eating Index-2005. In *Nutrition Insight*. Alexandria, VA: USDA, Center for Nutrition Policy and Promotion.

Ghirardelli, A., V. Quinn, and S. B. Foerster. 2010. Using geographic information systems and local food store data in California's low-income neighborhoods to inform community initiatives and resources. *Am J Public Health* 100 (11):2156–62.

Gittelsohn, J. and S. Sharma. 2009. Physical, consumer, and social aspects of measuring the food environment among diverse low-income populations. *Am J Prev Med* 36 (4 Suppl):S161–5.

Guenther, P. M., K. O. Casavale, J. Reedy, S. I. Kirkpatrick, H. A. Hiza, K. J. Kuczynski, L. L. Kahle, and S. M. Krebs-Smith. 2013. Update of the Healthy Eating Index: HEI-2010. *J Acad Nutr Diet* 113 (4):569–80.

Guenther, P.M., Reedy J, Krebs-Smith SM, Reeve BB, and Basiotis PP. 2007. Diet Quality of Americans in 1994–96 and 2001–02 as Measured by the Healthy Eating Index-2005. In *Nutrition Insight*. Alexandria, VA: USDA, Center for Nutrition Policy and Promotion.

Gustafson, A. A., J. Sharkey, C. D. Samuel-Hodge, J. Jones-Smith, M. C. Folds, J. Cai, and A. S. Ammerman. 2011. Perceived and objective measures of the food store environment and the association with weight and diet among low-income women in North Carolina. *Public Health Nutr* 14 (6):1032–8.

Gustafson, A., S. Lewis, S. Perkins, C. Wilson, E. Buckner, and A. Vail. 2013. Neighbourhood and consumer food environment is associated with dietary intake among Supplemental Nutrition Assistance Program (SNAP) participants in Fayette County, Kentucky. *Public Health Nutr* 16 (17):1229–37.

Guthrie, J. F., B. H. Lin, and E. Frazao. 2002. Role of food prepared away from home in the American diet, 1977–78 versus 1994–96: Changes and consequences. *J Nutr Educ Behav* 34 (3):140–50.

Hattori, A., R. An, and R. Sturm. 2013. Neighborhood food outlets, diet, and obesity among California adults, 2007 and 2009. *Prev Chronic Dis* 10:E35.

Havrankova, J. 2012. Is the treatment of obesity futile? YES. *Can Fam Physician* 58 (5):508, 510.

Heimendinger, J., M. A. Van Duyn, D. Chapelsky, S. Foerster, and G. Stables. 1996. The national 5 A Day for Better Health Program: A Large-Scale Nutrition Intervention. *J Public Health Manag Pract* 2 (2):27–35.

Hoehner, C.M., M. Schootman. 2010. Concordance of commercial data sources for neighborhood-effects studies. *J Urban Health* 87:713–25.

Honeycutt, S., E. Davis, M. Clawson, and K. Glanz. 2010. Training for and dissemination of the Nutrition Environment Measures Surveys (NEMS). *Prev Chronic Dis* 7 (6):A126.

Izumi, B. T., S. N. Zenk, A. J. Schulz, G. B. Mentz, and C. Wilson. 2011. Associations between neighborhood availability and individual consumption of dark-green and orange vegetables among ethnically diverse adults in Detroit. *J Am Diet Assoc* 111:274–9.

Jago, R., T. Baranowski, J. C. Baranowski, K. W. Cullen, and D. Thompson. 2007. Distance to food stores & adolescent male fruit and vegetable consumption. *Int J Behav Nutr Phys Act* 4:35.

Jeffery, R. W., J. Baxter, M. McGuire, and J. Linde. 2006. Are fast food restaurants an environmental risk factor for obesity? *Int J Behav Nutr Phys Act* 25 (3):2.

Kirkpatrick, S. I., K. W. Dodd, J. Reedy, and S. M. Krebs-Smith. 2012. Income and race / ethnicity are associated with adherence to food-based dietary guidance among US adults and children. *J Acad Nutr Diet* 112 (5):624–35.e6.

Krebs-Smith, S.M., J. Heimendinger, A.F. Subar, B.H. Patterson, and E. Pivonka. 1994. Estimating fruit and vegetable intake using food frequency questionnaires: A comparison of instruments. *Am J Clin Nutr* 59:283S.

Kubik, M. Y., L. A. Lytle, P. J. Hannan, C. L. Perry, and M. Story. 2003. The association of the school food environment with dietary behaviors of young adolescents. *Am J Public Health* 93 (7):1168–73.

Laraia, B. A., A. M. Siega-Riz, J. S. Kaufman, and S. J. Jones. 2004. Proximity of supermarkets is positively associated with diet quality index for pregnancy. *Prev Med* 39:869–75.

Laska, M. N., K. E. Borradaile, J. Tester, G. D. Foster, and J. Gittelsohn. 2010. Healthy food availability in small urban food stores: A comparison of four U.S. cities. *Public Health Nutr* 13 (7):1031–5.

Liese, A.D., N. Colabianchi, A.P. Lamichhane, T.L. Barnes, J.D. Hibbert, D.E. Porter, M.D. Nichols, A.B. Lawson. 2010. Validation of 3 food outlet databases: Completeness and geospatial accuracy in rural and urban food environments. *Am J Epidemiol* 172:1324–33.

Lopez, R. P. 2007. Neighborhood risk factors for obesity. *Obesity (Silver Spring)* 15 (8):2111–9.

Matthews, C. E., K. Y. Chen, P. S. Freedson, M. S. Buchowski, B. M. Beech, R. R. Pate, and R. P. Troiano. 2008. Amount of time spent in sedentary behaviors in the United States, 2003–2004. *Am J Epidemiol* 167 (7):875–81.

McGuire, S. 2011. Todd J.E., Mancino L., Lin B-H. The Impact of Food Away from Home on Adult Diet Quality. ERR-90, U.S. Department of Agriculture, Econ. Res. Serv., February 2010. *Adv Nutr* 2 (5):442–3.

Michimi, A. and M. C. Wimberly. 2010. Spatial patterns of obesity and associated risk factors in the conterminous U.S. *Am J Prev Med* 39:e1–12.

Monsivais, P. and A. Drewnowski. 2007. The rising cost of low-energy-density foods. *J Am Diet Assoc* 107 (12):2071–6.

Moore, L. V., A. V. Diez Roux, J. A. Nettleton, and D. R. Jacobs, Jr. 2008. Associations of the local food environment with diet quality—a comparison of assessments based on surveys and Geographic Information Systems: The multi-ethnic study of atherosclerosis. *Am J Epidemiol* 167:917–24.

Moore, L. V., A. V. Diez Roux, J. A. Nettleton, D. R. Jacobs, and M. Franco. 2009. Fast-food consumption, diet quality, and neighborhood exposure to fast food: The multi-ethnic study of atherosclerosis. *Am J Epidemiol* 170:29–36.

Moore, L. V. and A. V. Diez Roux. 2006. Associations of neighborhood characteristics with the location and type of food stores. *Am J Public Health* 96 (2):325–31.

Morland, K., S. Wing, A. Diez Roux, and C. Poole. 2002. Neighborhood characteristics associated with the location of food stores and food service places. *Am J Prev Med* 22 (1):23–9.

Nagata, J. M., M. B. Heyman, and J. M. Wojcicki. 2012. Evaluation of a Fresh Fruit Distribution Program in an Ethnically Diverse San Francisco High School. *ISRN Public Health* 2012 (2012): Article ID 252738.

Nelson, M. C., P. Gordon-Larsen, Y. Song, and B. M. Popkin. 2006. Built and social environments associations with adolescent overweight and activity. *Am J Prev Med* 31 (2):109–17.

Nestle, M. 2007. Introduction. In: *Food Politics: how the industry Influences Nutrition and Health*. University of California Press, Berkeley, California. p 16.

Neuhouser, M. L., S. Lilley, A. Lund, and D. B. Johnson. 2009. Development and validation of a beverage and snack questionnaire for use in evaluation of school nutrition policies. *J Am Diet Assoc* 109 (9):1587–92.

Neumark-Sztainer, D., S. A. French, P. J. Hannan, M. Story, and J. A. Fulkerson. 2005. School lunch and snacking patterns among high school students: Associations with school food environment and policies. *Int J Behav Nutr Phys Act* 2 (1):14.

Nielsen, S. J., A. M. Siega-Riz, and B. M. Popkin. 2002. Trends in food locations and sources among adolescents and young adults. *Prev Med* 35 (2):107–13.

Ogden, C. L., M. D. Carroll, B. K. Kit, and K. M. Flegal. 2012. Prevalence of obesity in the United States, 2009-2010. *NCHS Data Brief* (82):1–8.

Ollberding, N. J., C. R. Nigg, K. S. Geller, C. C. Horwath, R. W. Motl, and R. K. Dishman. 2012. Food outlet accessibility and fruit and vegetable consumption. *Am J Health Promot.* 26 (6):366–70.

Ornish, D. 1998. Serum lipids after a low-fat diet. *JAMA* 279 (17):1345–6.

Ornish, D. 2008. Weight loss with a low-carbohydrate, Mediterranean, or low-fat diet. *N Engl J Med* 359 (20):2170; author reply 2171–2.

Osypuk, T. L., A. V. Diez Roux, C. Hadley, and N. R. Kandula. 2009. Are immigrant enclaves healthy places to live? The multi-ethnic study of atherosclerosis. *Soc Sci Med* 69:110–20.

Pennington, J. A., P. J. Stumbo, S. P. Murphy, S. W. McNutt, A. L. Eldridge, B. J. McCabe-Sellers, and C. A. Chenard. 2007. Food composition data: The foundation of dietetic practice and research. *J Am Diet Assoc* 107 (12):2105–13.

Pereira, M. A., A. I. Kartashov, C. B. Ebbeling, L. Van Horn, M. L. Slattery, D. R. Jacobs, Jr, and D. S. Ludwig. 2005. Fast-food habits, weight gain, and insulin resistance (the CARDIA study): 15-year prospective analysis. *Lancet* 365 (9453):36–42.

Poti, J. M. and B. M. Popkin. 2011. Trends in energy intake among U.S. children by eating location and food source, 1977–2006. *J Am Diet Assoc* 111 (8):1156–64.

Powell, L. M. and E. Han. 2011. The costs of food at home and away from home and consumption patterns among U.S. adolescents. *J Adolesc Health* 48 (1):20–6.

Powell, L. M., E. Han, S. N. Zenk, T. Khan, C. M. Quinn, K. P. Gibbs, O. Pugach, et al.. 2011. Field validation of secondary commercial data sources on the retail food outlet environment in the U.S. *Health Place* 17 (5):1122–31.

Powell, L. M. et al. 2007. Associations between access to food stores and adolescent body mass index. *Am J Prev Med* 33:S301–S307.

Powell, L. M., Z. Zhao, and Y. Wang. 2009. Food prices and fruit and vegetable consumption among young American adults. *Health Place* 15 (4):1064–70.

Prochaska, J. J. and J. F. Sallis. 2004. Reliability and validity of a fruit and vegetable screening measure for adolescents. *J Adolesc Health* 34 (3):163–5.

Rose, D. and R. Richards. 2004. Food store access and household fruit and vegetable use among participants in the U.S. Food Stamp Program. *Public Health Nutr* 7:1081–8.

Rose, D., J. N. Bodor, P. L. Hutchinson, and C. M. Swalm. 2010. The importance of a multi-dimensional approach for studying the links between food access and consumption. *J Nutr* 140 (6):1170–4.

Rovner, A. J., T. R. Nansel, J. Wang, and R. J. Iannotti. 2011. Food sold in school vending machines is associated with overall student dietary intake. *J Adolesc Health* 48 (1):13–19.

Rundle, A., A. V. Diez Roux, L. M. Free, D. Miller, K. M. Neckerman, and C. C. Weiss. 2007. The urban built environment and obesity in New York City: A multilevel analysis. *Am J Health Promot* 21 (4 Suppl):326–34.

Sacks, F. M., L. P. Svetkey, W. M. Vollmer, L. J. Appel, G. A. Bray, D. Harsha, E. Obarzanek, et al.. 2001. Effects on blood pressure of reduced dietary sodium and the Dietary Approaches to Stop Hypertension (DASH) diet. DASH-Sodium Collaborative Research Group. *N Engl J Med* 344 (1):3–10.

Sebastian, R. S., C. Wilkinson Enns, and J. D. Goldman. 2009. US adolescents and MyPyramid: Associations between fast-food consumption and lower likelihood of meeting recommendations. *J Am Diet Assoc* 109 (2):226–35.

Seliske, L. M., W. Pickett, W. F. Boyce, and I. Janssen. 2009. Density and type of food retailers surrounding Canadian schools: Variations across socioeconomic status. *Health Place* 15 (3):903–7.

Sharkey, J. R., C. M. Johnson, and W. R. Dean. 2010. Food access and perceptions of the community and household food environment as correlates of fruit and vegetable intake among rural seniors. *BMC Geriatr* 10:32.

Song, H. J., J. Gittelsohn, M. Kim, S. Suratkar, S. Sharma, and J. Anliker. 2009. A corner store intervention in a low-income urban community is associated with increased availability and sales of some healthy foods. *Public Health Nutr* 12 (11):2060–7.

Srinath R. K. and M. B. Katan. 2004. Diet, nutrition and the prevention of hypertension and cardiovascular diseases. *Public Health Nutr* 7 (1A):167–86.

Steyn, N. P., J. Mann, P. H. Bennett, N. Temple, P. Zimmet, J. Tuomilehto, J. Lindström, and A. Louheranta. 2004. Diet, nutrition and the prevention of type 2 diabetes. *Public Health Nutr* 7 (1A):147–65.

Stimpson, J. P., A. C. Nash, H. Ju, and K. Eschbach. 2007. Neighborhood Deprivation is associated with lower levels of serum carotenoids among adults participating in the Third National Health and Nutrition Examination Survey. *J Am Diet Assoc* 107 (11):1895–902.

Sturm, R. 2008. Disparities in the food environment surrounding US middle and high schools. *Public Health* 122 (7):681–90.

Swinburn, B. A., I. Caterson, J. C. Seidell, and W. P. James. 2004. Diet, nutrition and the prevention of excess weight gain and obesity. *Public Health Nutr* 7 (1A):123–46.

Templeton, S. B., M. A. Marlette, and M. Panemangalore. 2005. Competitive foods increase the intake of energy and decrease the intake of certain nutrients by adolescents consuming school lunch. *J Am Diet Assoc* 105 (2):215–20.

Terry-McElrath, Y. M., P. M. O'Malley, J. Delva, and L. D. Johnston. 2009. The school food environment and student body mass index and food consumption: 2004 to 2007 national data. *J Adolesc Health* 45 (3 Suppl):S45–56.

Thompson, F. E., D. Midthune, A. F. Subar, L. L. Kahle, A. Schatzkin, and V. Kipnis. 2004. Performance of a short tool to assess dietary intakes of fruits and vegetables, percentage energy from fat and fibre. *Public Health Nutr* 7 (8):1097–105.

Thompson, F. E., D. Midthune, A. F. Subar, V. Kipnis, L. L. Kahle, and A. Schatzkin. 2007. Development and evaluation of a short instrument to estimate usual dietary intake of percentage energy from fat. *J Am Diet Assoc* 107 (5):760–7.

Thompson, F. E. A. F. Subar Dietary assessment methodology A. M. Coulston, C. J. Boushey, M. G. Ferruzzi (Eds.), *Nutrition in the prevention and treatment of disease* (3rd ed), Academic Press, New York (2012), pp. 5–46

USDA. 2010. Dietary Guidelines for Americans, 2010. In *Dietary Guidelines for Americans, 2010*. Washington, DC: U.S. Department of Agriculture and U.S. Department of Health and Human Services.

Wansink, B. and J. Sobal. 2007. Mindless eating—The 200 daily food decisions we overlook. *Environ Behav* 39 (1):106–123.

Wells, H. F. and J. C. Buzby. 2008. Dietary Assessment of Major Trends in US Food Consumption, 1970–2005. In *Economic Information Bulletin*, edited by U. D. o. A. Economic Research Service. Washington, DC.

Wiecha, J. L., D. Finkelstein, P. J. Troped, M. Fragala, and K. E. Peterson. 2006. School vending machine use and fast-food restaurant use are associated with sugar-sweetened beverage intake in youth. *J Am Diet Assoc* 106 (10):1624–30.

Wordell, D., K. Daratha, B. Mandal, R. Bindler, and S. N. Butkus. 2012. Changes in a middle school food environment affect food behavior and food choices. *J Acad Nutr Diet* 112 (1):137–41.

Yaroch, A. L., J. Tooze, F. E. Thompson, H. M. Blanck, O. M. Thompson, U. Colón-Ramos, A. R. Shaikh, S. McNutt, and L. C. Nebeling. 2012. Evaluation of three short dietary instruments to assess fruit and vegetable intake: The National Cancer Institute's food attitudes and behaviors survey. *J Acad Nutr Diet* 112 (10):1570–7.

Yaroch, A. L., K. Resnicow, A. D. Petty, and L. K. Khan. 2000. Validity and reliability of a modified qualitative dietary fat index in low-income, overweight, African American adolescent girls. *J Am Diet Assoc* 100 (12):1525–9.

Zenk, S. N., A. J. Schulz, B. A. Israel, S. A. James, S. Bao, and M. L. Wilson. 2005a. Neighborhood racial composition, neighborhood poverty, and the spatial accessibility of supermarkets in metropolitan Detroit. *Am J Public Health* 95 (4):660–7.

Zenk, S. N., A. J. Schulz, B. T. Izumi, G. Mentz, B. A. Israel, and M. Lockett. 2013. Neighborhood food environment role in modifying psychosocial stress-diet relationships. *Appetite* 65:170–7.

Zenk, S. N., A. J. Schulz, T. Hollis-Neely, R. T. Campbell, N. Holmes, G. Watkins, R. Nwankwo, and A. Odoms-Young. 2005b. Fruit and vegetable intake in African Americans income and store characteristics. *Am J Prev Med* 29:1–9.

Zenk, S. N. and L. M. Powell. 2008. U.S. secondary schools and food outlets. Health Place 14 (2):336–46.

Zenk, S. N., L. L. Lachance, A. J. Schulz, G. Mentz, S. Kannan, and W. Ridella. 2009. Neighborhood retail food environment and fruit and vegetable intake in a multiethnic urban population. *Am J Health Promot* 23:255–64.

6 Local Food Environments and Diet-Related Health Outcomes

A Systematic Review of Local Food Environments, Body Weight, and Other Diet-Related Health Outcomes

Shannon N. Zenk, Esther Thatcher, Margarita Reina, and Angela Odoms-Young

Countries that espouse neo-liberal economics tend to emphasize the primacy of individual choice in food policies. They often prefer to advise or educate consumers to 'choose wisely'. putting the onus of responsibility ideologically on choice, and existentially on the consumer. But is it reasonable to leave public health to individualized choice at the supermarket check-out points?

Tim Lang, David Barling, and Martin Caraher (2009)

Studies aimed as measuring how local food environments (LFEs) might influence disease progression and management are described in Chapters 4 and 5. This research has shown geographic disparities in the availability of healthy foods across the United States as well as provided empirical evidence of the relationship between these disparities and dietary intake among some U.S. populations. Results of these and other seminal studies on disease rates associated with area socioeconomic and racial/ethnic characteristics continue to challenge investigators to measure geographic disparities of disease patterns. Regarding the local food environment literature, investigators have heavily relied on obesity as a disease outcome. Part of the rationale for measuring the associations between local food environments and obesity is that like disparities in local food environments, racial/ethnic minorities, individuals of low socioeconomic status (SES), and rural residents are disproportionately affected by obesity. For example, in 2009–2010, the age-adjusted prevalence of obesity was 58.5% in African-American women compared to 32.2% in white women and 38.8% in African-American men (Flegal et al. 2012). Obesity rates are higher among rural residents of every race/ethnicity compared with urban whites (Patterson et al. 2004). Black et al. (2010) present geographic differences in obesity prevalence by neighborhood across the five boroughs of New York City, with some of the highest prevalence found in neighborhoods such as Bedford Stuyvesant in Brooklyn, Harlem in Manhattan, and the South Bronx, where people of color are concentrated (Figure 6.1).

Obesity is a risk factor for many debilitating chronic diseases including diabetes, coronary heart disease, stroke, and several cancers (Hu 2009; Pan and DesMeules 2009; Abdullah et al. 2010) with annual medical costs of obesity in the United States approaching $210 billion (20.6% of all national medical expenditures) (Cawley and Meyerhoefer 2012). Obesity is most directly and primarily a result of imbalance between energy intake and energy expenditure. Yet, despite tremendous investments in obesity treatment for individuals, obesity prevalence remains high and even continues to increase among certain subpopulations such as men and African-American boys (Flegal et al. 2012). Moreover, racial/ethnic, socioeconomic, and rural–urban disparities in obesity persist. This has turned attention to environmental contributors to energy imbalance (e.g., obesity), its rise, and other diet-related health outcomes (Sallis and Glanz 2009).

Early research on the environment, obesity, and related health outcomes focused on area socioeconomic characteristics and segregation. Several studies found that residing in a socioeconomically disadvantaged area was associated with poorer weight and disease outcomes (Cubbin et al. 2001; Diez Roux et al. 2001; Robert and Reither 2004; Boardman et al. 2005; Chang 2006). For example, Robert and Reither (2004) found that living in a socioeconomically disadvantaged area was associated with higher body mass index (BMI), independent of a range of individual characteristics. Another study showed that compared to those living in the most advantaged areas, whites in the most socioeconomically disadvantaged areas had a 70%–90% increased risk of coronary heart disease while African-Americans had a 30%–50% increased risk (Diez Roux et al. 2001). Boardman et al. (2005) found that living in an area with a relatively high proportion of African-Americans was associated with a 9% increase in the odds of obesity, controlling for individual characteristics and neighborhood socioeconomic characteristics. These findings have recently been supported by rare experimental evidence that showed that moving from a higher to a lower poverty neighborhood may have salutary effects on body weight and diabetes risk (Ludwig et al. 2011).

Results of these and other seminal studies on area socioeconomic and racial/ethnic characteristics and health outcomes renewed interest in identifying characteristics of disadvantaged communities that may lead to poorer health outcomes and contributed to the launch of a decade (to date) of research on how living in disadvantaged neighborhoods affects health. This included studies on local inequalities in the food environment (Morland et al. 2002; Sloane et al. 2003; Block et al. 2004; Horowitz et al. 2004; Zenk et al. 2005b; Moore and Diez Roux 2006; Zenk et al. 2006), as measured by availability of different types of stores and restaurants and by the availability, price, and quality of foods for sale. For example, in communities spanning four states, Morland et al. (2002) found that the wealthiest and white neighborhoods had three to four times more supermarkets than the poorest and African-American neighborhoods. In New Orleans, research established that there were 2.4 fast-food outlets per square mile in African-American neighborhoods compared to 1.5 outlets per square mile in white neighborhoods (Block et al. 2004).

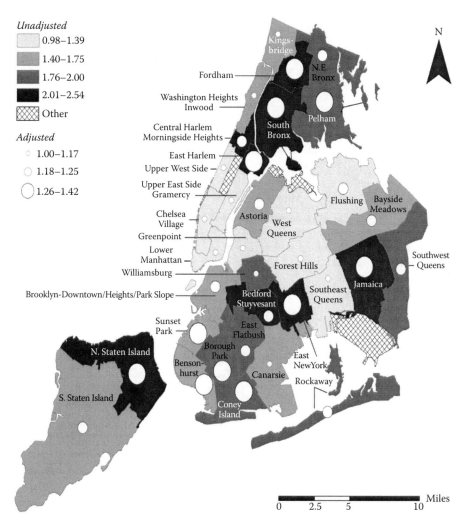

FIGURE 6.1 Neighborhood distribution of obesity, New York City, 2005. (From Black, J., et al., *Health and Place*, 16, 489–499, 2010.) *Data Source:* Community Health Survey 2005; the gray shading reflects the predicted neighborhood-level odds of obesity from a null model with no covariates in quartiles. These estimates are equivalent to the neighborhood-level obesity prevalence estimates, not adjusted for survey weights. The white circles reflect the predicted odds of obesity for each neighborhood relative to Chelsea-Village after controlling for the level-1 model; Neighborhoods with the largest white circles have a 52% to 84% higher odds of obesity compared to Chelsea-Village, after controlling for individual-level factors; Categories for predicted random effects are based on terciles. Level-1 covariates: female, annual income categories, racial/ethnic identity, age group, education, employment, smoking, marital status, and U.S. born.

In New York City, Upper East Side stores were significantly more likely to carry low-carbohydrate or high-fiber bread, low or nonfat milk, fresh fruits, and fresh green vegetables than East Harlem stores (Horowitz et al. 2004). In four Detroit area communities, although there was no overall difference in the selection or prices of fresh fruits and vegetables, the quality of fruits and vegetables was considerably lower in East Side Detroit, a low-income African-American community, compared to Southfield, a middle-income, racially heterogeneous community (Zenk et al. 2006). It is now well documented that the food environment varies considerably across communities and that economically disadvantaged, African-American, and rural communities—the same populations at highest risk for obesity and related health outcomes—tend to have poorer quality food environment than more economically advantaged, white, and some urban communities in the United States (Powell et al. 2007c; Beaulac et al. 2009; Larson et al. 2009).

Beyond describing differences in the local food environment, a growing number of researchers are directly testing associations with dietary behaviors, body weight, and related health outcomes such as diabetes risk. These studies aimed to understand whether variations in the local food environment translated into differences in health outcomes or contribute to disparities in obesity and related outcomes. The number of these studies has grown rapidly over the past several years, making it important to appraise the evidence on whether the local food environment affects body weight and related health outcomes. This will help to inform next steps in research and especially policies and other interventions to improve population health and reduce health disparities.

The purpose of this chapter is to systematically review evidence to date on the extent to which the local food environment is associated with diet-related health outcomes in the United States. Consistent with Glanz et al.'s (2005) widely used Model of Community Nutrition Environments, we considered the local food environment to include the *community* food environment (e.g., number, type, location, and accessibility of retail food outlets) and the *consumer* food environment (e.g., what consumers encounter inside retail food outlets such as food availability, price, promotion, placement, and quality, as well as nutrition information). This systematic review builds on prior reviews that addressed local food environments and body weight, or cardiometabolic risk, which covered literature as late as 2008 and some of which focused only on particular subpopulations such as African-Americans (Black and Macinko 2008; Casagrande et al. 2009; Lovasi et al. 2009; Feng et al. 2010; Fleischhacker et al. 2011; Leal and Chaix 2011). A recent review by Gustafson et al. (2011) included literature through 2011, but focused only on the *consumer food store environment*.

Specifically, researchers have aimed to develop mechanistic studies to measure specific features of local food environment that may impact the development of obesity and other diet-related health outcomes. In this research, it is important to distinguish between *exposure* to the local food environment and *utilization* of the local food environment because it affects study design and measurement, as well as the interpretation of study results. For example, auto ownership and availability of public transit or ride shares may be effect modifiers of the associations between local food environments and diet or health. But such factors do not change the targeted geographic boundary of interest to answer central research questions such as: "Are the features of the immediate local food environment sufficient to maintain the recommendations for a healthy diet?" In this chapter, we refer to exposure measures as measures of *potential access* and to utilization measures as *realized access* (Guagliardo 2004; Sharkey et al. 2010).

CAUSAL CONCEPTUAL MODEL

The goal of many studies on the local food environment is to measure how geographic patterns of disease may be attributed to disparities between local food environments. Individual level moderators may explain differences in effects between local food environments and health for some groups of people and therefore are important to include in statistical modeling. As such, measuring the effects of local food environments on health require specification of the causal pathways by which these disparities in food access may affect the diet-related health outcomes if interest. There are many health outcomes that could be investigated that may be impacted by inequalities between local food environments. For instance, hunger might be investigated as a health outcome because prolonged hunger results in comorbid conditions and potentially mortality, especially for vulnerable populations such as older adults. Similarly, it is conceivable that chronic exposure to restricted food environments might affect the progression of diabetes, hypertension, or metabolic syndrome. Also, for people experiencing chronic conditions such as diabetes, local food environments could potentially affect disease management of those conditions. And of course, the local availability of healthy affordable foods could potentially affect weight status. Each health outcome requires careful development of causal models to guide the study design, measurement, and data analysis.

Because the vast majority of studies to date have measured the effect of local food environments on obesity, the conceptual model in Figure 6.2 pertains to

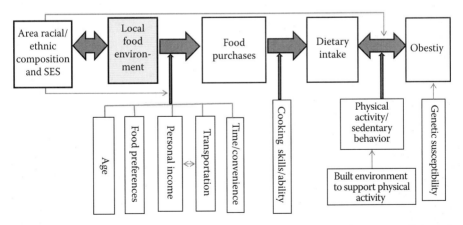

FIGURE 6.2 Hypothesized relationships between local food environments, diet, and obesity for adults.

that outcome specifically. Other investigators have proposed models that describe unidirectional relationships between macro and individual level factors on behaviors and health demonstrating the complicated relationships and intermediates between environmental exposures to local food environments on health (Black and Macinko 2008; Boehmer 2006). Here, it is proposed to use the causal diagram that has been presented in Chapters 4 and 5 and include additional component causes that would be necessary or sufficient to understand the relationship between local food environments and obesity. It is recognized with this diagram (and those presented by others) that disease is rarely developed by a single component cause; therefore it is essential, particularly for distal relationships such as health, that causal models are specific and well measured. Null findings from studies do not always represent a true null effect; rather null findings can be a result of lack of specificity of measured factors and/or variables missing entirely from equations. To the same extent, findings in the direction to support hypotheses can also develop erroneously from misclassification. Figure 6.2 depicts the hypothesized pathway by which exposure to restricted food environments may result in weight gain. The large unidirectional arrows between the local food environment, food purchases, and dietary intake are discussed in detail in Chapter 5.

It is important to note that food purchasing and dietary intake are intermediates of the relationship between local food environments and obesity, and therefore many would argue it is important to not adjust for those effects. Nevertheless, factors that may modify the relationship between the local food environment and diet remain potential effect modifiers of the relationship between the local food environment and obesity. Empirical evidence has been provided in Chapter 4 that local food environments in the United States vary by the race/ethnic composition of geographic areas as well as the SES of populations. The arrow remains bidirectional for the relationship, however, because the direction of how those geographic distributions have evolved remains to be studied. In other words, does area racial/ethnic composition influence where food retailers do business or do people of certain racial and ethnic groups specifically seek areas to live that have better food environments? This remains a question important to some investigators conducting this type of research and hence the call for longitudinal studies. This will be discussed in more detail later in this chapter. Unidirectional arrows between race/ethnicity or SES area also drawn to show the effect of differences in food purchasing that may be a function of differences in food purchasing between groups and also other pathways that may more directly interact with the diet and obesity relationship. Important also to note is that obesity is a function of energy intake and expenditure, therefore the interaction of sedentary behavior or levels of physical activity may modify the relationship between diet and obesity. Also note, the diagram does not consider time, which is an important variable when measuring disease initiation, progression, and management. It is believed that it is chronic exposure to segregated neighborhoods that contribute to poor health outcomes among residents. This is implied within the conceptual model, but the measurement of chronic exposure would strengthen the research.

Therefore, the purpose of this chapter is to discuss findings from all studies that have measured associations between local food environments and any health outcome. Because they represent another approach to understanding contributions of the local food environment to health outcomes, we also present findings for research on utilization of the food environment. Methodological challenges for estimating associations will also be addressed. The aim is for readers to not only understand the current state of evidence to support associations between local food environments and health, but also gain an understanding of how: (1) to measure disease risk in epidemiology and (2) to identify key methodological issues that may impact study findings. The literature for adults and children/adolescents will be presented separately because needs from local food environments are different and require specific considerations regarding study design for adults and children.

STUDY SELECTION

Peer-reviewed studies on relationships between local food environments and diet-related health outcomes published in English before October 2012 were selected for the review. Database searches completed in PubMed, CINAHL, and Web of Science using combinations of the following search terms: "neighborhood," "food environment," "grocery," "fast food," "body mass index," "waist circumference," "obesity," "stroke," "diabetes," and "blood pressure" yielded 5340 titles (including duplicates).

Inclusion criteria were a U.S.-based sample; quantitative data and a statistical analysis; a diet-related health outcome, specifically body mass index, waist circumference, blood pressure, diabetes (including hemoglobin A1C), cholesterol, or stroke as a dependent variable; an independent variable on the retail community or consumer food environment, tested separately (not as part of a composite with nonfood environment variables) and measured at a smaller geographic area than a county, metropolitan area, or state (as these were not considered "local"); and not an ecological analysis. In addition, we excluded studies that only examined relationships between fast-food consumption or eating out of home and a diet-related health outcome. An initial screening of each title and/or abstract was conducted to determine relevance. For those potentially relevant, a second level review of the article text was conducted to determine whether the article met the full inclusion criteria. Examination of previous literature reviews on related topics, reference lists of reviewed studies, and authors' personal collections led to the inclusion of additional articles. A total of 61 articles were ultimately included in the review.

Data on methods and results were abstracted from each article using a standardized form. Regular conversations among coauthors were used to resolve questions or discrepancies regarding eligibility and data abstraction. Abstracted data were checked by a second coauthor. In this chapter, we present information on design, sample characteristics, setting, key aspects of the food environment measurement, and attributes of the food environment for which any statistically significant results ($p < .05$) were found in the sample overall or a subgroup based on fully adjusted models.

SUMMARY OF STUDY FINDINGS

Table 6.1 summarizes key methodological aspects and results of the 61 studies. The data are organized first by outcome variable (body weight, other) and then by age group, study design, and finally alphabetically by the first author's last name. Fifty-six percent of the studies ($n = 34$) were published within the last 3 years (2010–2012). Eighty-four percent of the studies ($n = 51$) were published within the last 5 years (2008–2012). Ninety-three percent of the studies ($n = 57$) included body weight (BMI or weight status such as obesity) as an outcome. Studies also included blood pressure ($n = 4$), diabetes ($n = 3$), waist circumference ($n = 3$), cholesterol ($n = 1$), and stroke ($n = 1$) as outcomes. Forty-seven percent of studies ($n = 27$) measured body weight objectively (e.g., interviewer measured, medical record); the remaining studies ($n = 30$) measured body weight using self-report. In the studies including blood pressure, diabetes, waist circumference, cholesterol, and stroke, all the outcomes were measured objectively.

METHODS OVERVIEW

Design

With regard to the study design, 18.0% of the studies ($n = 11$) were longitudinal and 82.0% of the studies ($n = 50$) were cross-sectional (Table 6.1). The 11 longitudinal studies included repeated measures of the outcome, with the length of follow-up ranging from 1 to 30 years, but not necessarily repeated measures of the local food environment.

Sample

In terms of the study samples, 72.1% of the studies ($n = 44$) focused on adults (5 on older adults ages 50+ years only) and 27.9% ($n = 17$) on children or adolescents (six on children, six on adolescents, and five on children and adolescents). In 31.1% of the studies ($n = 19$), over half of the sample was racial/ethnic minorities (i.e., African-American, Hispanic, Asian, American-Indian). Studies for which the authors identified the sample as of low SES numbered 10 (16.4%).

Setting

The articles predominantly examined the residential food environment, or the environment surrounding the home residence. Of those studies on adults, all but one examined the food environment around the residence only; one study examined the food environment around both the residence and workplace. Of those studies on children or adolescents, 52.9% were based on the residence ($n = 9$), 35.3% were based on the school ($n = 6$), and 11.8% were based on the residence and school ($n = 2$). Four of the six studies involving only children were based on the residence; four of the six studies involving only adolescents were based on the school; and four of the five studies involving children and adolescents were based on the residence.

Potential or Realized Access

Most studies (86.9%; $n = 53$) assessed the food environment solely using a *potential* access measure. One study included only a *realized* access measure, or a measure of

TABLE 6.1

Studies Examining Relationships between the Local Food Environment and Diet-Related Health Outcomes ($n = 61$)

Author (Year)	Outcome[c]	Design[d]	Age[e]	Minority or Low-Income[f]	Setting[g]	Potential or Realized Access[h]	Food Environment Measure[i]	Geographic Unit[j]	Assessed Outlets[k]	Objective or Self-Report[l]	Positive Health Outcome[m]	Negative Health Outcome[n]
				Sample		**Food Environment Measurement**					**Statistically Significant Results**	
Adult						**Body Weight**						
Block et al. (2011)	Wt (Ob)	L (30)	Adult	NA	Res	P	Prox N	NA	Super, Groc, Conv, OthS, FF, FullR	Ob		FF, Groc
Gibson (2011)	Wt (SR)	L (6)	Adult	NA	Res	P	Dens	ZIP	Super, SMGr, OthS, FF, FullR	Ob	Super	SMGr
Han et al. (2012)	Wt (SR)	C, L (4)	Adult	Min	Res	P	Dens	ZIP	SupGr	Ob	SupGr	
Li et al. (2009b)	Wt (Ob)	L (1)	Older Adult	Oth	Res	P, R	Dens	CBG	FF	Ob		FF
Powell and Han (2011)	Wt (SR)	C, L (6)	Adult	Oth	Res	P	Dens	ZIP	Super, Groc, Conv, FF, FullR	Ob	Super, Groc, FullR	Groc, Conv, FF
Black et al. (2010)	Wt (SR)	C	Adult	Min	Res	P	Dens	Oth	Super, SMGr, OthS, FF, TotR	Ob	Super, OthS, FF, TotR	
Bodor et al. (2010)	Wt (SR)	C	Adult	Min	Res	P	Count	Buff (2 km N)	Super, SMGr, Conv, OthS, FF	Ob	Super	Conv, FF
Boehmer et al. (2006)	Wt (SR)	C	Adult	Oth	Res	P, R	Prox W, Avail, Qual	Walk	Super, OthS, FF, OhR	SR	Super	

(Continued)

TABLE 6.1 (Continued)
Studies Examining Relationships between the Local Food Environment and Diet-Related Health Outcomes ($n = 61$)

Author (Year)	Outcome[c]	Design[d]	Age[e]	Minority or Low-Income[f]	Setting[g]	Potential or Realized Access[h]	Food Environment Measure[i]	Geographic Unit[j]	Assessed Outlets[k]	Objective or Self-Report[l]	Positive Health Outcome[m]	Negative Health Outcome[n]
				Sample			Food Environment Measurement				Statistically Significant Results	
Brown et al. (2008)	Wt (SR)	C	Adult	Oth	Res	P, R	Dens, CommO	CT	Super, SupGr, SMGr, Conv	Ob, SR	Super	
Casagrande (2011)	Wt (Ob)	C	Adult	Min	Res	P	Avail	CT	NA	Ob		Avail
Casey et al. (2008)	Wt (SR)	C	Adult	Oth	Res	P, R	CommO, ConsO	Oth	NA	SR		
Cerin et al. (2011)	Wt (SR)	C	Adult	Oth	Res	P	Count, Prox N, Avail, Price, Qual	Buff (1 km N)	Groc, Conv, TotS, FF, FullR	Ob	Groc, Avail	
Chen et al. (2010)	Wt (SR)	C	Adult	Oth	Res	P	Dens	CT, Buff (1 mi. E)	Groc	Ob	Groc	Groc
Chen et al. (2012)	Wt (SR)	C	Adult	Oth	Res	P	Dens	CT, Buff (0.5 mi. E)	Groc, FF	Ob		
Drewnowski (2012)	Wt (SR)	C	Adult	Oth	Res	P, R	Prox N, Price	NA	Super	Ob, SR	Price	
Dubowitz et al. (2012)	Wt (Ob)	C	Older Adult	Oth	Res	P	Dens	Buff (0.75, 1.5, 3 mi. E)	SupGr, FF	Ob	SupGr	FF
Dunn et al. (2012)	Wt (SR)	C	Adult	Oth	Res	P	Dens, Prox N	Buff (1, 3 mi E)	FF	Ob		FF
Ford and Dzewaltowski (2010)	Wt (SR)	C	Adult	Low	Res	P	Dens	Buff (1, 3, 5 mi. E)	Super, SupGr, SMGr, Conv	Ob	Super	Super, SupGr, Groc, Conv

Study												
Ford and Dzewaltowski (2011)	Wt (SR)	C	Adult	Low	Res	P	Count	CT	Super, SMG, Conv	Ob		OthS
Gustafson et al. (2011)	Wt (Ob)	C	Adult	Low	Res	P, R	Count, Prox N, Avail	CT; Buff (5 mi.)	Super, Conv, OthS, TotS	Ob, SR		ConsO
Heinrich et al. (2012)	Wt (Ob)	C	Adult	Min, Low	Res	P	ConsO	Buff (800 m E)	NA	Ob		
Hickson et al. (2011)	Wt (Ob)	C	Adult	Min	Res	P	Dens	Buff (0.5, 1, 2, 5 mi. E)	FF	Ob	FF	
Hutchinson et al. (2012)	Wt (SR)	C	Adult	Oth	Res	P	Dens, Avail	Buff (500 m, 1, 2 km E)	Super, OthS	Ob	Avail	OthS
Inagami et al. (2006)	Wt (SR)	C	Adult	Min	Res	R	Prox E, CommO	CT	NA	Ob	Prox	CommO
Inagami et al. (2009)	Wt (SR)	C	Adult	Min	Res	P	Dens	CT	FF, TotR	Ob		FF, TotR
Janevic et al. (2010)	Wt (Ob)	C	Adult	NA	Res	P	Count	CT	HlthO, UnHlthO	Ob	HlthO, UnhlthO	
Jeffery et al. (2006)	Wt (SR)	C	Adult	Oth	Res, Work	P	Dens	Buff (0.5, 1, 2 mi. E)	FF, OthR, TotR	Ob		
Li et al. (2008)	Wt (Ob)	C	Older Adult	Oth	Res	P	Dens	CBG	FF	Ob		FF
Li et al. (2009b)	Wt (Ob)	C	Older Adult	Oth	Res	P	Dens	CBG	FF	Ob		FF
Michimi and Wimberly (2010)	Wt (SR)	C	Adult	Oth	Res	P	Prox E	NA	Super, OthS	Ob	Super, OthS	
Millstein et al. (2008)	Wt (Ob)	C	Adult	Min	Res	P	Count	CT	SupGr, Conv, OthS, FF, FullR	Ob		OthS
Mobley et al. (2006)	Wt (Ob)	C	Adult	Oth	Res	P	Dens	ZIP	Groc, Conv, FF, OthR	Ob		
Morland et al. (2006)	Wt (Ob)	C	Adult	Oth	Res	P	Count	CT	Super, SupGr, Groc, Conv, OthS	Ob	Super	Groc, Conv, OthS

(Continued)

TABLE 6.1 (Continued)
Studies Examining Relationships between the Local Food Environment and Diet-Related Health Outcomes ($n = 61$)

				Sample			Food Environment Measurement				Statistically Significant Results	
Author (Year)	Outcome[c]	Design[d]	Age[e]	Minority or Low-Income[f]	Setting[g]	Potential or Realized Access[h]	Food Environment Measure[i]	Geographic Unit[j]	Assessed Outlets[k]	Objective or Self-Report[l]	Positive Health Outcome[m]	Negative Health Outcome[n]
Morland and Evenson (2009)	Wt (SR)	C	Adult	Oth	Res	P	Count, Prox N	CT	Super, Groc, Conv, OthS, FF, FullR, OthR	Ob	Super, OthR	Groc, FF
Raja et al. (2010)	Wt (Ob)	C	Adult	Oth	Res	P	Count, Prox N, RatioO	Buff (5 min walk N, 5 min drive N)	TotS, TotR, Ratio	Ob	Ratio	TotR
Rose et al. (2009)	Wt (SR)	C	Adult	Oth	Res	P	Avail	Buff (500 m, 1, 2 km)	NA	Ob		Avail
Rundle et al. (2009)	Wt (Ob)	C	Adult	Oth	Res	P	Count	Buff (0.5 mi. N)	HlthO, UnhlthO, TotS	Ob	HlthO	
Truong et al. (2010)	Wt (SR)	C	Adult	NA	Res	P	RatioO	CT	RatioO	Ob		
Wang et al. (2007)	Wt (SR)	C	Adult	Oth	Res	P	Dens, Prox E	Oth	Super, SMGr, Conv, OthS, FF	Ob		Super, SMGr, OthS
Zick et al. (2009)	Wt (SR)	C	Adult	NA	Res	P	Count	CBG	Conv, TotS, FF, FullR, HlthO	Ob	Conv, FullR, HlthO, TotS	

Child or Adolescent

Lee (2012)	Wt (Ob)	L (6)	Child	Oth	Res	P	Dens	CT	SupGr, Conv, OthS, FF, FullR	Ob		
Leung et al. (2011)	Wt (Ob)	L (3)	Child	Oth	Res	P	Dens	Buff (0.25, 1 mi., N)	Super, SMGr, Conv, OthS, FF, FullR	Ob	Conv	
Shier et al. (2012)	Wt (Ob)	L (4)	Child, Teen	Oth	Res	P	Dens, RatioO	CT	Super, Groc, Conv, OthS, FF	Ob		
Sturm and Datar (2005)	Wt (Ob)	L (3)	Child	Oth	Res, Sch	P	Dens, RatioO	ZIP	Groc, Conv, FF, OthR, Ratio	Ob		
Burdette and Whitaker (2004)	Wt (Ob)	C	Child	Min, Low	Res	P	Prox N	NA	FF	Ob		
Elder et al. (2010)	Wt (Ob)	C	Child	Min, Low	Sch	P	Dens	Buff (1 mi. E)	Groc, TotR	Ob		
Davis and Carpenter (2009)	Wt (SR)	C	Teen	Min	Sch	P	Count, Prox E	Buff (0.25, 0.5, 0.75 mi. E)	Groc, Conv, FF	Ob	FF	
Galvez et al. (2009)	Wt (Ob)	C	Child	Min	Res	P	Count	CB	Super, Groc, Conv, OthS, FF, TotR	Ob	Conv	
Harris et al. (2011)	Wt (SR)	C	Teen	Oth	Sch	P	Count, Prox N	Buff (1 km N)	SupGr, OthS, TotS, TotR	Ob		
Hartley et al. (2011)	Wt (SR)	C	Child, Teen	Low	Res	P, R	Prox D, ConsO	Oth	NA	Ob, SR		
Jilcott et al. (2010)	Wt (Ob)	C	Child, Teen	Min, Low	Res	P	Count, Prox N and E	Buff (0.25, 0.5, 1, 5 mi. N and E)	Super, Groc, Conv, OthS, FF, FullR	Ob	Conv	OthS

(Continued)

TABLE 6.1 (Continued)
Studies Examining Relationships between the Local Food Environment and Diet-Related Health Outcomes ($n = 61$)

				Sample			Food Environment Measurement					Statistically Significant Results	
Author (Year)	Outcome[c]	Design[d]	Age[e]	Minority or Low-Income[f]	Setting[g]	Potential or Realized Access[h]	Food Environment Measure[i]	Geographic Unit[j]	Assessed Outlets[k]	Objective or Self-Report[l]	Positive Health Outcome[m]	Negative Health Outcome[n]
Lamicchane (2012)	Wt (Ob)	C	Child, Teen	Oth	Res	P	Count, Dens, Prox N	Buff (1, 2, 6 mi. N)	Super, FF	Ob	Super, FF	
Laska et al. (2010b)	Wt (Ob)	C	Teen	Oth	Res, Sch	P	Dens, Prox N	Buff (800,1600, 3000 m N)	Groc, Conv, FF, TotR, OthS	Ob	TotR	Conv
Powell et al. (2007a)	Wt (SR)	C	Teen	Oth	Sch	P	Dens	ZIP	FF, FullR	Ob		
Powell et al. (2007b)	Wt (SR)	C	Teen	Oth	Sch	P	Dens	ZIP	Super, Groc, Conv, OthS	Ob	Super	Groc, Conv
Sanchez (2012)	Wt (Ob)	C	Child, Teen	Min	Sch	P	Dens	Buff (0.5 mi E)	Conv, FF	Ob		Conv, FF
Wall et al. (2012)	Wt (Ob)	C	Teen	Min	Res	P	Dens, Prox N	Buff (400, 800, 1200, 1600 m N)	Super, Conv, FF, TotR	Ob		Conv, TotR
Other Health Outcomes												
Auchincloss et al. (2009)	Diab (Ob)	L (5)	Adult	Min	Res	P	Avail	Walk	NA	SR	Avail	
Li et al. (2009c)	BP (Ob)	L (1)	Older Adult	Oth	Res	P	Dens	CBG	FF	Ob		FF
Li et al. (2009b)[a]	Wcirc (Ob)	L (1)	Older Adult	Oth	Res	P, R	Dens	CBG	FF	Ob		FF

Study / Outcome[c]	Design[d]	Age[e]	Minority/ Low[f]	Setting[g]	Access[h]	Measure	Geography	Store type	Ob/SR	Sig.
Dubowitz et al. (2012)[a] — BP (Ob)	C	Older Adult	Oth	Res	P	Dens	Buff (0.75, 1.5, 3 mi. E)	SupGr, FF	Ob	SupGr
Hickson et al. (2011)[a] — Wcirc (Ob)	C	Adult	Min	Res	P	Dens	Buff (0.5, 1, 2, 5 mi. E)	FF	Ob	
Janevic et al. (2010)[a] — Diabetes (Ob)	C	Adult	NA	Res	P	Count	CT	HlthO, UnHlthO	Ob	
Lamicchane (2012)[a] — Wcirc (Ob)	C	Child, Teen	Oth	Res	P	Count, Dens, Prox N	Buff (1, 2, 6 mi. N)	Super, FF	Ob	Super
Morland et al. (2006)[b] — Diab (Ob)	C	Adult	Oth	Res	P	Count	CT	Super, SupGr, Groc, Conv, OthS	Ob	
Morland et al. (2006)[b] — BP (Ob)	C	Adult	Oth	Res	P	Count	CT	Super, SupGr, Groc, Conv, OthS	Ob	
Morland et al. (2006)[b] — Chol (Ob)	C	Adult	Oth	Res	P	Count	CT	Super, SupGr, Groc, Conv, OthS	Ob	
Morgenstern et al. (2009) — Stroke (Ob)	C	Adult	Min	Res	P	Count, Prox E	Buff (1 mi. E)	FF	Ob	FF
Mujahid et al. (2008) — BP (Ob)	C	Adult	Min	Res	P	Avail	CT	NA	SR	

[a] Study appears above under body weight (two outcomes were assessed).

[b] Study appears above under body weight; four outcomes assessed: body weight, diabetes, blood pressure, cholesterol.

[c] Outcome: Wt, body weight; Diab, diabetes; BP, blood pressure; Wcirc, waist circumference; Strok, stroke; Ob, objectively measured; SR, self-reported.

[d] Design: C, cross-sectional; L, longitudinal (Length of follow-up).

[e] Age: Older adult, Ages 50+ only; Adult, Ages 18–49 only or 18+; Teen, Ages 12–17 or middle/high school; Child, Ages < 12 or elementary school.

[f] Minority or low income: Min, >50% Black or African-American, Hispanic, American-Indian, or Asian; Low, Author identified as low-income or low SES sample. Includes WIC only samples, SNAP/food stamp recipient only samples, public housing residents.

[g] Setting: Res, residential; Sch, school; Work, workplace; Oth, other; NA, not applicable.

[h] Potential or realized access: P, potential spatial access measure; R, realized access or utilization measure.

(Continued)

TABLE 6.1 (*Continued*)
Studies Examining Relationships between the Local Food Environment and Diet-Related Health Outcomes (*n* = 61)

i   Food environment measure: Count, count (unadjusted) of outlets (including presence or absence); Dens, density of outlets (adjusted for land area, population, street network length); Prox W: W, walking distance, proximity of outlets (N, street network distance; E, Euclidean distance); Ratio, ratio of outlets (e.g., healthy to unhealthy); CommO, other community food environment measure; Avail, food availability or selection, including shelf space; Price, food prices; Qual, food quality; ConsO, Other consumer food environment measure.

j   Geographic unit: CB, census block; CBG, census block group; CT, census tract; ZIP, ZIP code; Buff, buffer (Size; N, street network distance; E, Euclidean distance); Walk, walking distance; Drive, driving distance; Oth, other; NA, not applicable or not specified.

k   Assessed outlets: Super, supermarket; SupGr, supermarket or grocery store; large grocery store; SMGr, small or medium grocery store; Groc, grocery store, all or size not specified; Conv, convenience store; OthS, other food store; TotS, total food stores; FF, fast-food stores; FullR, full service or sit-down restaurant; OthR, other restaurant (not fast-food or full service or not specified); TotR, Total restaurants; HlthO, healthy outlets; UnHlthO, unhealthy outlets; RatioO, Ratio of one outlet type to another; NA, not applicable or not specified.

l   Objective or self-report: Ob, objectively measured or observed food environment measure; SR, self-reported or perceived food environment measure.

m   Positive health outcome: Food environment measure associated with better health. Codes shown under Food Environment Measure and Assessed Outlets.

n   Negative health outcome: Food environment measure associated with poorer health. Codes shown under Food Environment Measure and Assessed Outlets.

utilization of the food environment. In that study, Inagami et al. (2006) assessed characteristics (proximity, socioeconomic characteristics of the surrounding neighborhood) of the store where survey respondents reported shopping. About 13% of studies ($n = 7$) included both potential and realized access measures.

Food Environment Measure: Community

Eighty percent of the studies ($n = 49$) examined the community food environment only, 8.2% ($n = 5$) the consumer food environment only, and 11.5% ($n = 7$) both the community and consumer food environment. Community food environment measures included classic measures of spatial accessibility: coverage or container measures (i.e., number of outlets within a geographic unit or specified distance) and proximity measures (i.e., distance or travel time between the origin—typically the place of residence—and food outlet). In this review, we divided coverage or container measures into density measures and count measures. Density measures were adjusted for population, land area (directly or indirectly through the use of a consistent size buffer), or roadway miles. Count measures were unadjusted or categorical (e.g., presence of one or more supermarkets) and included those unadjusted measures based on street network buffers because these buffers are of an inconsistent size, depending on street network connectivity.

Of the studies that examined the community food environment ($n = 56$), most used a density or count measure (83.9%; $n = 47$). Almost two-thirds of these studies used a density measure ($n = 30$), while the others used a count measure ($n = 16$) or both a density and a count measure ($n = 1$). Thirty-six percent of the studies ($n = 20$) measuring the community food environment included a proximity measure. Most of these studies ($n = 13$) measured proximity as the street network distance, six as Euclidean distance, and two as either walking or driving distance. (Two of the studies used both a street network and Euclidean distance measure.) Four studies used a *ratio* measure of the food environment; that is, the relative number of or distance to one type of food outlet as compared to another. Three studies included another measure of the community food environment: relative socioeconomic disadvantage of the surrounding neighborhood (Brown et al. 2008; Casey et al. 2008) and type of store at which the participant shopped (Inagami et al. 2006).

Of the 55 studies that measured counts, densities, or proximity of at least one food outlet, 63.6% ($n = 35$) included fast-food restaurants, 18.2% ($n = 1$) included full-service or sit-down restaurants, and 9.1% ($n = 5$) included another type of restaurant. Fifteen percent of studies ($n = 8$) included a measure of the total restaurants. Of the studies that measured counts, densities, or proximities, 41.8% ($n = 23$) included supermarkets and an additional 10.9% ($n = 6$) included a measure of supermarkets or grocery stores. (We consider these two groups together when discussing relationships with health outcomes.) Twenty-seven percent of studies ($n = 15$) measured *grocery stores*, and another 14.5% ($n = 8$) measured small- or medium-sized grocery stores specifically. Forty percent of studies ($n = 22$) measured convenience stores. Three studies included grouping of outlets that they considered *healthy* or *unhealthy*. Thirty-five percent of studies ($n = 19$) included another type of food store, such as fruit and vegetable markets, meat markets, specialty stores, and bakeries. Most studies (81.8%; $n = 45$) included more than one type of outlet.

Food Environment Measure: Consumer

Of the studies that examined the consumer food environment ($n = 12$), most included a measure of food availability ($n = 8$). Two measured food prices, two measured food quality, and three measured other aspects of the consumer food environment: marketing (Heinrich et al. 2012) and composite measures of the consumer food environment (Casey et al. 2008; Hartley et al. 2011).

Adjustment for Physical Activity

Relatively few studies adjusted for physical activity/energy expenditure or an indicator of the built environment that is related to physical activity. Only 26.2% of studies ($n = 16$) adjusted for physical activity, and only 26.2% ($n = 16$) adjusted for an indicator of the built environment that is related to physical activity (e.g., walkability, proximity to a park or indoor recreation facility, safety, population density). About half of all studies (49.2%; $n = 30$) adjusted for neither, and only 13.1% of studies ($n = 8$) adjusted for both physical activity and at least one related measure of the built environment.

Geographic Unit

Almost all studies ($n = 57$) measured an aspect of the food environment within a geographic unit; the other studies used proximity measures only. Of the studies that measured an aspect of the food environment within a geographic unit ($n = 57$), 38.6% of the studies ($n = 22$) included a food environment measure based on a buffer only. Fourteen of these studies tested relationships for more than one buffer size. One-third of studies ($n = 19$) measuring the food environment within a geographic unit used census geography only; the census tract was the most common geographic unit ($n = 13$), with the other studies including measures based on census block groups ($n = 5$) and census blocks ($n = 1$). Seven studies used ZIP codes, two walking distance, four another geography, and three both a buffer and census geography. Overall, 39.8% of studies ($n = 17$) tested more than one geography.

Objective or Self-Report Measure

Almost all the studies (88.5%; $n = 54$) relied solely on *objective* (from a secondary source) or observed measures (e.g., collected via direct observations or audits) of the food environment; 6.6% of the studies ($n = 4$) relied solely on self-reported or perceived measures of the food environment; and 4.9% of the studies ($n = 3$) included at least one objective and one self-reported measure.

EVIDENCE FOR BODY WEIGHT BY AGE

ADULTS

Forty studies examined the relationships between aspects of the local food environment and body weight among adults. Five of these studies were longitudinal, all of which found at least one statistically significant association. The community food environment was included in almost all of these studies ($n = 37$), with the accessibility of fast-food restaurants ($n = 20$), supermarkets or supermarket/grocery stores ($n = 19$), and convenience stores ($n = 14$) most commonly examined. Half of the studies ($n = 10$) on fast-food restaurants found better accessibility was associated with less healthy weights (higher BMI, overweight, or obesity), while 40% ($n = 8$) found no significant associations and two studies found better accessibility was associated with healthier weights (lower BMI, normal, or underweight). Four of the studies with significant findings were based on the same sample (Li et al. 2008; Li et al. 2009a,b,c). For example, a one standard deviation increase in the density of fast-food restaurants in the census block group was associated with a 7% increase in the odds of overweight/obesity in Portland, Oregon (Li et al. 2008), while fast-food restaurant availability in the census block group was not associated with BMI in the sample overall or among residents of low- or high-income neighborhoods in Salt Lake City, UT (Zick et al. 2009). The vast majority of studies on full-service or sit-down restaurants, other restaurants, or total restaurants found no relationships with body weight. In a sample of African-Americans with type 2 diabetes participating in a diabetes management intervention, Millstein et al. (2008) found no relationship, for example, between full-service restaurant availability and BMI.

Composite Scores for Local Food Environments

With regard to other measures of the community food environment, each of the three studies using groupings of healthy and/or unhealthy outlet found some evidence, in the expected direction, with weight outlets. In New York City, for example, Rundle et al. (2009) examined the number of healthy outlets (i.e., supermarkets, fruit and vegetable markets, natural food stores), unhealthy outlets (seven outlets including fast-food restaurants, pizza restaurants, convenience stores), or *intermediate* outlets (four outlets including nonfast-food restaurants and specialty food stores) within a half-mile street network buffer of the residential address. They found that the prevalence ratio for obesity was 0.87 when comparing those in the highest quintile for healthy outlets to those in the lowest two quintiles (Rundle et al. 2009). Ratios of different types of food outlets have also been used. Using the physical food environment indicator (PFEI), adapted from the retail food environment index proposed by the California Center for Public Advocacy and calculated as the ratio of counts of fast-food restaurants, convenience stores, and small food stores to counts of supermarkets, produce markets and these other three outlet types, Truong et al. (2010) found that a census tract-level measure of PFEI was associated with higher BMI and obesity risk among adults in California. In a Los Angeles sample, Inagami et al. (2006) found that living in a neighborhood in which the average person shops in more economically disadvantaged neighborhoods was positively associated with BMI, which the authors indicated may reflect social norms around food purchasing.

Food Availability

Concerning the consumer food environment, six studies included a measure of food availability. Two studies found no relationship with weight outcomes. One of these studies examined perceptions of fruit and vegetable availability at the store where the participant shopped in a sample of physical activity intervention participants in three states (Boehmer et al. 2007); the other examined perceptions of healthy food availability both at the primary store where participants shopped and in the residential neighborhood among low-income women participating in a weight loss intervention (Gustafson et al. 2012). Two studies used measures derived from the Nutrition Environment Measurement Surveys (NEMS). One study found that healthy food availability at grocery stores was associated with 18% lower odds of overweight/obesity, and that vegetable availability at sit-down restaurants was associated with 54% lower odds of overweight/obesity (Cerin et al. 2011). Contrary to hypotheses, the other study in Baltimore found that living in a predominately white census tract with medium or high availability of healthy foods was associated with a 3.9 and 3.2 unit increase in BMI, respectively (Casagrande et al. 2011). Two studies used the same telephone survey and food audit data in New Orleans. One found that greater shelf space for a variety of snacks (candy, salty snacks, cookies, soda) were positively associated with BMI, although there were no relationships between shelf space for fruits and vegetables and BMI (Rose et al. 2009). In the other study, a high ratio of shelf space for healthy foods (fruits, vegetables) to junk food (snacks) shelf space in 1 km of home was associated with a lower risk of overweight (relative risk [RR] 0.55) and obesity (RR 0.50 [Hutchinson et al. 2012]).

Food Prices

Two studies examined food prices. Cerin et al. (2011) found no relationship between the prices of healthier food options as measured by the NEMS in stores and body weight outcomes. In Seattle Drewnowski et al. (2012) found that shopping at a high-priced supermarket was associated with a lower risk of obesity (RR 0.34), which the authors suggested may indicate economic access to healthy foods.

Food Quality

Few studies examined other aspects of the consumer food environment. Two of these studies examined food quality, neither of which found a significant relationship with weight (Boehmer et al. 2007; Cerin et al. 2011). Heinrich et al. (2012) examined relationships between store and restaurant advertisements for alcohol and high-calorie and low-calorie food products and BMI in public housing residents. They found that each additional store alcohol sign was associated with a 0.10 unit increase in BMI although each additional restaurant alcohol sign was associated with a 1.26 unit increase in BMI.

Summary of Adult Studies

The most consistent evidence in favor of a relationship between the food environment and body weight in adults was found for supermarkets. Fifty-eight percent of studies (n = 11) that examined supermarkets found that better accessibility of supermarkets was associated with healthier weight outcomes. In a longitudinal study using data from the Panel Study for Income Dynamics, for example, Powell and Han (2011) found that each additional population-adjusted number of supermarkets in the ZIP code was associated with a 0.13 unit reduction in BMI in poor women, but not in nonpoor women or men (poor or nonpoor). Thirty-two percent of studies (n = 6) found no statistically significant associations, whereas one study found a negative association and one study found evidence of both positive and negative associations. Results were quite mixed for grocery stores, with three studies finding better accessibility to be associated with less healthy weights, one study finding better accessibility to be associated with healthier weights, two studies finding evidence of both positive and negative effects, and two studies finding no association. Morland et al. (2006) found that the presence of a grocery store (i.e., non-chain grocer) in the census tract was associated with a 3% increase in the prevalence of overweight in the Atherosclerosis Risk in Communities Study, whereas Mobley et al. (2006) found no association between ZIP code-level grocery store availability and BMI in WISEWOMAN participants in five states. For small–medium grocery stores and convenience stores, included in eight and six studies respectively, the vast majority found no association with body weight (66.7%, 64.3% respectively). In a 30-year longitudinal study of the Framingham Heart Study Offspring Cohort, no association was found between convenience store proximity and BMI (Block et al. 2011). One-third of studies on small–medium grocery stores found that they were related to less healthy weight outcomes, while 28.6% of studies including convenience stores found that they were associated with less healthy weights.

Children or Adolescents

Seventeen studies examined the relationships between aspects of the food environment and body weight among children or adolescents. Four of these studies were longitudinal, only one of which found a statistically significant association with body weight. At least one measure of the community food environment was included in all 17 studies; one study included a measure of the consumer food environment. The accessibility of fast-food restaurants ($n = 13$) and convenience stores ($n = 11$) were most commonly assessed. All but two studies included at least one measure of restaurant accessibility. Of the studies that examined fast-food restaurants ($n = 13$), only 23.1% ($n = 3$) found that better accessibility to the residence or school was associated with less healthy weight outcomes. One study found better accessibility to fast food was associated with healthier weight; the others found no statistically significant associations. In a sample of youth in Greenville, North Carolina and surrounding Pitt County, Jilcott et al. (2010) found no association between proximity of fast-food restaurants and BMI.

Four studies examined full-service or sit-down restaurants, one study examined other restaurants, and five examined total restaurants. Of these 10 studies, only two found statistically significant associations. Laska et al. (2010b) found that presence of any restaurant within 800 m of the school, but not the home residence, was associated with a 0.28 unit decrease in BMI z-score in an adolescent sample in the Minneapolis-St. Paul metropolitan area. On the other hand, also in Minneapolis-St. Paul but with a different sample, Wall et al. (2012) found that presence of any restaurant within 1200 m of the home was associated with a 0.20 unit increase in adolescent girls' BMI z-score.

Of the studies that examined supermarkets ($n = 9$), only two found statistically significant relationships with weight outcomes. Using national data from the Monitoring the Future survey with eighth and tenth graders, Powell et al. (2007b) found that each additional population-adjusted number of chain supermarkets in the school ZIP code was associated with a 0.11 unit decrease in adolescent BMI. In a sample of children and adolescents in the SEARCH for Diabetes in Youth study,

Lamichhane et al. (2012) found that each additional supermarket within 2 km of the residence was associated with a 0.05 unit reduction in BMI z-score. Only one of the seven studies that included a measure of grocery store accessibility found a significant relationship with body weight. Of the 11 studies that examined convenience stores, seven (63.6%) found that greater accessibility was associated with less healthy weight outcomes. In a 3-year longitudinal study, for example, Leung et al. (2011) found that presence of a convenience store within 0.25 mi. of home was associated with a 3.38 increase in the odds of overweight/obesity.

As the only study of children or adolescents that included a measure of the consumer food environment, Hartley et al. (2011) examined a composite measure of the store food environment (capturing good availability, prices, and quality based on the NEMS in stores) and found no relationship with obesity risk in a sample of low-income rural children.

SUPERMARKETS AND OBESITY, ADULTS 2006–2012

As suggested above, the most consistent evidence in favor of a relationship between the food environment and body weight in adults was found for supermarkets. The effect estimates of associations and 95% confidence intervals for those estimates are presented in Figure 6.3. Studies are presented chronologically and there is a consistent small protective effect of supermarkets on obesity. Estimates in most studies are quite precise and in many cases if confidence intervals do cross the null, it is at the tail end of the interval. Readers are to be reminded that although the confidence interval presents all possible values representing the association at $\alpha = 0.05$, the effect estimate is the most likely association. All studies that measured supermarkets are included in Figure 6.2, regardless of statistical significance of those estimates. One of the many criteria epidemiologists and others use as evidence of causal relationships is the consistency of findings across studies (Hofler 2005). Quite

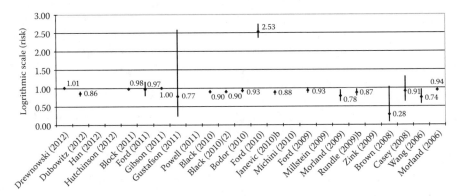

FIGURE 6.3 Measured associations and 95% confidence intervals between supermarkets and obesity.[a] The presence of supermarkets was measured in a number of different ways by investigators and for some measured within composite scored for healthy local food environments. Studies that presented findings in nonlogrithmic statistics that could not be converted for the figure. *Note:* Many effects in all of the above studies were measured. Selected here are the effects with supermarkets specifically.

remarkably, across 18 U. S. studies, (1) nearly all measure effects between supermarkets and obesity show supermarkets to be protective of obesity (estimates are below 1.0); (2) the size of the effect is quite consistently around 0.9; and (3) again for the most part, confidence intervals are precise. These findings are supported by positive linear associations and also found by Zick et al. (2009), Michini et al. (2010), Han et al. (2012), and Hutchinson et al. (2012).

EVIDENCE FOR OTHER HEALTH OUTCOMES

Ten studies examined relationships between the local food environment and a diet-related health outcome other than body weight. Two of these studies were based on the same sample: one examined blood pressure and one examined waist circumference (Li et al. 2009b,c). One of the 10 studies examined three health outcomes: diabetes, blood pressure, and cholesterol (Morland et al. 2006). Nine of the 10 studies had adult samples. Eight of the 10 studies measured the community food environment exclusively. Of the five studies that examined fast-food outlets, three found significant associations with poorer health outcomes: diabetes, blood pressure, and stroke. In Nueces County, TX, for example, Morgenstern et al. (2009) found that each additional fast-food restaurant within 1-mi. of the residential census tract was associated with a 1% increase in the risk of ischemic stroke. On the other hand, among African-American participants in the Jackson Heart Study, local fast-food restaurant availability was not associated with waist circumference (Hickson et al. 2011). Of the five studies that examined supermarkets, two found that better accessibility was associated with better health outcomes: blood pressure and waist circumference. Using national data from the Women's Health Initiative Clinical Trial, for example, Dubowitz et al. (2012) found an inverse association between residential supermarket density and diastolic blood pressure. The very few studies assessing other types of food outlets, including healthy outlets, grocery stores, and convenience stores, found no statistically significant associations.

Two studies examined the consumer food environment; both measured perceptions of healthy food availability in the neighborhood. One longitudinal study found that greater perceived healthy food availability was associated with 37% lower type 2 diabetes incidence (Auchincloss et al. 2008). The other study found no statistically significant association between perceived neighborhood healthy food availability and blood pressure (Mujahid et al. 2008).

DISCUSSION

Research on the local food environment and body weight and other diet-related health outcomes has increased rapidly over the past 8 years. One study per year was published in 2004 and 2005; 12 studies were published in 2011 (the last full year of data included in this review). Overall evidence in the United States is quite mixed regarding the relationship between the local food environment and diet-related health outcomes, with only some tested associations being statistically significant, many nonsignificant, and others in an unexpected direction. When statistically significant relationships were found they were often small in magnitude and confined to particular subpopulations (e.g., women [Wang et al. 2007]) or settings (e.g., low-income neighborhoods [Chen and Florax 2010]). This is not necessarily surprising given that health outcomes such as obesity and blood pressure are complex and shaped by a multitude of factors including genetics, nondietary behaviors, and social/cultural contexts. We would expect stronger relationships between the local food environment and dietary behaviors, although contributions to health outcomes are arguably of most interest. Nonetheless, three-quarters of the studies reported at least one significant relationship between the local food environment and a health outcome, although publication bias in favor of studies with significant results may contribute to this finding.

LIMITATIONS

This review has limitations that are worth noting. Many of the limitations stem from wide variation in study methods, including measurement of outcomes and especially the local food environment as well as the analysis, which is a well-recognized challenge in comparing studies and summarizing results on the local food environment and health (Mozaffarian et al. 2012). First, given this challenge, we relied on conventional levels of statistical significance to identify studies that found a relationship between the local food environment and a diet-related health outcome. However, we recognize that statistical significance does not equate with practical importance. Second, our reports of significant relationships are based on analyses with different covariates and samples. The studies included quite different sets of control variables, both at the individual level and area level. Further, some studies conducted subgroup analyses or tested interactions to determine whether associations were found only in some segments of the population, whereas other studies only tested for associations in the overall sample. We indicated there was a relationship if any statistically significant association was detected in a fully adjusted model (if more than one model with different sets of covariates were presented) for either the entire sample or a subsample. Third, comparability of findings on the community food environment by outlet type is limited. Because studies used a large number of operational definitions for a single type of food outlet (e.g., *supermarket*), we generally used the outlet label provided by the authors. Thus, outlet types we used often capture several different operational definitions. Fourth, we focused only on relationships with diet-related health outcomes and not more direct and proximal relationships with diet, which provides only a partial picture of the potential importance of the food environment. Researchers, policy makers, advocates, and community members should consider evidence in this chapter in conjunction with that presented in Chapter 5 to inform interventions and future research. Fifth, we summarized results by published paper, rather than by sample. Finally, this review did not specifically examine evidence in populations at highest risk for obesity (e.g., African-Americans, low SES individuals, residents of high poverty neighborhoods, rural residents), for which the local food environment may have stronger effects. Despite these limitations, this review provides an up-to-date report on the state of the science on relationships between the local food environment and diet-related health outcomes in the United States. Later we discuss implications for interventions and future research.

IMPLICATIONS FOR POLICY AND OTHER INTERVENTIONS

A number of influential reports have called for policies and other environmental interventions directed at improving local food environments (Ver Ploeg et al. 2009; Flournoy 2011; Glickman et al. 2012). Policies to expand access to healthy foods in underserved communities (e.g., Fresh Food Financing Initiative and its state and local-level equivalents) and to limit access to unhealthy options (e.g., fast-food moratoriums) are in early stages of implementation. These efforts are justifiable from a social justice perspective given convincing evidence in the United States of inequalities in access to healthy and unhealthy food sources and products by area racial/ethnic and socioeconomic characteristics. Nonetheless, experiences in the United Kingdom illustrate how policies related to the local food environment that aim to improve population health can outpace the evidence base (Wrigley 2002; Cummins et al. 2008). As highlighted later, additional research is needed to advance understanding of the role of the local food environment in diet-related health outcomes. The produced evidence can help identify the most promising targets (e.g., increasing access to supermarkets or reducing access to fast-food restaurants) and locations (e.g., supermarket within 3 miles just as beneficial as having one within 1 mile) of interventions and thus inform the best investment of finite public resources to improve diet-related population health and reduce health disparities. In the interim, based on findings to date on the local food environment and diet-related health outcomes, what are the implications for policy and other types of interventions that address the local food environment?

Our findings support the American Heart Association's recommendation of increased availability of supermarkets near home as a priority population approach to improve diet and related health outcomes (Mozaffarian et al. 2012). Over half of studies (57.8%) that assessed supermarkets and body weight in adults found a significant association; we also showed—across all studies including measures of supermarket access regardless of statistical significance—consistency that points to a salubrious effect on body weight. Thus, having better spatial access to supermarkets, which are associated with a wide selection of healthy foods and possibly lower prices, may facilitate healthier eating and consequently body weights. Given that African-American and economically disadvantaged areas often have fewer supermarkets than more advantaged areas (Morland et al. 2002; Zenk et al. 2005b; Beaulac et al. 2009), these areas should be prioritized for intervention.

Almost two-thirds of studies (63.6%) that assessed convenience stores and body weight in children or adolescents found a significant association. Results to date suggest that convenience stores, which predominately sell and market energy-dense, nutrient poor snacks and sugar sweetened beverages (Farley et al. 2009; Laska et al. 2010a; Lucan et al. 2010; Sharkey et al. 2012; Cavanaugh et al. 2013), may be deleterious to children and adolescents' body weights. Research shows that children and adolescents frequent convenience stores or *corner* stores, for example on their way to or from school, and purchase large amounts of calories from these venues (Borradaile et al. 2009; Cannuscio et al. 2010; Dennisuk et al. 2011). Convenience stores may be disproportionately located in African-American and economically disadvantaged neighborhoods (Hilmers et al. 2012). Changing the product mix and marketing at convenience or corner stores have shown some promise and should continue to be advanced and evaluated (Song et al. 2009; Bleich et al. 2012; Dannefer et al. 2012; Gittelsohn et al. 2012).

Half of adult studies and a quarter of studies with adolescents or children found that better spatial access to fast-food restaurants were associated with less healthy weight outcomes. Fast-food restaurants tend to sell energy-dense, nutrient poor foods, although they may not differ from other restaurants in availability of healthy alternatives (Saelens et al. 2007). Research to date is still inconclusive regarding contributions of fast-food restaurant accessibility to health outcomes. They may be more relevant for adults than youth. Extant evidence does not support prioritization of interventions targeting fast-food restaurants.

Of the small number of studies examining the consumer food environment in adults, about half of studies including a direct measure of food availability found hypothesized associations with weight outcomes. Studied food products differed across these studies and included overall availability of fruits and vegetables, low-fat options, snacks, and sugar-sweetened beverages, as well as relative availability of healthy to unhealthy foods. There is growing recognition of the potential need to not only increase healthy food availability but also restrict availability of energy-dense, nutrient poor snacks and sugar-sweetened beverages. However, it remains unclear which approach or whether a combination of the two will be most effective in promoting healthier diets and related health outcomes.

IMPLICATIONS FOR FUTURE RESEARCH

Results of this systematic review have multiple implications for future research with regard to study design, measurement, and analysis, as well as research questions that could be addressed to strengthen the evidence base.

Design

Given that extant research is overwhelmingly cross-sectional, more longitudinal and quasi-experimental designs are needed (Mozaffarian et al. 2012). The small number of longitudinal studies on body weight in adults all found at least one significant relationship, suggesting that results may be more consistent for longitudinal studies, but this pattern was not observed for studies on body weight in children. Nonetheless, studies with repeated measures on both the local food environment and health outcomes are needed to establish temporal ordering and rule out self-selection. Such studies should carefully consider length of follow up to take advantage of environmental changes stemming from both residential moves (to a different environment) and especially changes in attributes within environments (e.g., supermarket closing), both of which may not be observable in studies with a short follow-up period. Quasi-experimental and experimental studies should be explored, such as evaluating effects of natural or planned changes in the local food environment on health outcomes. Building on work in the United Kingdom (Wrigley 2002; Cummins et al. 2008), for example, studies in Philadelphia and Pittsburgh are currently underway to evaluate effects of the opening of new full-service supermarkets on health outcomes among residents in low-income communities. However, length of the follow-up period is an important consideration in these studies as well because it is unlikely that we can detect changes in dietary behaviors, let alone health outcomes, within 12 months, when they are shaped over the life course. Other designs such as those using ecological momentary assessment that take advantage of real-time, repeated observations of food environments and behaviors may also prove useful, though these designs are most relevant for understanding relationships between the environment and dietary behaviors.

Measurement

Given that the majority of studies are still based on self-reported health outcomes, research with measured outcomes is greatly needed. Measurement error from self-reported outcomes can distort relationships and thus lead to erroneous conclusions regarding relationships between the local food environment and health outcomes (Leal and Chaix 2011).

With the preponderance of research focused on community food environments (e.g., accessibility of food outlets), more attention should be directed at measuring aspects of the consumer food environment, including food availability, quality (which may be particularly relevant in low SES and African-American communities), and prices. Although retail food outlet type is a reasonably good proxy for the availability and to some extent quality and prices of healthy and unhealthy food products, there is variation within outlet types (Zenk 2004; Glanz et al. 2007; Liese et al. 2007; Farley et al. 2009). Some research has shown, for example, that food and beverage availability, prices, and quality are poorer in low SES and African-American communities than higher SES and white communities among stores of the same type (Zenk et al. 2006; Franco et al. 2008). To inform policy, research is needed to identify the effects of both increasing healthy food availability and restricting unhealthy food availability in improving weight and other health outcomes. Research using absolute measures as well as relative measures of healthy to unhealthy food availability may be informative. However, studies using these relative measures should consider how such results can inform environmental changes. Extant evidence on relationships between food prices and health outcomes largely comes from large-scale studies, in which prices are measured at the metropolitan area level or state level. Because they were not considered *local*, these studies were not included in this review. A 2012 review of studies published between 2007 and 2012 by Powell et al. (2013) showed, however, that higher fast-food prices and lower fruit and vegetable prices were associated with lower weight outcomes in adolescents and both adults and children, respectively. That review concluded that there was little evidence of relationships between sugar-sweetened beverage prices and body weight, but noted that studies were based on existing state-level sales taxes that were relatively low. Because prices can vary at the local level, more research on local food prices and health outcomes would be beneficial. Beyond food availability and prices, very little work has been done on other aspects of the local consumer food environment, such as food quality and marketing, which may influence food purchasing and dietary behaviors and ultimately health outcomes. These are important directions for future research (Zenk et al. 2006; Cummins et al. 2009; Grier and Kumanyika 2010; Glanz et al. 2012).

Incorporating food environment exposures beyond the residential neighborhood may improve the measurement accuracy in future studies. We found that only one study examined food environment exposures in settings beyond the residential neighborhood in adults. Jeffrey et al. (2006) examined relationships between fast-food restaurant density around both the home and workplace and body weight. In children and adolescents, more studies measured nonresidential food environments, particularly school food environments, though only two of these studies measured the food environment around both the home and school. Yet, most people, adults and youth, travel and spend considerable time outside their residential neighborhood as part of day-to-day activities such as work, school, and socializing. These nonresidential settings and broader *activity space* may expose them to food environments that differ from their residential neighborhood (Golledge and Stimson 1997; Kwan and Weber 2003; Zenk et al. 2011b) and impact their dietary behaviors and health outcomes. Measuring the food environment in these other nonresidential settings or in the activity space may more accurately capture exposures. Studies that incorporate both residential and nonresidential food environments would be particularly valuable to examine relative and joint effects and to ensure that the residential food environment does not confound any significant findings for the nonresidential food environment.

More research is needed that assesses relationships between food environment utilization or realized access and outcomes, including the extent to which utilization moderates relationships between local food environment exposures and outcomes and contributes to inconsistencies in findings. Most research on the local food environment has tested relationships between potential spatial access to an element of the food environment and outcomes. Yet, there is rapidly growing qualitative and quantitative research on how individuals interact with, or use, the food environment which is revealing important information on food shopping behaviors such as the type of store where they shop, how far they travel, perceptions of foods where they shop, and factors that influence their choices (Rose and Richards 2004; Zenk et al. 2005a; Inagami et al. 2006; Hillier et al. 2011; Zenk et al. 2011a; Chaix et al. 2012 Zenk et al. 2013b). This research shows that many individuals shop outside their residential neighborhood, particularly if it lacks healthy food options. For example, Inagami et al. (2006) in a study included in this review found that 21.8% of a Los Angeles, California sample shopped within their census tract. In a racially/ethnically diverse sample in Detroit, Michigan, Zenk et al. (2013b) found that individuals travelled, on average, 3.1 miles from home to shop. In that study, those without a local large grocery and living farther from a supermarket travelled farther to shop. However, as evidenced by this review in which only 13% of studies included a realized access (utilization) measure, few studies have yet examined the implications of realized food access for health outcomes. Of those studies that have, some linked longer travel distance, perceived food availability, and measured food prices to health outcomes, but overall utilization research is also mixed.

As highlighted in previous reviews (Charreire et al. 2010), the geography for which the food environment may matter for dietary behaviors and health outcomes remains unclear. There is general consensus that administrative units (e.g., ZIP code, census tract) are not ideal conceptually, but are sometimes the only option due to data availability. Ultimately, until the appropriate geography is determined, we recommend that researchers conduct sensitivity analyses to measures derived for multiple geographies and/or spatial accessibility measures (e.g., density, proximity).

Analysis

Testing multiple aspects of the local food environment simultaneously in adequately powered studies would be beneficial in future research. Local food environment measures can be correlated; therefore, researchers should determine relationships between attributes of interest while controlling for other aspects of the local food environment to avoid confounding. For example, because fast-food restaurant availability and full-service restaurant availability can be correlated, it is important to account for full-service restaurant availability when attempting to pinpoint the contribution of fast-food restaurant availability to health outcomes. Similarly, researchers should test for multi-collinearity when simultaneously including multiple food environment measures.

To the extent possible, future studies should control for other behavioral and social pathways by which the environment may influence body weight and related health outcomes. Body weight and related health outcomes are influenced by multiple behavioral and social factors (e.g., physical activity, sleep, stress) that are correlated with diet. Moreover, the local food environment is correlated with environmental attributes that affect these other behavioral and social pathways. Without appropriate controls, relationships between the local food environment and outcomes may be confounded. Thus, controlling for these other environmental attributes and nondietary behaviors can help to isolate relationships between local food environment and health outcomes. Nonetheless, Controlling for behaviors alone may be insufficient because many behavioral measures are notorious for error. Alternatively, models that explicitly test dietary behaviors as mediators in relationships between the local food environment and health outcomes may be useful, but residual confounding due to measurement error in dietary behaviors is still a concern.

Research should continue attempts to identify subgroups for which the local food environment may matter. This is often accomplished through subgroup analysis or inclusion of statistical interactions. Most commonly, researchers have focused on subgroups based on individual demographics (e.g., age, gender, race/ethnicity, SES), area demographics (e.g., racial composition, socioeconomic characteristics, urbanicity), and to a lesser extent psychosocial factors (e.g., mastery, reward sensitivity, stress) (Paquet et al. 2010a,b; Ledoux et al. 2012). Identifying contributions of the food environment for those at highest risk for obesity and poor diet-related health outcomes (e.g., African-Americans, rural residents, low-income individuals, residents of poor neighborhoods) is particularly important to identify policies and environmental changes to improve health outcomes in these groups and reduce disparities.

New Research Questions

As the field evolves, new questions emerge regarding the role of local food environments in health outcomes and factors that mediate or moderate these relationships. Conceptual models of food access published to date have helped to outline dimensions of the local food environment, its macro-level determinants, and mechanisms by which it may affect diet and related health outcomes (Glanz et al. 2005; Kumanyika et al. 2007; Story et al. 2008; Rose et al. 2010). Building on these models, further theoretical innovations will help to advance the field, including greater incorporation of social determinants of health perspectives into these models, multilevel mediators and moderators of food environment-health relationships (and the food environment as a moderator of other risk factor-health relationships), and multiple pathways by which the food environment may affect health (Zenk et al. 2013b).

Models that explicitly contextualize local food environments as shaped by unequal distribution of resources and power can keep the nonrandom nature of differences in local food environments at the forefront and reinforce the local food environment as a social determinant of health (Schulz et al. 2002; Diez Roux and Mair 2010). Equivocal results to date may partially reflect the fact that the local food environment only matters for some subgroups and in some contexts. Identifying these moderators will help to clarify the role of the local food environment. Synergistic effects between the food environment and social environment (e.g., stress) are also possible (Diez Roux and Mair 2010). For example, it is possible that the local food environment has stronger effects on diet and health outcomes among those under stress (Ledoux et al. 2012) or that it triggers or exacerbates the effects of stress on diet (Zenk et al. 2013a). Concerning the possibility of multiple potential pathways, most research to date assumes that food access (e.g., availability, prices, quality, and marketing) and its effects on food choice is the primary pathway by which the local food environment affects health outcomes. Yet, other pathways are also possible. The local food environment, for example, can be a source of stress, such as discrimination for racial/ethnic minorities, which may have indirect effects via diet as well as direct effects on health outcomes (Zenk et al. 2013b).

Finally, another potentially fruitful area of research is testing the extent to which the local food environment moderates the effectiveness of behavioral and weight management interventions. With more research to date conducted on physical activity interventions (King et al. 2006; Zenk et al. 2009; Kerr et al. 2010; McAlexander et al. 2011), we identified one study that tested whether the local food environment moderated the effectiveness of a weight loss intervention (Samuel-Hodge et al. 2012). The authors found, for example, a larger increase in fruit and vegetable intake among intervention participants than controls who perceived low availability of produce where they shopped at baseline and suggested that the intervention may have helped these individuals learn where to obtain these foods. Research demonstrating that the local food environment impacts success in weight management interventions would have major implications for the design of future interventions.

CONCLUSIONS

Research on the local food environment and diet-related health outcomes has unfolded quickly over the past decade, with increasingly sophisticated questions and better methods. Yet, while this early research is promising, there remains no consensus on the importance of the local food environment in Americans' health. This includes what aspects of the food environment are likely to produce the largest improvements in population health and reduction in health disparities and at what spatial scale. Further research with longitudinal and quasi-experimental designs, more accurate measurement of the local food environment, and analyses with stricter controls on potential confounders, for example, will help to advance the field and provide greater clarity on promising targets for policy and other interventions.

REFERENCES

Abdullah, A., A. Peeters, M. de Courten, and J. Stoelwinder. 2010. The magnitude of association between overweight and obesity and the risk of diabetes: A meta-analysis of prospective cohort studies. *Diab Res Clin Pract* 89: 309–311.

Auchincloss, A. H., A. V. Diez Roux, D. G. Brown, C. A. Erdmann, and A. G. Bertoni. 2008. Neighborhood resources for physical activity and healthy foods and their association with insulin resistance. *Epidemiology* 19: 146–157.

Auchincloss, A. H., A. V. Diez-Roux, M. S. Mujahid, M. Shen, A. G. Bertoni, and M. R. Carnethon. 2009. Neighborhood resources for physical activity and healthy foods and incidence of type 2 diabetes mellitus: The multi-ethnic study of atherosclerosis. *Arch Intern Med* 169: 1698–1704.

Beaulac, J., E. Kristjansson, and S. Cummins. 2009. A systematic review of food deserts, 1966–2007. *Prev Chron Dis* 6: 1–10.

Black, J. L. and J. Macinko. 2008. Neighborhoods and obesity. *Nutr Rev* 66: 2–20.

Black, J. L., J. Macinko, L. B. Dixon, and G. E. Fryer Jr. 2010. Neighborhoods and obesity in New York City. *Health Place* 16: 489–499.

Bleich, S. N., B. J. Herring, D. D. Flagg, and T. L. Gary-Webb. 2012. Reduction in purchases of sugar-sweetened beverages among low-income black adolescents after exposure to caloric information. *Am J Public Health* 102: 329–335.

Block, J. P., N. A. Christakis, A. J. O'Malley, and S. V. Subramanian. 2011. Proximity to food establishments and body mass index in the Framingham heart study offspring cohort over 30 years. *Am J Epidemiol* 174: 1108–1114.

Block, J. P., R. A. Scribner, and K. B. DeSalvo. 2004. Fast-food, race/ethnicity, and income: A geographic analysis. *Am J Prev Med* 27: 211–217.

Boardman, J. D., J. M. Saint Onge, R. G. Rogers, and J. T. Denney. 2005. Race differentials in obesity: The impact of place. *J Health Soc Behav* 46: 229–243.

Bodor, J. N., J. C. Rice, T. A. Farley, C. M. Swalm, and D. Rose. 2010. The association between obesity and urban food environments. *J Urban Health* 87: 771–781.

Boehmer, T. K., C. M. Hoehner, A. D. Deshpande, L. K. Brennan Ramirez, and R. C. Brownson. 2007. Perceived and observed neighborhood indicators of obesity among urban adults. *Int J Obes* 31: 968–977.

Borradaile, K. E., S. Sherman, S. S. Vander Veur, T. McCoy, B. Sandoval, J. Nachmani, A. Karpyn, and G. D. Foster. 2009. Snacking in children: The role of urban corner stores. *Pediatrics* 124: 1293–1298.

Brown, A. F., R. B. Vargas, A. Ang, and A. R. Pebley. 2008. The neighborhood food resource environment and the health of residents with chronic conditions: The food resource environment and the health of residents. *J Gen Intern Med* 23: 1137–1144.

Burdette, H. L., and R. C. Whitaker. 2004. Neighborhood playgrounds, fast food restaurants, and crime: Relationships to overweight in low-income preschool children. *Prev Med* 38: 57–63.

Cannuscio, C. C., E. E. Weiss, and D. A. Asch. 2010. The contribution of urban foodways to health disparities. *J Urban Health* 87: 381–393.

Casagrande, S. S., M. Franco, J. Gittelsohn, A. B. Zonderman, M. K. Evans, M. Fanelli
    Kuczmarski, and T. L. Gary-Webb. 2011. Healthy food availability and the association
    with BMI in Baltimore, Maryland. *Public Health Nutr* 14: 1001–1007.
Casagrande, S. S., M. C. Whitt-Glover, K. J. Lancaster, A. M. Odoms-Young, T. L. Gary. 2009.
    Built environment and health behaviors among African Americans: A systematic review.
    Am J Prev Med 36: 174–181.
Casey, A. A., M. Elliott, K. Glanz, D. Haire-Joshu, S. L. Lovegreen, B. E. Saelens, J. F.
    Sallis, and R. C. Brownson. 2008. Impact of the food environment and physical activity
    environment on behaviors and weight status in rural U. S. communities. *Prev Med* 47:
    600–604.
Cavanaugh, E., G. Mallya, C. Brensinger, A. Tierney, and K. Glanz. 2013. Nutrition environ-
    ments in corner stores in Philadelphia. *Prev Med* 56: 149–151.
Cawley, J., and C. Meyerhoefer. 2012. The medical care costs of obesity: An instrumental
    variables approach. *J Health Econ* 31: 219–230.
Cerin, E., L. D. Frank, J. F. Sallis, B. E. Saelens, T. L. Conway, J. E. Chapman, and K. Glanz.
    2011. From neighborhood design and food options to residents' weight status. *Appetite*
    56: 693–670.
Chaix, B., K. Bean, M. Daniel, S. N. Zenk, Y. Kestens, H. Charreire, C. Leal, et al. 2012.
    Associations of supermarket characteristics with weight status and body fat: A multilevel
    analysis of individuals within supermarkets (RECORD study). *PloS One* 7: e32908.
Chang, V. W. 2006. Racial residential segregation and weight status among U. S. adults. *Soc
    Sci Med* 63: 1289–1303.
Charreire, H., R. Casey, P. Salze, C. Simon, B. Chaix, A. Banos, D. Badariotti, C. Weber, and
    J. M. Oppert. 2010. Measuring the food environment using geographical information
    systems: A methodological review. *Public Health Nutr* 13: 1773–1785.
Chen, S., R. J. Florax, S. Snyder, and C. C. Miller. 2010. Obesity and access to chain grocers.
    Econ Geogr 86: 431–452.
Chen, S. E. and R. J. Florax. 2010. Zoning for health: The obesity epidemic and opportunities
    for local policy intervention. *J Nutr* 140: 1181–1184.
Chen, S. E., R. J. Florax, and S. D. Snyder. 2012. Obesity and fast food in urban markets:
    A new approach using geo-referenced micro data. *Health Econ* 22: 835–856.
Cubbin, C., W. C. Hadden, and M. A. Winkleby. 2001. Neighborhood context and cardiovascu-
    lar disease risk factors: The contribution of material deprivation. *Ethn Dis* 11: 687–700.
Cummins, S., A. Findlay, C. Higgins, M. Petticrew, L. Sparks, and H. Thomson. 2008.
    Reducing inequalities in health and diet: Findings from a study on the impact of a food
    retail development. *Environ Plan A* 40: 402–422.
Cummins, S., D. M. Smith, M. Taylor, J. Dawson, D. Sparks Marshall L., and A. S. Anderson.
    2009. Variations in fresh fruit and vegetable quality by store type, urban-rural setting
    and neighbourhood deprivation in Scotland. *Public Health Nutr* 12: 2044–2050.
Dannefer, R., D. A. Williams, S. Baronberg, and L. Silver. 2012. Healthy bodegas: Increasing
    and promoting healthy foods at corner stores in New York City. *Am J Public Health* 102:
    e27–e31.
Davis, B. and C. Carpenter. 2009. Proximity of fast-food restaurants to schools and adolescent
    obesity. *Am J Public Health* 99: 505–510.
Dennisuk, L. A., A. J. Coutinho, S. Suratkar, P. J. Surkan, K. Christiansen, M. Riley, J. A.
    Anliker, et al. 2011. Food expenditures and food purchasing among low-income, urban,
    African-American youth. *Am J Prev Med* 40: 625–628.
Diez Roux, A. V. and C. Mair. 2010. Neighborhoods and health. *Ann N Y Acad Sci* 1186:
    125–145.
Diez Roux, A. V., S. S. Merkin, D. Arnett, L. Chambless, M. Massing, F. J. Nieto, P. Sorlie,
    M., et al. 2001. Neighborhood of residence and incidence of coronary heart disease. *N
    Engl J Med* 345: 99–106.

Drewnowski, A., A. Aggarwal, P. M. Hurvitz, P. Monsivais, and A. V. Moudon. 2012. Obesity and supermarket access: Proximity or price? *Am J Public Health* 102: 74–80.

Dubowitz, T., M. Ghosh-Dastidar, C. Eibner, M. E. Slaughter, M. Fernandes, E. A. Whitsel, C. E. Bird, et al. 2012. The women's health initiative: The food environment, neighborhood socioeconomic status, BMI, and blood pressure. *Obesity* 20: 862–871.

Dunn, R. A., J. R. Sharkey, and S Horel. 2012. The effect of fast-food availability on fast-food consumption and obesity among rural residents: An analysis by race/ethnicity. *Econ Hum Biol* 10: 1–13.

Elder, J. P., E. M. Arredondo, N. Campbell, B. Baquero, S. Duerksen, G. Ayala, N. C. Crespo, D. Slymen, and T. McKenzie. 2010. Individual, family, and community environmental correlates of obesity in Latino elementary school children [corrected] [published erratum appears in *J Sch Health* 2010 Mar;80(3):159]. *J Sch Health* 80: 20–30.

Farley, T. A., J. Rice, J. N. Bodor, D. A. Cohen, R. N. Bluthenthal, and D. Rose. 2009. Measuring the food environment: Shelf space of fruits, vegetables, and snack foods in stores. *J Urban Health* 86: 672–682.

Feng, J., T. A. Glass, F. C. Curriero, W. F. Stewart, and B. S. Schwartz. 2010. The built environment and obesity: A systematic review of the epidemiologic evidence. *Health Place* 16: 175–190.

Flegal, K. M., M. D. Carroll, B. K. Kit, and C. L. Ogden. 2012. Prevalence of obesity and trends in the distribution of body mass index among U. S. adults, 1999–2010. *JAMA* 307: 491–497.

Fleischhacker, S. E., K. R. Evenson6, D. A. Rodriguez, and A. S. Ammerman. 2011. A systematic review of fast food access studies. *Obes Rev* 12: e460–e471.

Flournoy, R. 2011. *Healthy Food, Healthy Communities: Promising Strategies to Improve Access to Fresh, Healthy Food and Transform Communities (Expanded Version).* Oakland, CA: PolicyLink.

Ford, P. and D. Dzewaltowski. 2011. Neighborhood deprivation, supermarket availability, and BMI in low-income women: A multilevel analysis. *J Community Health* 36: 785–796.

Ford, P. B., and D. A. Dzewaltowski. 2010. Limited supermarket availability is not associated with obesity risk among participants in the Kansas WIC program. *Obesity* 18: 1944–1951.

Franco, M., A. V. Diez Roux, T. A. Glass, B. Caballero, and F. L. Brancati. 2008. Neighborhood characteristics and availability of healthy foods in Baltimore. *Am J Prev Med* 35: 561–567.

Galvez, M. P., L. Hong, E. Choi, L. Liao, J. Godbold, and B. Brenner. 2009. Childhood obesity and neighborhood food-store availability in an inner-city community. *Acad Pediatr* 9: 339–343.

Gibson, D. M. 2011. The neighborhood food environment and adult weight status: Estimates from longitudinal data. *Am J Public Health* 101: 71–78.

Gittelsohn, J., M. Rowan, and P. Gadhoke. 2012. Interventions in small food stores to change the food environment, improve diet, and reduce risk of chronic disease. *Prev Chronic Dis* 9: 110015.

Glanz, K., J. F. Sallis, B. E. Saelens, and L. D. Frank. 2005. Healthy nutrition environments: Concepts and measures. *Am J Health Promot* 19: 330–333, ii.

Glanz, K., J. F. Sallis, B. E. Saelens, and L. D. Frank. 2007. Nutrition environment measures survey in stores (NEMS-S): Development and evaluation. *Am J Prev Med* 32: 282–289.

Glanz, K., M. D. M. Bader, and S. Iyer. 2012. Retail grocery store marketing strategies and obesity: An integrative review. *Am J Prev Med* 42: 503–512.

Glickman, D., L. Parker, L. J. Sim, H. Del Valle Cook, and E. A. Miller. 2012. *Accelerating Progress in Obesity Prevention: Solving the Weight of the Nation.* Washington, DC: The National Academies Press.

Golledge, R. G. and R. J. Stimson. 1997. *Spatial Behavior: A Geographic Perspective.* New York: Guilford Press.

Grier, S. A., and S. Kumanyika. 2010. Targeted marketing and public health. *Annu Rev Public Health* 31: 349–369.

Guagliardo, M. F. 2004. Spatial accessibility of primary care: Concepts, methods and challenges. *Int J Health Geogr* 3: 3.

Gustafson, A. A., J. Sharkey, C. D. Samuel-Hodge, J. C. Jones-Smith, J. Cai, and A. S. Ammerman. 2012. Food store environment modifies intervention effect on fruit and vegetable intake among low-income women in North Carolina. *J Nutr Metab*. 932653.

Gustafson, A., S. Hankins, and S. Jilcott. 2011. Measures of the consumer food store environment: A systematic review of the evidence 2000–2011. *J Commun Health* 37: 897–911.

Han, E., L. M. Powell, and Z. Isgor. 2012. Supplemental nutrition assistance program and body weight outcomes: The role of economic contextual factors. *Soc Sci Med* 74: 1874–1881.

Harris, D. E., J. W. Blum, M. Bampton, L. M. O'Brien, C. M. Beaudoin M. Polacsek, and K. A. O'Rourke. 2011. Location of food stores near schools does not predict the weight status of Maine high school students. *J Nutr Educ Behav* 43: 274–278.

Hartley, D., N. Anderson, K. Fox, and J. Lenardson. 2011. How does the rural food environment affect rural childhood obesity? *Child Obes* 7: 450–461.

Heinrich, K. M., D. Li, G. R. Regan, H. H. Howard, J. S. Ahluwalia, and R. E. Lee. 2012. Store and restaurant advertising and health of public housing residents. *Am J Health Behav* 36: 66–74.

Hickson, D. A., A. V. Diez Roux, A. E. Smith, K. L. Tucker, L. D. Gore, L. Zhang, and S. B. Wyatt. 2011. Associations of fast food restaurant availability with dietary intake and weight among African Americans in the Jackson heart study, 2000–2004. *Am J Public Health* 101 (Suppl 1): S301–S309.

Hillier, A., C. C. Cannuscio, A. Karpyn, J. McLaughlin, M. Chilton, and K. Glanz. 2011. How far do low-income parents travel to shop for food? Empirical evidence from two urban neighborhoods. *Urban Geogr* 32: 712–729.

Hilmers, A., D. C. Hilmers, and J. Dave. 2012. Neighborhood disparities in access to healthy foods and their effects on environmental justice. *Am J Public Health* 102: 1644–1645.

Hofler, M. 2005. The Bradford Hill consideration on causality: A counterfactual perspective. *Emerg Themes Epidemiol* 2: 1–9.

Horowitz, C. R., K. A. Colson, P. L. Hebert, and K. Lancaster. 2004. Barriers to buying healthy foods for people with diabetes: Evidence of environmental disparities. *Am J Public Health* 94: 1549–1554.

Hu, F. B. 2009. Diet and lifestyle influences on risk of coronary heart disease. *Curr Atheroscler Rep* 11: 257–263.

Hutchinson, P. L., J. Nicholas Bodor, C. M. Swalm, J. C. Rice, and D. Rose. 2012. Neighbourhood food environments and obesity in Southeast Louisiana. *Health Place* 18: 854–860.

Inagami, S., D. A. Cohen, A. F. Brown, and S. M. Asch. 2009. Body mass index, neighborhood fast food and restaurant concentration, and car ownership. *J Urban Health* 86: 683–695.

Inagami, S., D. A. Cohen, B. K. Finch, and S. M. Asch. 2006. You are where you shop: Grocery store locations, weight, and neighborhoods. *Am J Prev Med* 31: 10–17.

Janevic, T., L. N. Borrell, D. A. Savitz, A. H. Herring, and A. Rundle. 2010. Neighbourhood food environment and gestational diabetes in New York City. *Paediatr Perinat Epidemiol* 24: 249–254.

Jeffery, R. W., J. E. Baxter, M. T. McGuire, and J. A. Linde. 2006. Are fast food restaurants an environmental risk factor for obesity? *Int J Behav Nutr Phys Act* 3: 1–6.

Jilcott, S. B., J. T. McGuirt, S. Imai, and K. R. Evenson. 2010. Measuring the retail food environment in rural and urban North Carolina counties. *J Public Health Manage Pract* 16: 432–440.

Kerr, J., G. J. Norman, M. A. Adams, S. Ryan, L. Frank, J. F. Sallis, K. J. Calfas, and K. Patrick. 2010. Do neighborhood environments moderate the effect of physical activity lifestyle interventions in adults? *Health Place* 16: 903–908.

King, A. C., D. Toobert, D. Ahn, K. Resnicow, M. Coday, D. Riebe, C. E. Garber, S. Hurtz, J. Morton, and J. F. Sallis. 2006. Perceived environments as physical activity correlates and moderators of intervention in five studies. *Am J Health Promot* 21: 24–35.

Kumanyika, S., M. C. Whitt-Glover, T. L. Gary, T. E. Prewitt, A. M. Odoms-Young, J. Banks-Wallace, B. M. Beech, et al. 2007. Expanding the obesity research paradigm to reach African American communities. *Prev Chron Dis* 4: A112.

Kwan, M. P. and J. Weber. 2003. Individual accessibility revisited: Implications for geographical analysis in the twenty-first century. *Geogr Analysis* 35: 341–354.

Lamichhane, A. P., E. Mayer-Davis, R. Puett, M. Bottai, D. E. Porter, and A. D. Liese. 2012. Associations of built food environment with dietary intake among youth with diabetes. *J Nutr Edu Behav* 44: 217–224.

Lang, T., D. Barling, M. Caraher. 2009. Chapter 1: Introduction and Themes. In: Food Policy: Integrating health, environment and society. Oxford University Press, New York.

Larson, N. I., M. T. Story, and M. C. Nelson. 2009. Neighborhood environments disparities in access to healthy foods in the U. S. *Am J Prev Med* 36: 74–81.

Laska, M. N., K. E. Borradaile, J. Tester, G. D. Foster, and J. Gittelsohn. 2010a. Healthy food availability in small urban food stores: A comparison of four U. S. cities. *Public Health Nutr* 13: 1031–1035.

Laska, M. N., M. O. Hearst, A. Forsyth, K. E. Pasch, and L. Lytle. 2010b. Neighbourhood food environments: Are they associated with adolescent dietary intake, food purchases and weight status? *Public Health Nutr* 13: 1757–1763.

Leal, C. and B. Chaix. 2011. The influence of geographic life environments on cardiometabolic risk factors: A systematic review, a methodological assessment and a research agenda. *Obes Rev* 12: 217–230.

Ledoux, T. A., S. K. Mama, D. P. O'Connor, H. Adamus, M. L. Fraser, and R. E. Lee. 2012. Home availability and the impact of weekly stressful events are associated with fruit and vegetable intake among African American and Hispanic/Latina women. *J Obes* 2012: 737891.

Lee, H. 2012. The role of local food availability in explaining obesity risk among young school-aged children. *Soc Sci Med* 74: 1193–1203.

Leung, C. W., B. A. Laraia, M. Kelly, D. Nickleach, N. E. Adler, L. H. Kushi, and I. H. Yen. 2011. The influence of neighborhood food stores on change in young girls' body mass index. *Am J Prev Med* 41: 43–51.

Li, F., P. Harmer, and B. J. Cardinal. 2008. Built environment, adiposity, and physical activity in adults aged 50-75. *Am J Prev Med* 35: 38–46.

Li, F., P. Harmer, B. J. Cardinal, M. Bosworth, and D. Johnson-Shelton. 2009a. Obesity and the built environment: Does the density of neighborhood fast-food outlets matter? *Am J Health Promot* 23: 203–209.

Li, F., P. Harmer, B. J. Cardinal, M. Bosworth, D. Johnson-Shelton, J. J. M. Moore, A. Acock, and N. Vongjaturapat. 2009b. Built environment and 1-year change in weight and waist circumference in middle-aged and older adults: Portland neighborhood environment and health study. *Am J Epidemiol* 169: 401–408.

Li, F., P. Harmer, B. J. Cardinal, N. Vongjaturapat. 2009c. Built environment and changes in blood pressure in middle aged and older adults. *Prev Med* 48: 237–241.

Liese, A. D., K. E. Weis, D. Pluto, E. Smith, and A. Lawson. 2007. Food store types, availability, and cost of foods in a rural environment. *J Am Diet Assoc* 107: 1916–1923.

Lovasi, G. S., M. A. Hutson, M. Guerra, and K. M. Neckerman. 2009. Built environments and obesity in disadvantaged populations. *Epidemiol Rev* 31: 7–20.

Lucan, S. C., A. Karpyn, and S. Sherman. 2010. Storing empty calories and chronic disease risk: Snack-food products, nutritive content, and manufacturers in Philadelphia corner stores. *J Urban Health* 87: 394–409.

Ludwig, J., L. Sanbonmatsu, L. Gennetian, E. Adam, G. J. Duncan, L. F. Katz, R. C. Kessler, et al. 2011. Neighborhoods, obesity, and diabetes: —A randomized social experiment. *N Engl J Med* 365: 1509–1519.

McAlexander, K. M., S. K. Mama, A. Medina, D. P. O'Connor, and R. E. Lee. 2011. The concordance of directly and indirectly measured built environment attributes and physical activity adoption. *Int J Behav Nutr Phys Act* 8: 72.

Michimi, A. and M. C. Wimberly. 2010. Associations of supermarket accessibility with obesity and fruit and vegetable consumption in the conterminous United States. *Int J Health Geogr* 9: 49–63.

Millstein, R. A., S. A. Carlson, J. E. Fulton, D. A. Galuska, J. Zhang, H. M. Blanck, and B. E. Ainsworth. 2008. Relationships between body size satisfaction and weight control practices among U. S. adults. *Medscape J Med* 10: 119.

Mobley, L. R., E. D. Root, E. A. Finkelstein, O. Khavjou, R. P. Farris, and J. C. Will. 2006. Environment, obesity, and cardiovascular disease risk in low-income women. *Am J Prev Med* 30: 327–332.

Moore, L. V. and A. V. Diez Roux. 2006. Associations of neighborhood characteristics with the location and type of food stores. *Am J Public Health* 96: 325–331.

Morgenstern, L. B., J. D. Escobar, B. N. Sánchez, R. Hughes, B. G. Zuniga, N. Garcia, and L. D. Lisabeth. 2009. Fast food and neighborhood stroke risk. *Ann Neurol* 66: 165–170.

Morland, K., A. V. Diez Roux, and S. Wing. 2006. Supermarkets, other food stores, and obesity: The atherosclerosis risk in communities study. *Am J Prev Med* 30: 333–339.

Morland, K., S. Wing, A. V. Diez Roux, and C. Poole. 2002. Neighborhood characteristics associated with the location of food stores and food service places. *Am J Prev Med* 22: 23–29.

Morland, K. B. and K. R. Evenson. 2009. Obesity prevalence and the local food environment. *Health Place* 15: 491–495.

Mozaffarian, D., A. Afshin, N. L. Benowitz,, V. Bittner, S. R. Daniels, H. A. Franch, D. R. Jacobs Jr., et al. 2012. Population approaches to improve diet, physical activity, and smoking habits: A scientific statement from the American Heart Association. *Circulation* 126: 1514–1563.

Mujahid, M. S., A. V. Diez Roux, M. Shen, D. Gowda, B. Sánchez, S. Shea, D. R. Jacobs Jr., and S. A. Jackson. 2008. Relation between neighborhood environments and obesity in the multi-ethnic study of atherosclerosis. *Am J Epidemiol* 167: 1349–1357.

Pan, S. Y. and M. DesMeules. 2009. Energy intake, physical activity, energy balance, and cancer: Epidemiologic evidence. *Methods Mol Biol* 472: 191–215.

Paquet, C., L. Dube, L. Gauvin, Y. Kestens, and M. Daniel. 2010a. Sense of mastery and metabolic risk: Moderating role of the local fast-food environment. *Psychosom Med* 72: 324–331.

Paquet, C., M. Daniel, B. Knauper, L. Gauvin, Y. Kestens, and L. Dube. 2010b. Interactive effects of reward sensitivity and residential fast-food restaurant exposure on fast-food consumption. *Am J Clin Nutr* 91: 771–776.

Patterson, P. D., C. G. Moore, J. C. Probst, and J. A. Shinogle. 2004. Obesity and physical inactivity in rural America. *J Rural Health* 20: 151–159.

Powell, L. M. and E. Han. 2011. Adult obesity and the price and availability of food in the United States. *Am J Agr Econ* 93: 378–384.

Powell, L. M., J. F. Chriqui, T. Kahn, R. Wada, and F. J. Chaloupka. 2013. Assessing the potential effectiveness of food and beverage taxes and subsidies for improving public health: A systematic review of prices, demand and body weight outcomes. *Obes Rev* 14: 110–128.

Powell, L. M., M. C. Auld, F. J. Chaloupka, P. M. O'Malley, and L. D. Johnston. 2007a. Access to fast-food and food prices: Relationship with fruit and vegetable consumption and overweight among adolescents. *Adv Health Econ Health Serv Res* 17: 23–48.

Powell, L. M., M. C. Auld, F. J. Chaloupka, P. M. O'Malley, and L. D. Johnston. 2007b. Associations between access to food stores and adolescent body mass index. *Am J Prev Med* 33: S301–S307.

Powell, L. M., S. Slater, D. Mirtcheva, Y. Bao, and F. J. Chaloupka. 2007c. Food store availability and neighborhood characteristics in the United States. *Prev Med* 44: 189–195.

Raja, S., L. Yin, J. Roemmich, C. Ma, L. Epstein, P. Yadav, and A. B. Ticoalu. 2010. Food environment, built environment, and women's BMI: Evidence from Erie County, New York. *J Plan Ed Res* 29: 444–460.

Robert, S. A. and E. N. Reither. 2004. A multilevel analysis of race, community disadvantage, and body mass index among adults in the U. S. *Soc Sci Med* 59: 2421–2434.

Rose, D., J. N. Bodor, P. L. Hutchinson, and C. M. Swalm. 2010. The importance of a multidimensional approach for studying the links between food access and consumption. *J Nutr* 140: 1170–1174.

Rose, D., P. L. Hutchinson, N. Bodor, C. M. Swalm, T. A. Farley, D. A. Cohen, and J. C. Rice. 2009. Neighborhood food environments and body mass index: The importance of in-store contents. *Am J Prev Med* 37: 214–219.

Rose, D. and R. Richards. 2004. Food store access and household fruit and vegetable use among participants in the U. S. food stamp program. *Public Health Nutr* 7: 1081–1088.

Rundle, A., K. M. Neckerman, L. Freeman, G. S. Lovasi, M. Purciel, J. Quinn, C. Richards, N. Sircar, and C. Weiss. 2009. Neighborhood food environment and walkability predict obesity in New York City. *Environ Health Perspect* 117: 442–447.

Saelens, B. E., K. Glanz, J. F. Sallis, and L. D. Frank. 2007. Nutrition environment measures study in restaurants (NEMS-R): Development and evaluation. *Am J Prev Med* 32: 273–281.

Sallis, J. F. and K. Glanz. 2009. Physical activity and food environments: Solutions to the obesity epidemic. *Milbank Q* 87: 123–154.

Samuel-Hodge, C. D., B. A. Garcia, L. F. Johnston, J. L. Kraschnewski, A. A. Gustafson, A. F. Norwood, R. E. Glasgow, et al. 2012. Rationale, design, and sample characteristics of a practical randomized trial to assess a weight loss intervention for low-income women: The Weight-wise II Program. *Contemp Clin Trials* 33: 93–103.

Sánchez, B., N., E. Sanchez-Vaznaugh, A. Uscilka, J. Baek, and L. Zhang. 2012. Differential associations between the food environment near schools and childhood overweight across race/ethnicity, gender, and grade. *Am J Epidemiol* 175: 1284–1293.

Schulz, A. J., D. R. Williams, B. A. Israel, and L. B. Lempert. 2002. Racial and spatial relations as fundamental determinants of health in Detroit. *Milbank Q* 80: 677–707.

Sharkey, J. R., H. Horel, and W. R. Dean 2010. Neighborhood deprivation, vehicle ownership, and potential spatial access to a variety of fruits and vegetables in a large rural area in Texas. *Int J Health Geogr* 9: 26.

Sharkey, J. R., W. R. Dean, and C. Nalty. 2012. Convenience stores and the marketing of foods and beverages through product assortment. *Am J Prev Med* 43: S109–S115.

Shier, V., R. An, and R. Sturm. 2012. Is there a robust relationship between neighbourhood food environment and childhood obesity in the USA? *Public Health* 126: 723–730.

Sloane, D. C., A. L. Diamant, L. V. B. Lewis, A. K. Yancey, G. Flynn, L. M. Nascimento, W. J. McCarthy, et al. 2003. Improving the nutritional resource environment for healthy living through community-based participatory research. *J Gen Intern Med* 18: 568–575.

Song, H. J., J. Gittelsohn, M. Kim, S. Suratkar, S. Sharma, and J. Anliker. 2009. A corner store intervention in a low-income urban community is associated with increased availability and sales of some healthy foods. *Public Health Nutr* 12: 2060–2067.

Story, M., K. M. Kaphingst, R. Robinson-O'Brien, and K. Glanz. 2008. Creating healthy food and eating environments: Policy and environmental approaches. *Annu Rev Public Health* 29: 253–272.

Sturm, R. and A. Datar. 2005. Body mass index in elementary school children, metropolitan area food prices and food outlet density. *Public Health* 119: 1059–1068.

Truong, K., M. Fernandes, R. An, V. Shier, and R. Sturm. 2010. Measuring the physical food environment and its relationship with obesity: Evidence from California. *Public Health* 124: 115–118.

Ver Ploeg, M., V. Breneman, T. Farrigan, K. Hamrick, D. Hopkins, P. Kaufman, B. Lin, et al. 2009. *Access to Affordable and Nutritious Food—Measuring and Understanding Food Deserts and Their Consequences: Report to Congress.* Washington, DC: USDA Economic Research Service, Administrative Publication No. 036.

Wall, M. M., N. I. Larson, A. Forsyth, D. C. Van Riper, D. J. Graham, M. T. Story, and D. Neumark-Sztainer. 2012. Patterns of obesogenic neighborhood features and adolescent weight: A comparison of statistical approaches. *Am J Prev Med* 42: E65–E67.

Wang, M. C., C. Cubbin, D. Ahn, and M. A. Winkleby. 2007. Changes in neighborhood environment food behavior and body mass index, 1981–1990. *Public Health Nutr* 11: 963–970.

Wrigley, N. 2002."Food deserts" in British cities: Policy context and research priorities. *Urban Stud* 39: 2029–2040.

Zenk, S. N. 2004. *Neighborhood Racial Composition, Neighborhood Poverty, and Food Access in Metropolitan Detroit: Geographic Information Systems and Spatial Analysis.* University of Michigan.

Zenk, S. N., A. J. Schulz, B. Izumi, G. Mentz, B. A. Israel, and M. Lockett. 2013a. Neighborhood food environment role in modifying psychosocial stress-diet relationships. *Appetite* 65: 170–177.

Zenk, S. N., A. J. Schulz, B. A. Israel, G. Mentz, P. Y. Miranda, A. Opperman, and A. Odoms-Young. 2014. Food shopping behaviors and exposure to unfair treatment. *Public Health Nutr* 17: 1167–1176.

Zenk, S. N., A. J. Schulz, B. A. Israel, S. A. James, S. Bao, and M. L. Wilson. 2006. Fruit and vegetable access differs by community racial composition and socioeconomic position in Detroit, Michigan. *Ethn Dis* 16: 275–280.

Zenk, S. N., A. Odoms-Young, C. Dallas, E. Hardy, A. Watkins, J. Hoskins-Wroten, and L. Holland. 2011a. "You have to hunt for the fruits, the vegetables": Environmental barriers and adaptive strategies to acquire food in a low-income African–American community. *Health Educ Behav* 38: 282–292.

Zenk, S. N., A. J. Schulz, S. A. Matthews, A. Odoms-Young, J. Wilbur, L. Wegrzyn, K. Gibbs, C. Braunschweig, and C. Stokes. 2011b. Activity space environment and eating and physical activity behaviors: A pilot study. *Health Place* 17: 1150–1161.

Zenk, S. N., A. J. Schulz, T. Hollis-Neely, R. T. Campbell, N. Holmes, G. Watkins, R. Nwankwo, and A. Odoms-Young. 2005a. Fruit and vegetable intake in African Americans: Income and store characteristics. *Am J Prev Med* 29: 1–9.

Zenk, S. N., A. J. Schulz, T. Hollis-Neely, R. T. Campbell, N. Holmes, G. Watkins, R. Nwankwo, and A. Odoms-Young. 2005b. Neighborhood racial composition, neighborhood poverty, and the spatial accessibility of supermarkets in metropolitan Detroit. *Am J Public Health* 95: 660–667.

Zenk, S. N., J. Wilbur, E. Wang, J. McDevitt, A. Oh, R. Block, S. McNeil, and N. Savar. 2009. Neighborhood environment and adherence to a walking intervention in African–American women. *Health Educ Behav* 36: 167–181.

Zick, C. D., K. R. Smith, J. X. Fan, B. B. Brown, I. Yamada, and L. Kowaleski-Jones. 2009. Running to the store? The relationship between neighborhood environments and the risk of obesity. *Soc Sci Med* 69: 1493–1500.

7 Measurement and Analytical Issues Involved in the Estimation of the Effects of Local Food Environments on Health Behaviors and Health Outcomes

Latetia V. Moore and Ana V. Diez-Roux

Small area variations in morbidity, mortality and health related behavior have been documented consistently during the last 150 years in many countries.…. If we observe differences in health between places, these differences could be because of difference in the kinds of people who live in these places (a compositional explanation), or because of differences between the places (a contextual explanation).

Sally Macintyre and Anne Ellaway (2003)

Diet-related health conditions such as cardiovascular disease, diabetes, hypertension, some cancers, and obesity have been concerns of public health professionals for many years (U.S. Department of Agriculture and U.S. Department of Health and Human Services 2012). More recently, these professionals have been asking questions about how environmental factors may contribute to these conditions. As researchers, policymakers, practitioners, and others think about how to change the environment to support diet and health and how different features of local food environments (LFEs) affect dietary behaviors and related health outcomes, determining how the LFE varies by area and what drives that variability is not easy. The difficulty in answering these questions arises from a myriad of study design, measurement, and analytical issues. Each of these issues can significantly affect inferences regarding what influence the LFE has on purchasing behaviors, diet, and health. In this chapter, the reader is introduced to common design, measurement, and analytical issues in the research of food environments. The strengths and limitations of various design and analytical approaches with respect to their ability to estimate the causal effects of the LFE on health behaviors and health outcomes are detailed. Both established and newer methods are also discussed.

CONCEPTUAL MODELS

The fundamental questions that food environment studies are trying to address are as follows: (1) What is it about areas that matters or what are the specific area characteristics relevant to diet and health?; (2) how does it matter or what are the specific processes through which these characteristics affect diet and health?; (3) what are the spatial scales at which these processes operate, and are different scales relevant for different diet and health outcomes?; and finally, (4) can we change area characteristics and show an effect on diet and health? Fundamental to answering these questions is the development of conceptual models of the specific processes through which neighborhoods or areas may affect a given behavior or health outcome. Food environment work is frequently criticized for lacking these theoretical frameworks. These models are crucial to developing operational hypotheses that can be tested with empirical data. They are also crucial for laying out which variables of interest should be addressed as confounders, effect modifiers, or both. Greater specificity in the hypotheses carried out to date is necessary to strengthen inferences regarding causal effects of environments on health.

As in any type of research, research on the effects of LFE on health must begin with a clear articulation of the research question and the broader conceptual model within which the question is embedded. This implies specifying the spatial scale assumed to be relevant, the specific features of the LFE that are believed to be most important, the processes or mechanisms through which these features affect specific behaviors (including what behaviors they affect), and, in some cases, the links between behaviors and other outcomes such as obesity or dietary patterns. A clear articulation of the underlying conceptual models is fundamental to selecting the study design and measures, understanding the limitations of the selected study design and measures, and developing the most appropriate analytical strategy once data are collected. Graphical approaches, such as directed acyclic graphs (DAGs), can be very useful to identify the variables that must be statistically controlled to identify the causal effect of interest (Greenland et al. 1999). DAGs can also be used to identify unintended consequences of conditioning on a given variable through adjustment or situations in which intuition about what variables need to be controlled for is simply wrong (Fleischer and Diez-Roux 2008).

STUDY DESIGN

Various study designs have been used to explore the relationship between the food environment and health and behavior. A combination of factors determines what the most appropriate design is for any given context including the question to be answered, feasibility, budget, and time. The strengths and limitations of several broad types of designs that have been used in the food environment literature are discussed in this section.

Experimental Studies

Experimental studies yield the strongest causal inferences because they most closely approximate controlled laboratory experiments where the exposure is assigned, other conditions held constant, and outcomes observed. In the case of experimental studies of the LFE on diet and health, the investigator would randomly assign individuals or communities to receive improved access to healthy foods and observe whether the expanded access measurably improves diet and health. Randomization ensures that, on average, the control group is similar to the intervention groups in terms of most factors other than the intervention itself. This allows any observed effects of improved access on diet and health to be attributed to the intervention rather than to other factors.

For several reasons, including logistical and ethical issues related to the feasibility of randomization of the LFE, as well as the high cost, this type of design has rarely been used to date to assess the relationship between food environments and health. One example includes studies of specific aspects of the LFE, such as the presence of signage (Bleich et al. 2012). John Hopkins University researchers evaluated the extent to which in-store signage differentially impacts the volume of sugar-sweetened beverage purchases. Investigators randomly assigned corner stores in Baltimore into 4 groups: (1) controls, (2) those provided with calorie information, (3) those provided with calorie information relative to total recommended daily intake, and (4) those provided with calorie information relative to physical activity equivalents (Bleich et al. 2012). The authors found that providing caloric information particularly relative to a physical activity equivalent significantly reduced the odds of sugar-sweetened beverage purchases.

Another example of the use of randomization to investigate neighborhood health effects is the Moving to Opportunity study, a randomized controlled trial in which families in high-poverty neighborhoods were randomized to receive vouchers and assistance allowing them to move into nonpoor neighborhoods (Leventhal and Brooks-Gunn 2003). Notably, adults (mostly women) randomized to move to nonpoor areas experienced improvements in some mental and physical health outcomes (such as weight and diabetes risk). Although diet was not specifically evaluated, randomized studies such as this could allow for opportunities to determine whether improvements in the LFE lead to improvements in diet and health, if there was sufficient variation in environments. However, because the intervention tested in the Moving to Opportunity study was allowing families to move to other neighborhoods, rather than effecting changes in the neighborhoods themselves, the trial has limited ability to identify the specific neighborhood conditions related to the changes observed. For example, it is unclear whether observed weight reductions are attributable to better access to healthier foods, improved access to recreational resources, or some combination of these along with other contextual factors. Identifying and disentangling these specific features is fundamental to the development of place-based policies.

Although desirable, trials more directly relevant to place-based policies (including policies to affect the LFE) are challenging for several reasons. These trials require randomization of a large number of distinct areas. A large number of areas are necessary to have sufficient power to detect an association, but also to ensure that the comparison and intervention groups are similar. In addition, areas need to be distinct enough to avoid contamination of the intervention across areas. However, before undertaking randomized trials, there needs to be a clear understanding of how to select the appropriate intervention for implementation (Diez-Roux 2007). In the absence of clear evidence of what specific features of the food environment are the most influential, rigorous observational studies are still needed.

OBSERVATIONAL STUDIES

Observational studies heavily dominate the study of food environments. These designs allow investigators to explore a wider range of exposures than experimental studies at the expense of complete control over the distribution of extraneous factors that may confound the effects of the intervention. The types of observational studies most commonly used in the study of the LFE are briefly summarized in this section.

Ecologic studies are those in which the units of analysis are aggregates, such as geographic areas. Most ecologic studies are cross-sectional in that they investigate associations between independent and dependent variables at the aggregate level at a single point in time. Ecologic studies are most appropriate when both the dependent and independent variables are conceptualized as group-level constructs. For example, Reidpath et al. (2002) used an ecologic design to examine whether area socioeconomic context is associated with access to fast-food outlets. The poorest districts had 2.5 times more fast-food outlets than the wealthiest districts. This provides useful information about spatial inequities in the LFE and contextual factors associated with this spatial distribution. However, ecologic studies are more limited when interest centers on identifying factors associated with interindividual variability in an outcome. For example, an ecologic study investigating whether density of fast-food outlets across counties is related to the mean body mass index (BMI) of the county (to draw inferences about how access to fast foods affects individuals' BMI) would be subject to the ecologic fallacy because of the absence of cross-classified information on individual-level variables within counties (Aschengrau and Seage 2003).

Observational studies with individuals as units of analysis can be cross-sectional studies, cohort studies, or case–control studies. Cross-sectional and cohort studies have been most commonly used to investigate the effect of the LFE on health. Cross-sectional studies examine the relationship between the environment and other factors at one particular point in time. For example, Moore et al. (2008a) investigated the relation between two global diet indices and three complementary measures of the LFE: (1) supermarket density, (2) participant-reported assessments, and (3) aggregated survey responses of independent informants. Participants with no supermarkets near their homes were 25%–46% less likely to have a healthy diet than those with the most stores, after adjustment for age, sex, race/ethnicity, and socioeconomic indicators. Similarly, participants living in areas with the worst-ranked food environments (by participants or informants) were 22%–35% less likely to have a healthy diet than those in the best-ranked food environments. Cross-sectional studies are relatively low-cost compared to other designs as they can often be done linking existing data collected at one point in time. The major limitation of this type of design is the inability to draw causal inferences because it is not possible to determine whether the LFE exposure preceded the development of the outcome in question. This makes this design especially vulnerable to confounding because of the selection of individuals into neighborhoods (e.g., individuals predisposed to better diets seek out neighborhoods with a better LFE) and reverse causation (e.g., if the dietary preferences of residents influence the LFE).

Cohort studies are observational studies in which a sample of individuals is followed over time to assess how a given exposure, or a change in a given exposure, relates to the development of an outcome (e.g., incidence of diabetes) or to a change in an outcome over time (e.g., change in weight). A major advantage of cohort studies over other observational study designs is the ability to clearly establish whether the *exposure* preceded the development of the outcome, or whether a change in an exposure is related to a simultaneous change in the outcome. However, because of their observational nature, cohort studies are still subject to residual confounding by mismeasured or omitted variables. Auchincloss et al. (2009) examined whether neighborhood resources supporting physical activity and healthy diets are associated with a lower incidence of type 2 diabetes using 5 years of follow-up data from the Multi-Ethnic Study of Atherosclerosis. Better neighborhood resources were associated with a 38% lower incidence of type 2 diabetes. Gibson examined changes in the food environment in relation to changes in weight using data from the National Longitudinal Survey of Youth (begun in 1979) in 8770 households in the United States (Gibson 2011; U.S. Department of Labor 2012). Follow-up interviews were conducted annually until 1994 and biennialy thereafter. Gibson (2011) used individual-level data on adults from 1998 to 2004 to examine the relationship between the neighborhood food environment and adult weight status. She found that for individuals who moved from a rural area to an urban area over a 2-year period, changes in neighborhood supermarket density, small grocery store density, and full-service restaurant density were significantly related to changes in BMI over that period. Another example of a cohort study design is a study published in 2011, which used 15 years of longitudinal data to track diet quality and adherence to fruit and vegetable recommendations over time in relation to fast food and supermarket availability (Boone-Heinonen et al. 2011). In this cohort, a 1% increase in fast-food availability within 1.00 km and from 1.00 to 2.99 km was related to a 0.13% and 0.34% increase in fast-food consumption among low-income men only, but greater supermarket availability was generally unrelated to diet quality and fruit and vegetable intake.

NATURAL OR QUASI EXPERIMENTS

Because of the limitations of most observational studies in drawing causal inferences, several researchers have called for increasing the use of *natural* or quasi experiments to study the effects of neighborhood context (including the LFE) on health. Although still a type of observational study, natural experiments capitalize on changes in the LFE (e.g., store openings and closings) by strategically measuring outcomes preceding the exposure change and evaluating its impact by repeating the measurement after the change has been implemented. For example, two of the often-cited natural experiments are from the United Kingdom. Wrigley et al. (2003) found a positive but modest impact of the addition of a superstore on diet. Cummins et al. (2005) also assessed the impact of the addition of a hypermarket on diet. Although there were also positive but modest increases in fruit and vegetable intake in the intervention community, the authors did not find evidence for a net intervention effect on fruit and vegetable consumption because of equivalent increases in intake in a matched comparison community. Although randomization is not involved, this approach allows for the evaluation of a naturally occurring intervention (i.e., an intervention without the interference of the investigator) that may approximate a randomized experiment. Although potentially very useful, natural experiments are often difficult to find and may be difficult to evaluate because of the extremely time-sensitive nature of the data collection needed and the fact that often the time frame of the LFE changes is hard to reliably predict. For these reasons, most existing quasi-experimental evaluations of the LFE have been of limited scope and sample size. Nevertheless, their advantages in terms of causal inference makes them a potentially very useful approach in increasing evidence on the effect of the LFE on a range of outcomes (Diez-Roux 2007; Lytle 2009).

MEASUREMENT OF THE LOCAL FOOD ENVIRONMENT

A major challenge in studies of the LFE is the operationalization and measurement of the LFE.

As in any study, the first step is to define conceptually what aspects of the LFE are hypothesized to be related to the outcome in question. This requires defining the specific features that are thought to be of interest (e.g., local availability of different types of foods, price, quality) as well as the spatial scale within which the LFE is hypothesized to affect behavior and health (e.g., is it the local narrowly defined neighborhood or the broader geographic area within which individuals travel in their daily life?). We briefly discuss each of these two issues and then review the data sources that can be used to characterize key constructs of interest.

THEORETICALLY RELEVANT LOCAL FOOD ENVIRONMENT FEATURES

Many studies of the LFE use the phrase *access to healthy foods* to encompass a range of different features that may affect behavior and diet. Four major aspects are (1) proximity to different types of retailers, (2) selection of goods within those retailers, (3) affordability of items, and (4) quality of goods. The domain of access that is most commonly measured when investigating the food environment is proximity to different types of stores, as a proxy for proximity to retailers offering healthy food items. Of the 27 studies Larson reviewed that examined inequalities in access to food stores and healthful food products in the United States, only one study is listed as including all four major aspects of access above in the summary of findings (Larson et al. 2009). Ten summaries indicate that both proximity and selection of food items available were assessed, whereas the remainder only discusses proximity. Proximity is typically measured because it is the least burdensome and costly to assess, especially on a large scale as it can be characterized using secondary data on the geographic location of different types of stores. Collecting information on any of the other three components (i.e., selection of food items actually available in stores and their cost and quality) involves obtaining complex and often expensive price data or primary data collection, such as conducting in-store assessments, or administering a survey. Proximity is used so often to measure access that the two words are often used interchangeably in food environment research.

There is an empirical basis for using proximity to different types of stores as a proxy measure for broader access to healthy foods. Various studies indicate that the selection, quality, and affordability of healthy items vary significantly by store type. Supermarkets, supercenters, and large grocery stores tend to offer a wider selection of high-quality healthy options at affordable prices than smaller retailers, although not always consistently (Larson et al. 2009). Franco et al. (2008) conducted a cross-sectional study in 2006 to determine differences in the availability of healthy foods across 159 contiguous neighborhoods (census tracts) in Baltimore City and Baltimore County and in the 226 food stores within them. Supermarkets on average scored 75%–89% of possible points on a healthy food availability index, whereas grocery stores and convenience stores scored 14%–23% and 14%–19% of all possible points, respectively. Similarly, in a study of the selection of 5 types of healthier foods in New York City, over 90% of large stores carried all 5 types of healthier foods studied versus 63%–64% of medium stores and 13%–47% of small stores (Horowitz et al. 2004). At the same time, there is also evidence that stores classified as supermarkets can offer very different types of products in different areas. For example, Franco et al. (2008) found that supermarkets in wealthier, predominantly white areas scored better than supermarkets in predominantly black, poor areas. These results highlight the limitations of measures based on proximity to different types of stores as a proxy for overall access to healthy foods and further suggest that complementary approaches that can specifically characterize the foods available (through direct observation or surveys) are needed.

As mentioned earlier, selection of goods—often operationalized as counts of different types of healthy foods within stores—is related to the size of the store. Likewise, the rated quality of healthier options may be fairly consistent across store type and may be reasonably approximated by store type (Glanz et al. 2007; Krukowski et al. 2010). Quality has been measured as the rated appearance and freshness of perishables, such as whether or not the majority of a given type of fruit or vegetable is clearly bruised, old looking, overripe, or spotted (Glanz et al. 2007). However, with the increasing popularity of healthy corner store initiatives (Food Trust 2012) and changes to minimum stocking requirements for federal food assistance programs like the Women, Infants, and Children program (Gleason et al. 2011), it is becoming more difficult to rationalize that only larger stores typically offer a wide selection of high-quality healthier items. Affordability or price of goods within stores may be more variable. Affordability is typically operationalized as the average price of a market basket of goods or relative price differences between healthy and unhealthy choices. Some studies have reported larger stores offering more favorable pricing (Krukowski et al. 2010), whereas others have observed the inverse (Glanz et al. 2007) and variation within larger stores (Jetter and Cassady 2006).

Although a large part of access involves proximity, selection, affordability, and quality, other store characteristics can also influence purchasing behavior and diet and health. A store that offers a wide selection of affordable and high-quality fruits and vegetables, but is lacking in service or safety, may be perceived as just as inaccessible as one that has none of the traditional elements of access. For example, qualitative interviews in two Detroit neighborhoods indicated that the majority (96%) of residents were dissatisfied with at least one of their local grocery stores in regard to prices (87%), food quality (68%), selection (66%), service (34%), and cleanliness (30%) (Rose 2011). Interventions aimed at improving traditional access may not be successful in encouraging better dietary habits if these other factors are also not addressed. To date there is little empirical information on whether and how these factors are important.

SPATIAL SCALE

A fundamental problem in all research related to how residential contexts affect health is that there is still relatively little theory on the spatial scale likely to be relevant to a specific health outcome. It is very plausible that areas of different size (some of which may not be thought of as *neighborhoods* at all) could be relevant for different processes and different health outcomes. In fact, the area that a person thinks of as his or her *neighborhood* may not even be the relevant area for the outcome being studied. A priori theorizing on the links between spatial scale, mediating processes, and health outcomes is therefore a key element. Measuring the relevant attributes of these areas (many of which may not coincide with commonly used administrative areas such as census tracts) is a major challenge, but is likely to be facilitated by the growing availability of geographic information system (GIS) software and spatial analysis methods. In the absence of strong theory on the spatial scale relevant to a particular health-related process, exploratory analyses will continue to be important. At minimum, whenever possible, work should test the sensitivity of results to different spatial scales.

The vast majority of existing work has assumed that only the local area or immediate area around a person's residence is relevant to health, ignoring the possible impact of features or resources of more distant areas. However, it is unlikely that only features of the local area are relevant to a person's health. For example, poor areas spatially isolated from resource-rich, wealthy areas may be substantially worse for health than poor areas near resource-rich areas. Failure to investigate these spatial effects may result in substantial underestimation of the hypothesized area effects on health. A growing body of work has begun to investigate these spatial effects much more broadly through the incorporation of distance measures and through spatial methods that allow the simultaneous investigation of the effects of both distal and proximal areas.

Although it is not known what spatial scale is most relevant to food shopping or diet, spatial scale has been operationalized in a variety of ways. Researchers have used a range of scales from 0.25 square miles to approximate what may be considered to be an easy walking distance, to 10 miles to approximate travel patterns in less densely populated areas. Additional research on the spatial scale that is relevant to food shopping behaviors in varying contexts and for different populations will help enhance understanding of how various features of the food environment affects diet. A challenge in identifying the relevant spatial context based on observations of individuals' actual shopping behavior is the possibility that realized behavior is itself a function of spatial access (i.e., if the spatial context were different, the places where a person shops, and hence for which relevant food environment measures need to be obtained, would also be different).

DATA SOURCES USED TO CHARACTERIZE LOCAL FOOD ENVIRONMENTS

A variety of data sources can be used to assess the retail food environment. The most common are secondary data from public and commercial entities, survey data, and data derived from direct observation. Although some data sources may be better suited to measurement of some aspect of the LFE than others, there is also some overlap in the domains that can be assessed with different data sources, allowing for the evaluation of the robustness of results using alternate measures of the same construct.

Data on Location of Different Types of Stores

Commercial data directories (Centers for Disease Control and Prevention 2011) provide many relevant characteristics of stores including name, address, square footage, number of employees on payroll, whether the store is franchised, geographic coordinates, and North American Industry Classification System (NAICS) codes. Data from local, state, and federal departments of health or agriculture, telephone directories, and internet searches are also frequently used (Liese et al. 2010; USDA 2013). The benefit of using this type of data is that the exact point location of stores can be obtained, allowing investigators to link stores to a variety of geographic measures of the environment (Guagliardo 2004). For example, stores can be assigned to census tracts to investigate area-level differences in proximity (Moore and Diez-Roux 2006), used to generate densities around individuals homes (Moore et al. 2008a), or estimate nearest distance to one or more stores from an individual's home (Zenk et al. 2009). In addition to the limits of using proximity to measure access discussed previously, major disadvantages of secondary data are the amount of data reduction required to estimate access, the cost of data, and data validity concerns. To generate access estimates, data from secondary sources must often be cleaned by checking for geocoding errors, classifying businesses into relevant store types, and importing data into mapping software to assign stores to areas. Each of these steps is labor intensive and is described later in the section "Common Sources of Error When Using Locational Data." Costs vary widely based on provider, how many records are purchased, and the level of detail needed. For example, obtaining the phone numbers of establishments may cost more than only obtaining the addresses. Also, geocoding in-house versus purchasing address data that has been geocoded may lower the cost. Finally, secondary data is also limited by data validity because evidence suggests that this type of data may only capture 52%–68% of food outlets that truly exist in an area and store type misclassification is common (Paquet et al. 2008; Hoehner and Schootman 2010; Lake et al. 2010; Liese et al. 2010; Powell et al. 2011; Han et al. 2012). Combining data sources and supplementing the information provided in this data source is one solution for improving the accuracy of secondary data (Ohri-Vachaspati et al. 2011; Auchincloss et al. 2012b; Grimm et al. 2013).

An example of how secondary data can be cleaned and aggregated to explore the food environment is shown by Grimm et al. (2013), who estimated access to venues that typically sell a variety of fruits and vegetables, or healthier food retailers, across the United States and regionally, using census tracts as the unit of analysis (Grimm et al. 2013). A list of 54,622 healthier food retailers was derived from two directories, InfoUSA (2011) and Supplemental Nutrition Assistance Program (SNAP) authorized stores (USDA 2013). Healthier food retailers were identified from each source using several criteria including 2007 NAICS codes, annual sales volume, annual employees on payroll, and chain store name lists. Sixty-seven percent of the healthier food retailers identified in InfoUSA were also in SNAP ($n = 23{,}732$). The remaining 30,890 stores appeared only in one data source (11,514 InfoUSA stores, and 19,376 SNAP stores). Although measures of proximity to different types of stores have and will continue to be useful as imperfect proxies of access to healthy foods, these results highlight some of the challenges inherent in using these data sources to characterize healthy food access.

Survey Data

Surveys can also be used to obtain information on the availability of healthy food items in local areas. As mentioned earlier, stores with the same classification, such as supermarkets, may offer different goods depending on neighborhood characteristics. Survey measures may be helpful in detecting variation in healthy food availability, affordability, and quality that is not captured by proximity measures. By definition any self-reported measure reflects a combination of the objective reality and a person's perception of that objective reality, as affected by his/her knowledge and subjectivity. Survey measures can be used in two distinct ways in research on neighborhoods and health: (1) as indicators of perceptions and (2) as measures of aspects of objective reality. Survey measures are used primarily as indicators of perceptions when it is hypothesized that perception of environmental features rather than the objective reality of the environmental feature affects behavior. For example, perceptions of neighborhood safety may be more important than objective crime rates if it prevents individuals from entering local stores they perceive as unsafe. In this case, it is appropriate to relate each person's perception of his/her neighborhood to that person's behavior or health outcome. However, survey respondents can also be treated as *informants* of neighborhood conditions. In this case, the interest centers in identifying variations in objective realities across areas using the survey measure. The question of interest is not about how individual perceptions affect behavior but about how objective reality (e.g., are healthy food options available?) affects behavior. In this case, it is common to create the survey-based measure for a given area by aggregating across various respondents using empirical Bayes estimation or spatial smoothing techniques (see the next paragraph) to smooth out the influence of individual subjectivities and obtain a survey-derived measure of real variations across space. The use of measures created by aggregating the responses of multiple respondents (as opposed to individual reports) also avoids the same source bias that may arise. For example, this problem could occur if individuals that adhere to a healthier diet are more likely than those who have a poorer diet quality to report resources in their neighborhood, irrespective of the actual condition of the neighborhood.

A growing body of work has begun to focus on assessing the properties of area measures constructed by aggregating the responses of survey participants or the observations of raters. This field has been referred to as ecometrics (Raudenbush and Sampson 1999). Traditionally, psychometrics has evaluated the measurement properties of scales administered to individuals (e.g., the extent to which an individual's responses to different items of a scale are consistent with each other). Ecometrics moves beyond the individual level to an assessment of the measurement properties at the area level. If the construct of interest differs in a systematic manner across areas (and if the scale used appropriately captures this variation), respondents or raters within a given area should arguably be more likely to agree in their assessment than respondents or raters from different areas. Thus, a key indicator of the measurement properties of the area-level measure is the within-neighborhood intraclass correlation coefficient for the scale of interest, which quantifies the extent to which respondents or raters agree in their assessment of a given neighborhood. The assessment of the measurement properties of neighborhood-level measures can be assessed using three-level multilevel models (scale items nested within person nested within neighborhoods). Another issue is the construction of the aggregate measures itself, especially when the number of observations differs substantially by neighborhoods and some neighborhoods have few observations. In the case of neighborhoods with small numbers of observations, measures based simply on aggregating the observed data may have an important measurement error. The use of shrinkage estimates, such as empirical Bayes estimates, as well as the potential use of other area level covariates to improve the estimate for a given area (as in conditional empirical Bayes estimates) have been used increasingly in health research (Mujahid et al. 2007; Curl et al. 2013).

Area-level measures constructed using surveys or raters are usually estimated for predefined (and often somewhat arbitrary) geographic areas, such as census tracts. However, it may be unreasonable to think that these attributes change dramatically across these arbitrary geographic borders. More novel approaches have begun to use geostatistical methods and point data (e.g., from surveys or rater observations) to model and estimate smooth surfaces of the distribution of these attributes over space (Auchincloss et al. 2007, 2012a). This modeling takes advantage of the spatial patterning in the data and may also make use of colocated covariate information to improve predictions. For example, data on the location of supermarkets can be used to improve survey-derived estimates of the availability of healthy foods. These surfaces can be used to obtain estimates for unobserved locations and also to obtain summary measures for areas of varying size (e.g., for a given radius around each participant's home), which can then be examined in relation to health outcomes.

Few studies have compared survey-derived measures with other measures of the LFE. One study that compared survey measures with objectively measured data from store audits found no evidence that participants' perceptions differed from the reality of their LFE in terms of the availability of fresh fruits and vegetables, in particular, and healthy foods, in general, within an urban community context with high levels of household food insecurity (Freedman and Bell 2009). Another study found that survey- and GIS-based characterizations of the environment are associated, but not identical (Moore et al. 2008b). On average, respondents who lived in areas with the lowest densities of supermarkets around their home (less than 0.5 supermarkets per square mile) rated the availability of healthy foods 17% lower than those in areas with the highest densities of supermarkets. Among persons living in areas with no supermarkets, having higher densities and a larger variety of smaller stores within close proximity of the home was associated with improved perceived availability of healthy foods. Moore et al. (2012) examined the validity of reported availability using directly measured availability of healthful choices as a *gold standard*. Persons in areas with above average directly measured availability reported above-average availability 70%–80% of the time (sensitivity = 79.6% for all stores within 1 mile (1.6 km) of participants' homes and 69.6% for the store with the highest availability within 1 mile). Those with below average directly measured availability reported low availability only half the time (Moore et al. 2012). Differences between survey-derived and other measures of the LFE (based on store locations or direct observation) are difficult to interpret because all measures are likely to have substantial error. Survey measures are undoubtedly affected by resident's knowledge of the area, but may also tap into aspects that are very imperfectly captured using proximity or even direct observation data. Given the challenges in measuring the LFE, different approaches to measurement can be thought of as complementary and studies may benefit from evaluating the robustness of results to different forms of measurement (Moore et al. 2008a).

Direct Observation

Directly measuring what is available in stores is thought to be a more valid indicator of availability. Directly observing what is available in the environment allows the investigator to ensure that all types of venues are open and accurately classified and include them in assessments. Venues often omitted from secondary data, such as mobile vending, can also be included to get more comprehensive assessments of the environment. Various validated instruments and methods have been developed for the systematic direct observation of access to foods (McKinnon et al. 2009), with some designed to capture all aspects of access. The National Collaborative on Childhood Obesity Research (NCCOR) Measures Registry, a searchable database of diet and physical activity measures relevant to childhood obesity research, currently lists 93 direct observation tools (McKinnon et al. 2012). One such example is the Nutrition Environment Measures Survey for stores and restaurants (Glanz et al. 2007). This tool assesses the availability, quality, and price of healthier and less-healthy options including milk, fresh fruits and vegetables, ground beef, hot dogs, frozen dinners, baked goods, beverages (soda/juice), whole grain bread, baked chips, and cereal. The tool was found to have a high degree of inter-rater and test–retest reliability (Glanz et al. 2007). Also, it showed construct validity in that it was able to detect significant differences across store types and neighborhoods of high and low socioeconomic status (Glanz et al. 2007). However, the tool may require modifications to appropriately assess the variety of foods offered in stores in different contexts and may not be applicable to other types of stores that sell goods in communities.

Direct observation is often costly, requires training of raters, and is labor and time intensive. For these reasons, both survey measures and measures derived from secondary data are often far more feasible for studies spanning large geographic areas and will likely continue to be used in food environment research.

Types of Measures Used

Examples of the types of measures that can be created using locational, survey, and direct observation data include densities of stores per square mile (Moore et al. 2008b), reported availability of fruits and vegetables within 1 mile of home (Moore et al. 2008b), and mean linear shelf space dedicated to fruits and vegetables within stores (Bodor et al. 2008), respectively. Over 300 food environment measures are catalogued in the NCCOR Measures Registry, including the broad categories mentioned earlier and several others derived from document/sales records reviews (McKinnon et al. 2012b). Because of earlier mentioned limitations of locational or GIS-based measures, aggregating multiple data sources may help to improve accuracy. Supplementing GIS measures with survey data or direct observation data may help to improve the ability of GIS measures to assess the environment; for example, a method to weight stores differently based on empirically determined average product selection, quality, and affordability within different store types. Like GIS measures, reported measures are not perfect, but are useful for identifying areas with above average availability of healthy foods, and may feasibly offer additional insights into what foods are available in areas (Moore et al. 2012). However, they may be subject to same source bias and often lack validity and reliability testing. Both GIS-based and survey measures can be advantageous in terms of efficiency when investigating effects in a large geographic area. Direct observation tools can capture all aspects of access when appropriately designed, but at a higher cost than administering a survey or relying on GIS-based measures derived from secondary data. Which type of tool is most appropriate depends largely on the research question being asked and the population to be studied. Some tools have been tested specifically in urban contexts or only among adolescents. Of the 308 instruments catalogued in the Measures Registry to date, 216 are listed as being administered in metropolitan or urban contexts. The size of an area that needs to be assessed is often one of the most influential factors when determining what tool to select to assess the environment. For example, direct observational instruments may be used to determine how shelf space allotted to healthy foods differs between four contiguous neighborhoods (Bodor et al. 2008), whereas GIS-based measures may be more efficient when assessing differences in the availability of stores across a large number of diverse neighborhoods (Moore and Diez-Roux 2006).

Because of time and resource limitations, the best choice of food environment measurement tool can also vary from study to study. However, some key concepts should be incorporated depending on which type of measure is selected. GIS-based measures may benefit from the combination of several different data sources to improve the locational data available and the classification of stores into types. Survey measures should ideally have been tested in the target population in which they will be used. Finally, regardless of whether using secondary data, survey data, or data from direct observations, validity and reliability testing is necessary. The state of the science regarding the psychometric and ecometric standards for environmental measures is in its infancy (Lytle 2009). In a review of 48 instruments that assess the food environment, only 39% were tested for validity or reliability (Ohri-Vachaspati and Leviton 2010). Another review by McKinnon et al. (2009) concluded only 13.1% of the 137 articles that measured the community-level food environment mentioned psychometric properties of measures.

Instruments used to characterize food options in a community generally report good to excellent reliability, particularly when documenting the presence of foods in a store or restaurant (Lytle 2009). The most commonly cited psychometric properties of food environment tools are inter-rater and test–retest reliability and internal consistency. For example, Glanz et al. (2007) assessed inter-rater reliability by having two trained raters independently visit food outlets to complete the same set of assessments on the same day. To assess test–retest reliability, outlets were reassessed within 1 month after the initial observations by one of the same raters. In the Nutrition Environment Measures Survey in Stores (NEMS-S) tool, construct validity was evaluated by testing the tool's ability to discriminate between types of stores (grocery stores vs. convenience stores) and between the healthfulness of foods in stores (Glanz et al. 2007). Using NEMS-S as a pseudo-gold standard, Moore et al. (2012) examined how different survey measures performed. The sensitivity and specificity of self-reported measures of availability compared with direct measures were 69.6%–79.6% and 46.8–50.9%, respectively. The lack of a gold standard that quantifies relevant features of the food environment and which can be used to gauge the accuracy of newly developed instruments continue to limit the field and validity testing.

ANALYTICAL ISSUES

Key analytical issues when investigating the effect of the LFE on diet and health include (1) measurement error in exposure and outcome, (2) accounting for confounding at the area and individual level, (3) effect modification, (4) time lags and time-dependent confounding, and (5) dynamic relations and reverse causation.

MEASUREMENT ERROR IN EXPOSURE AND OUTCOME

Measurement error is an important source of bias in LFE research. Although often nondifferential measurement error will result in bias toward the null, this may not always be the case and differential measurement error that can result in bias away from or toward the null is also possible. In the case of measures based on surveys or raters assessments, measurement error may arise from poor psychometric or ecometric properties of scales or rating instruments (such as, low internal consistency of a scale, low inter-rater reliability, or low intra-class correlation for reports within a neighborhood). Other sources of measurement error that may arise when locational data are used include store type misclassification, operational status errors, and geocoding errors.

Common Sources of Error When Using Locational Data

Store type misclassification, operational status errors, and geocoding errors may lead an investigator to assume a store is operational when it is not, assign it to the wrong area because of geocoding variability, or not count a store because it is incorrectly classified, respectively. Each has the potential to distort the association between the environment and diet and health, thus data cleaning is necessary. In regard to store misclassification, Han et al. (2012) found Dun & Bradstreet (D&B) had a higher classification match rate than InfoUSA for supermarkets and grocery stores (91% of supermarkets and 75% of grocery stores on the ground were similarly classified in D&B vs. 81% of supermarkets and 69% of grocery stores on the ground were listed as supermarkets and grocery stores in InfoUSA). However, InfoUSA had a higher classification match rate than D&B for convenience stores with approximately half of convenience stores on the ground classified correctly in InfoUSA versus 24% of convenience stores in D&B. Both lists were more likely to correctly classify large supermarkets, grocery stores, and convenience stores with more cash registers and different types of service counters (supermarkets and grocery stores only). The likelihood of a correct classification match for supermarkets and grocery stores did not vary systemically by tract characteristics, whereas convenience stores were more likely to be misclassified in predominantly black tracts. On the other hand, Bader et al. (2010) found that although most business types were more likely to be reported by direct observations than in the commercial database listings, disagreement between the two sources was not significantly correlated with the socioeconomic and demographic characteristics of neighborhoods. The authors concluded researchers should have reasonable confidence using whichever method (or combination of methods) is most cost-effective and theoretically appropriate for their research design. Conflicting evidence as the field continues to develop should prompt all investigators to cautiously use store type classification information from one source. A more robust practice is to use at least two sources to verify store information (Auchincloss et al. 2012b; Grimm et al. 2013).

Operational status errors, or misclassifying whether a store exists and is open, are also common. Secondary data have been shown to represent only 52%–68% of food outlets that truly exist in an area (Hoehner et al. 2005; Paquet et al. 2008; Lake et al. 2010; Liese et al. 2010; Powell et al. 2011; Han et al. 2012). Given that a store appears on a commercial database list, one can expect it is both present and open 45%–90% of the time (i.e., positive predictive values ranged from 0.45 in some urban areas to 0.89 in a study of rural areas) (Liese et al. 2010; Powell et al. 2011). Values were even lower when stratified by type of store. Using midpoints from ranges of sensitivities and positive predictive values reported by Han and Liese (Han et al. 2012; Liese et al. 2010), the probability that a store is both operational and classified appropriately is only about 53%. This further emphasizes the earlier point that using data from one source may no longer be a good practice. Methods for systematically handling disagreement between sources area are still needed.

Finally, geospatial accuracy also varies. Liese et al. (2010) reported that more than 80% of outlets were geocoded to the correct U.S. census tract, but only 29%–39% were correctly allocated within 100 m. Because food environment work using secondary data largely depends on accurately assigning environmental exposures to locations of people to investigate the impact of the environment on diet and health, geocoding errors can introduce a significant amount of measurement error depending on the spatial scale chosen. Although likely not as problematic when looking at larger spatial scales such as census tracts (as indicated by the results of Liese et al.), when examining smaller areas it may be good practice to check a random sample of geocoded stores to identify the magnitude of any bias that could be introduced.

Sources of Error in Survey Data

Same source bias, that is the possibility of a spurious association between self-reported exposure and a self-reported outcome, is one possible manifestation of error in survey measures. This can occur because the measurement error in both reports is correlated or because the outcome affects the perception or report of the neighborhood attribute (Diez-Roux 2007). For example, persons who report eating healthier diets may be more likely to report healthy food resources in their neighborhood than those who report consuming a less healthy diet, irrespective of the actual condition of the neighborhood. The same source bias problem is obviously not present when the health outcome is directly measured by the investigator as opposed to self-reported. But even in the case of directly measured outcomes, a limitation of the use of participant reports is that each measure is based on the report of a single participant, and individual reports of neighborhood conditions may have substantial error. This bias may arise from the simple lack of knowledge on the resident's part of certain conditions in the neighborhood, and from the necessarily subjective nature of perceptions. Of course, if it is hypothesized that an individual's perception of neighborhood conditions is the construct relevant to health (as opposed to the objective condition), then participant self-reports are the measure of choice, although the interpretation of results may be rendered complex by the same source bias issue alluded to earlier.

An alternative to the use of each participant's self-report of neighborhood characteristics is to combine the responses of several residents of the same neighborhood (Moore et al. 2008a). Theoretically, by averaging over measurement error in individual responses, this aggregation process may yield a more valid measure of the *objective* neighborhood construct of interest. This approach can be implemented by aggregating responses of participants in a health study to characterize a given neighborhood represented in the study, or by conducting a separate survey colocated with health study participants to derive measures for areas that can then be linked to health study participants based on their place of residence. The rationale for conducting a separate survey is twofold: (1) the focus of the survey is assessment of area or neighborhood characteristics and hence a more detailed assessment can be included than is possible in the health study itself (where neighborhoods are only one of several domains being assessed), and (2) the separate survey allows for denser sampling in space, which is likely to improve estimation of the area-level construct of interest.

In some cases, it may be advantageous to combine separate survey approach with a similar data collection approach targeted at the health study participants themselves. This would allow simultaneous investigation of the self-reported, individual-level perceived measure and the aggregate (potentially more *objective*) neighborhood-level measure. An alternative to conducting a separate survey is to employ trained raters to evaluate neighborhoods in systematic manner on prespecified dimensions. It has the advantage that raters can be trained and assessments can be conducted in a systematic and quality-controlled manner. A disadvantage is that some constructs (e.g., social cohesion) may not be measurable using this approach because their assessment necessitates the knowledge and perceptions of residents. The logistics and cost of systematic social observation also make it a difficult approach to implement across very broad geographic areas. Other sources of error in survey and rater measures include poor psychometric or ecometric properties of the scales or assessment instruments being used.

Measurement Errors in Outcomes

The NCCOR Measures Registry currently lists 250 individual dietary behavior assessment tools including 24-hour recalls, food frequency questionnaires, and other types of surveys and logs (McKinnon et al. 2012). Despite the abundance of tools, there is no error-free way to objectively assess dietary intake. Even direct observation of diet is prone to observer bias in that subjects may change their dietary habits while under observation making the recorded observations unrepresentative of their usual intake. When measuring the association between LFE and diet, in addition to the measurement error inherent in dietary assessment tools themselves, it is unclear whether global dietary patterns, individual foods, or nutrients should be the dietary outcome of interest. Moore et al. (2008a) used two measures of global dietary quality when assessing the link between diet and the food environment. The first, the Alternate Healthy Eating Index, is based on dietary behaviors that have been shown to be associated with a lower risk of chronic disease (McCullough et al. 2002). This index also encompasses many federal dietary guidance recommendations thus offering a way to compare what people are eating versus what they should be eating. The second index, an empirically derived dietary pattern characterized by high consumption of fats and processed meats, on the other hand, represents a constellation of actual dietary practices observed in the study population. Each provides a unique perspective on eating behaviors, and each was differentially associated with other individual-level characteristics, such as race/ethnicity and income in the study. In spite of these differences, better diet quality was associated with living in better food environments. On the other hand, utilizing intake of individual foods such as fruits and vegetables or nutrients such as fat rather than aggregate dietary patterns may be more readily interpretable (i.e., Black Americans' fruit and vegetable intake increased by 32% for each additional supermarket in the census tract) (Morland et al. 2002). Examining consumption of individual foods and nutrients such as fruits and vegetables (Morland et al. 2002) or fat (French et al. 2000) may also be advantageous when investigating access to specific food groups. For example, it may make more sense to examine fat intake rather than global diet when examining access to energy-dense foods in convenience stores near schools. Ideally, the specific outcome being investigated should be driven by the underlying theoretical model of what specific features of the LFE are the most relevant and how they may affect specific or general features of diet.

An important issue in the study of how the LFE affects diet is establishing the correct functional form of the relationship. Evidence has been mixed of whether there is a linear dose–response relationship of the LFE with diet or whether there are threshold effects. Morland and Rose both reported greater produce consumption for each additional supermarket in neighborhoods (Morland et al. 2002; Rose and Richards 2004). Moore found evidence of a dose–response relation between the LFE and diet quality for only one of the two dietary patterns examined (Moore et al.

2008a). Laraia et al. (2004) found that intake was lower only among persons who lived farthest from a supermarket. If a dose–response relationship is expected, then a continuous measure of diet can be modeled as a function of continuous environmental variables. Anticipated threshold effects require categorical modeling techniques or splines. The dietary outcome can also be treated as a continuous or categorical outcome, depending on the research question at hand and the way in which the LFE is hypothesized to operate (e.g., is it expected to shift the whole distribution of a given dietary parameter in one direction, or is it expected to affect the probability of achieving a certain threshold of intake on the diet).

ACCOUNTING FOR CONFOUNDING AT THE AREA AND INDIVIDUAL LEVELS

The majority of work on food environment effects has been observational. The fundamental critique of this type of analysis has been that persons exposed and unexposed to the neighborhood characteristic of interest differ in other factors related to the outcome, which will confound any associations of neighborhood characteristics with health outcomes. This issue of confounding has also been referred to as *the selection problem* (because persons are selected or select themselves into neighborhoods based on individual characteristics related to the outcome) and nonexchangeability of exposed and unexposed. Nonexchangeability implies that the observational comparison does a poor job of approximating the counterfactual contrast necessary for drawing causal inferences.

The traditional approach to this problem in epidemiology is to estimate associations after adjusting for individual-level confounders using stratification or regression approaches, such as multilevel models. Critics have argued that this approach often relies on extrapolations beyond the range observed in the data because of the limited overlap in individual-level characteristics for persons living in different types of neighborhoods. The extent to which persons living in *exposed* and *unexposed* neighborhoods are comparable in individual-level characteristics, as well as the extent to which distributions overlap, can be (and should be) empirically examined in the data before any adjustment is performed. The amount of overlap in the distributions necessary for the adjusted estimate to be *valid* ultimately depends on the assumptions one is willing to make. Reporting the actual distributions, and therefore making the assumptions explicit, is important. The extent to which nonexchangeability and nonoverlapping distributions are a problem may also differ substantially depending on the sample and on the specific neighborhood characteristic being examined. For example, nonoverlapping distributions in individual-level socioeconomic indicators may be a problem when extreme categories of neighborhoods classified based on aggregate socioeconomic position measures are compared. However, it may be less of a problem when specific environmental features are examined.

Propensity score approaches have increasingly been used as an alternative to regression adjustment in studies of neighborhood effects (Rubin 1997; Joffe and Rosenbaum 1999). An advantage of propensity score matching is that it allows estimates to be derived from subgroups of the sample, which are directly comparable. A limitation is that propensity score matching estimates the association of interest using a selected subgroup; hence, it may not be generalizable to the full sample of interest. In addition, propensity score approaches obviously do not solve the problem of mismeasured or unmeasured confounders. Another causal inference technique that may be useful is instrumental variables (Glymour 2006; Martens et al. 2006). A valid instrument is a variable that is associated with the exposure (in this case the LFE) but is not linked to the outcome through any other mechanism—it is linked to the outcome only through its association with the exposure. For example, to the extent that zoning laws affect the location of healthy food stores but are otherwise unrelated to the diets of residents, zoning laws can be used as an instrument for the LFE. A recent article has used proximity to highways as an instrument for exposure to restaurants (Anderson and Matsa 2011). The use of instruments avoids the bias generated by confounders (i.e., a cause of both diet and exposure to a certain kind of LFE), as well as reverse causation (diet affects the LFE). Unfortunately, valid instruments are often difficult to find because it is challenging to identify a variable that is associated with the exposure, yet has no other links to the outcome (e.g., if zoning laws were related to area race composition and related to diet through other mechanisms, then zoning laws would not be a valid instrument).

An additional complexity in studying the effects of the LFE on health is that other area-level variables may also operate as confounders. For example, a study investigating the impact of the LFE on BMI may need to adjust for neighborhood characteristics related to physical activity that could also affect BMI. An important challenge is that area features may often be highly correlated, making it difficult to estimate their *independent* effects. Yet another challenge in estimating environmental effects pertains to identifying which variables are true confounders (and hence should be adjusted for) and which are mediators (and hence should not). Some variables could conceivably be both confounders and mediators (see section on time lags and time-dependent confounding). Developing a plausible theoretical model or causal diagram is likely to be helpful when determining which variables are confounders and which are mediators.

Studies adjusting for a variety of neighborhood and individual factors when examining LFE associations with diet and health still face the possibility of residual confounding by mismeasured or omitted variables. No amount of standard statistical adjustment is likely to control for all individual life course and neighborhood factors. Alternative study designs that may capitalize on natural experiments or even randomized experiments wherever possible are needed.

EFFECT MODIFICATION

In addition to adjusting for extraneous factors to rule out alternative explanations of the association between LFE and outcomes of interest, exploring effect modification is also important. For example, does the relationship between spatial proximity to healthy food stores and diet vary by car ownership? Sometimes showing effect modification that would be expected if the association were causal is one way of strengthening the causal conclusions that can be drawn. For example, it might be reasonable to expect that if spatial access to healthy stores is causally associated with diet, the association will be stronger in persons with limited access to transportation.

Effect modification can be explored through stratified analyses or by incorporating interactions into regression models. Effect modification by individual characteristics (e.g., car ownership) and area-level characteristics (e.g., urbanicity) are both possible. For example, Moore and Diez-Roux (2006) found city-specific differences in the association of the LFE with neighborhood racial/ethnic composition and neighborhood income, suggesting that broader contextual features that vary from city to city may affect the extent to which the LFE is associated with other social characteristics. In another example of effect modification by area characteristics, area transportation features could modify the relation between proximity to healthy stores and dietary patterns. In an example of interaction between the LFE and individual characteristics, Boone-Heinonen found that fast-food consumption was related to fast-food availability among low-income men but not women (Boone-Heinonen et al. 2011).

TIME LAGS AND TIME-DEPENDENT CONFOUNDING

In studying the effects of the LFE on diet it is important to consider the expected time lag between the exposure and the manifestation of its potential diet or health effect. This is especially important in longitudinal studies that investigate how changes in the LFE may be related to changes in health-related outcomes. For example, effects on dietary behavior may occur relatively quickly when the environment changes, whereas other effects (such as effects on BMI, hypertension, or diabetes) may take much longer to manifest themselves.

The fact that the LFE is dynamic and changes over time also has important measurement implications, especially when the exposure and the outcome are not measured at the same time. Many studies use a single measure of the LFE to characterize exposure over an often much longer causally relevant exposure period. Relatively few studies have investigated the stability of the LFE or how this may be patterned by other area characteristics. In one study of three sites, overall, 62% of stores did not change names or locations in adjacent years (Moore 2007). The average number of stores in census tracts also did not change significantly. This would suggest that a measure at one point in time is a relatively stable measure of exposure over a longer time frame. More work is needed to characterize the extent to which changes are occurring on the LFE and whether these changes can be adequately characterized using available measures.

As discussed earlier, it is important for researchers to carefully consider what variables may be confounders and what variables may be mediators of the effects they are attempting to estimate. However, in the context of longitudinal studies, it is possible for a variable to be simultaneously a confounder and a mediator. For example, in a study of how the LFE affects BMI, diet may be in the causal pathway (i.e., a mediator), but may also affect future residential locations and exposure to the LFE (if persons with better diets choose to live in areas with better food access) making it also a confounder. By controlling for individual-level diet, traditional regression analytic techniques may underestimate the effects of the LFE on BMI (because they control for a mediator), but failure to control for diet may result in confounding. One solution to this conundrum is marginal structural modeling. When contextual exposures, outcomes, and confounders vary over time, marginal structural models can be used to properly account for time-dependent covariates that act simultaneously as confounders and as intermediate variables in the causal pathway between the neighborhood exposure of interest and the outcome (Robins et al. 2000). For example, marginal structural models have been used to estimate the causal relationship between a time-varying exposure such as neighborhood poverty and alcohol use allowing for control of time-varying confounders without conditioning on these variables (Cerda et al. 2010). Although highly applicable to LFE research, these models have not been used to date.

REVERSE CAUSATION AND DYNAMIC RELATIONS

Reverse causation is a common limitation of LFE studies because of the cross-sectional nature of most of these studies. Cross-sectional analyses cannot rule out the possibility that ill-health causes people to see their neighborhoods in a more negative light or that health consciousness prompts people to move to healthier neighborhoods. Studies with a prospective design are needed to address this common limitation.

An important challenge in estimating the causal effects of neighborhood characteristics on health is that the spatial patterning of health emerges from the functioning of a system in which individuals interact with each other and their environment and in which both individuals and environments adapt and change over time. Thus, neighborhood spatial patterning of health results from a web of conditions, dependencies, and feedback loops. Persons are sorted (or selected) into neighborhoods based on external constraints related to socioeconomic resources and discrimination, as well as preferences for neighborhoods with particular features. These selection processes lead to spatial clustering by individual-level attributes (e.g., income) that are related to health behaviors. Health behaviors are, in turn, affected by features of residential environments, such as whether the environment has recreational resources and places to purchase healthy foods. Norms may emerge in the context of places as a result of the predominant health behaviors in the area and individual health behaviors may in turn change in response to these norms. Neighborhoods also change in response to residents' characteristics and preferences, and in response to the features of surrounding or related neighborhoods. Neighborhood differences in health behaviors (and health more generally) emerge from the simultaneous operation of all these processes making it challenging to empirically isolate one from the other.

In general, regression approaches are not well suited to investigate processes embedded in complex systems characterized by dynamic interactions between heterogeneous individuals and interactions between individuals and their environment with multiple feedback loops and adaptation (Auchincloss and Diez-Roux 2008). Aside from logistical difficulties, experimental approaches (which attempt to isolate the effect of changing a single factor while holding all other features of the system constant) may not yield easily generalizable results in the context of dynamic interactions and feedback loops. Identifying the interventions most likely to be effective under different circumstances requires understanding the processes involved. Experiments and their observational approximations yield little insights into these processes, particularly when they involve feedback loops and adaptation. Yet, understanding these processes may be important for predicting the effects of the intervention under other scenarios, and for identifying alternate interventions that may achieve the desired effect.

For these reasons, it has been argued that complex systems methodologies, such as agent-based models, may be a useful complement to existing observational and experimental studies (Auchincloss and Diez-Roux 2008). Systems methodologies raise their own sets of nontrivial challenges (Auchincloss and Diez-Roux 2008). Although all types of modeling should hypothesize processes to help in the selection of variables or understanding whether variables should be considered modifiers, confounders, or mediators, agent-based models force investigators to specify and model processes. Aside from the utility of these models in simulating outcomes under different scenarios, the simple formulation of these models may yield new insights into what is known and unknown about the processes involved and point to the need for new types of data. These approaches have been increasingly used to examine how neighborhood environments shape behaviors (Yang et al. 2011). In an application of these tools, Auchincloss et al. (2011) used an agent-based model to examine the contribution of segregation and spatial inequities in the distribution of food access to inequalities in diet, as well as the impact of intervention strategies (related to cost and health education) on these inequalities. The use of these methodologies as a complement to existing approaches is an exciting new direction in this field.

As in other complex public health questions, understanding the impact of the LFE on diet and related outcomes will require using a variety of complementary methods, including rigorous observational studies (especially longitudinal studies), state-of-the-art analytical approaches to improve causal inference, evaluations of natural experiments, or experiments when possible, and simulation approaches as well as qualitative studies.

REFERENCES

Anderson, M.L. and D.A. Matsa. 2011. Are restaurants really supersizing America? *Am Econ J App Econ* 3(1): 152–188.

Aschengrau, A. and G.R. Seage III. 2003. Overview of epidemiologic study designs. In *Essentials of Epidemiology in Public Health*, pp. 135–162. Sudbury, MA: Jones and Bartlett.

Auchincloss, A.H., A.V. Diez-Roux, D.G. Brown, T.E. Raghunathan, and C.A. Erdmann. 2007. Filling the gaps: Spatial interpolation of residential survey data in the estimation of neighborhood characteristics. *Epidemiology* 18(4): 469–478.

Auchincloss, A.H. and A.V. Diez-Roux. 2008. A new tool for epidemiology: The usefulness of dynamic-agent models in understanding place effects on health. *Am J Epidemiol* 168(1): 1–8.

Auchincloss, A.H., A.V. Diez-Roux, M.S. Mujahid, M.W. Shen, A.G. Bertoni, and M.R. Carnethon. 2009. Neighborhood resources for physical activity and healthy foods and incidence of type 2 diabetes mellitus: The multi-ethnic study of atherosclerosis. *Arch Intern Med* 169(18): 1698–1704.

Auchincloss, A.H., R.L. Riolo, D.G. Brown, J. Cook, and A.V. Diez-Roux. 2011. An agent-based model of income inequalities in diet in the context of residential segregation. *Am J Prev Med* 40(3): 303–311.

Auchincloss, A.H., S.Y. Gebreab, C. Mair, and A.V. Diez-Roux. 2012a. A review of spatial methods in epidemiology, 2000–2010. *Annu Rev Public Health* 33: 107–122.

Auchincloss, A.H., K.A.B. Moore, L.V. Moore, and A.V. Diez-Roux. 2012b. Improving retrospective characterization of the food environment for a large region in the United States during a historic time period. *Health Place* 18(6): 1341–1347.

Bader, M.D., J.A. Ailshire, J.D. Morenoff, and J.S. House. 2010. Measurement of the local food environment: A comparison of existing data sources. *Am J Epidemiol* 171(5): 609–617.

Bleich, S.N., B.J. Herring, D.D. Flagg, and T.L. Gary-Webb. 2012. Reduction in purchases of sugar-sweetened beverages among low-income Black adolescents after exposure to caloric information. *Am J Public Health* 102(2): 329–335.

Bodor, J.N., D. Rose, T.A. Farley, C. Swalm, and S.K. Scott. 2008. Neighbourhood fruit and vegetable availability and consumption: The role of small food stores in an urban environment. *Public Health Nutr* 11(4): 413–420.

Boone-Heinonen, J., P. Gordon-Larsen, C.I. Kiefe, J.M. Shikany, C.E. Lewis, and B.M. Popkin. 2011. Fast food restaurants and food stores: Longitudinal associations with diet in young to middle-aged adults: The CARDIA study. *Arch Intern Med* 171(13): 1162–1170.

Centers for Disease Control and Prevention. 2011. Healthier Food Retail: Beginning the Assessment Process in Your State or Community. www.cdc.gov/obesity/downloads/hfrassessment.pdf (Accessed September 12, 2013).

Cerda, M., A.V. Diez-Roux, E.T. Tchetgen, P. Gordon-Larsen, and C. Kiefe. 2010. The relationship between neighborhood poverty and alcohol use: Estimation by marginal structural models. *Epidemiology* 21(4): 482–489.

Cummins, S., M. Petticrew, C. Higgins, A. Findlay, and L. Sparks. 2005. Large scale food retailing as an intervention for diet and health: Quasi-experimental evaluation of a natural experiment. *J Epidemiol Community Health* 59(12): 1035–1040.

Curl, C.L., S.A.A. Beresford, A. Hajat, J.D. Kaufman, K. Moore, J.A. Nettleton, and A.V. Diez-Roux. 2013. Associations of organic produce consumption with socioeconomic status and the local food environment: Multi-ethnic study of atherosclerosis (MESA). *PLoS One* 8(7): e69778.

Diez-Roux A.V. 2007. Neighborhoods and health: Where are we and where do we go from here? *Rev Epidemiol Sante Publique* 55(1): 13–21.

Fleischer, N.L. and A.V. Diez-Roux. 2008. Using directed acyclic graphs to guide analyses of neighbourhood health effects: An introduction. *J Epidemiol Community Health* 62(9): 842–846.

Food Trust. 2012. What we do: In corner stores. http://thefoodtrust.org/what-we-do/corner-store (Accessed September 12, 2013).

Franco, M., A.V. Diez-Roux, T.A. Glass, B. Caballero, and F.L. Brancati. 2008. Neighborhood characteristics and availability of healthy foods in Baltimore. *Am J Prev Med* 35(6): 561–567.

Freedman, D.A. and B.A. Bell. 2009. Access to healthful foods among an urban food insecure population: Perceptions versus reality. *J Urban Health* 86(6): 825–838.

French, S.A., L. Harnack, and R.W. Jeffery. 2000. Fast food restaurant use among women in the Pound of Prevention study: Dietary, behavioral and demographic correlates. *Int J Obes Relat Metab Disord* 24(10): 1353–1359.

Gibson, D.M. 2011. The neighborhood food environment and adult weight status: Estimates from longitudinal data. *Am J Public Health* 101(1): 71–78.

Glanz, K., J.F. Sallis, B.E. Saelens, and L.D. Frank. 2007. Nutrition environment measures survey in stores (NEMS-S): Development and evaluation. *Am J Prev Med* 32(4): 282–289.

Gleason, S., R. Morgan, L. Bell, and J. Pooler. 2011. Impact of the Revised WIC Food Package on Small WIC Vendors: Insights From a Four-State Evaluation. Washington, DC: Altarum Institute.

Glymour, M. 2006. Natural experiments and instrumental variable analyses in social epidemiology. In *Methods in Social Epidemiology*, edited by J.M. Oakes and J.S. Kaufman. San Francisco: Jossey Bass.

Greenland, S., J. Pearl, and J.M. Robins. 1999. Causal diagrams for epidemiologic research. *Epidemiology* 10(1): 37–48.

Grimm, K., L.V. Moore, and K. Scanlon. 2013. Access to healthier food retailers—United States, 2011. *MMWR* 62(3): 20–26.

Guagliardo, M.F. 2004. Spatial accessibility of primary care: Concepts, methods and challenges. *Int J Health Geogr* 3(1): 3.

Han, E., L. Powell, S. Zenk, L. Rimkus, P. Ohri-Vachaspati, and F. Chaloupka. 2012. Classification bias in commercial business lists for retail food stores in the U.S. *Int J Behav Nutr Phys Act* 9(1): 46.

Hoehner, C.M., L.K.B. Ramirez, M.B. Elliott, S.L. Handy, and R.C. Brownson. 2005. Perceived and objective environmental measures and physical activity among urban adults. *Am J Prev Med* 28(2): 105–116.

Hoehner, C.M. and M. Schootman. 2010. Concordance of commercial data sources for neighborhood-effects studies. *J Urban Health* 87(4): 713–725.

Horowitz, C.R., K.A. Colson, P.L. Hebert, and K. Lancaster. 2004. Barriers to buying healthy foods for people with diabetes: evidence of environmental disparities. *Am J Public Health* 94(9): 1549–1554.

InfoUSA. 2011. Database of U.S. businesses, vol. 2011. http://www.infousa.com/business-lists/ (Accessed October 28, 2013).

Jetter, K.M. and D.L. Cassady. 2006. The availability and cost of healthier food alternatives. *Am J Prev Med* 30(1): 38–44.

Joffe, M.M. and P.R. Rosenbaum. 1999. Invited commentary: Propensity scores. *Am J Epidemiol* 150(4): 327–333.

Krukowski, R.A., D.S. West, J. Harvey-Berino, and T.E. Prewitt. 2010. Neighborhood impact on healthy food availability and pricing in food stores. *J Community Health* 35(3): 315–320.

Lake, A.A., T. Burgoine, F. Greenhalgh, E. Stamp, and R. Tyrrell. 2010. The foodscape: Classification and field validation of secondary data sources. *Health Place* 16(4): 666–673.

Laraia, B.A., A.M. Siega-Riz, J.S. Kaufman, and S.J. Jones. 2004. Proximity of supermarkets is positively associated with diet quality index for pregnancy. *Prev Med* 39(5): 869–875.

Larson, N.I., M.T. Story, and M.C. Nelson. 2009. Neighborhood environments: Disparities in access to healthy foods in the U.S. *Am J Prev Med* 36(1): 74–81.

Leventhal, T. and J. Brooks-Gunn. 2003. Moving to opportunity: An experimental study of neighborhood effects on mental health. *Am J Public Health* 93(9): 1576–1582.

Liese, A.D., N. Colabianchi, A.P. Lamichhane, T.L. Barnes, J.D. Hibbert, D.E. Porter, M.D. Nichols, and A.B. Lawson. 2010. Validation of 3 food outlet databases: Completeness and geospatial accuracy in rural and urban food environments. *Am J Epidemiol* 172(11): 1324–1333.

Lytle, L.A. 2009. Measuring the food environment: State of the science. *Am J Prev Med* 36(4): S134–S144.

Macintyre, S. and A. Ellaway. 2003. Neighborhoods and health: An overview. In *Neighborhoods and Health*, p. 24, edited by I. Kawachi and L. F. Berkman. New York: Oxford University Press.

Martens, E.P., W.R. Pestman, A. de Boer, S.V. Belitser, and O.H. Klungel. 2006. Instrumental variables: Application and limitations. *Epidemiology* 17(3): 260–267.

McCullough, M.L., D. Feskanich, M.J. Stampfer, E.L. Giovannucci, E.B. Rimm, F.B. Hu, D. Spiegelman, D.J. Hunter, G.A. Colditz, and W.C. Willett. 2002. Diet quality and major chronic disease risk in men and women: Moving toward improved dietary guidance. *Am J Clin Nutr* 76(6): 1261–1271.

McKinnon, R.A., J. Reedy, D. Berrigan, and S.M. Krebs-Smith. 2012. The national collaborative on childhood obesity research catalogue of surveillance systems and measures registry: New tools to spur innovation and increase productivity in childhood obesity research. *Am J Prev Med* 42(4): 433–435.

McKinnon, R.A., J. Reedy, M.A. Morrissette, L.A. Lytle, and A.L. Yaroch. 2009. Measures of the food environment: A compilation of the literature, 1990–2007. *Am J Prev Med* 36(4): S124–S133.

Moore, L.V., A.V. Diez-Roux, and M. Franco. 2012. Measuring availability of healthy foods: Agreement between directly measured and self-reported data. *Am J Epidemiol* 175(10): 1037–1044.

Moore, L.V., A.V. Diez-Roux, J.A. Nettleton, and D.R. Jacobs. 2008a. Associations of the local food environment with diet quality—a comparison of GIS and survey assessments: The multi-ethnic study of atherosclerosis. *Am J Epidemiol* 167(8): 917–924.

Moore, L.V., A.V. Diez-Roux, and S. Brines. 2008b. Comparing perception-based and geographic information system (GIS)-based characterizations of the local food environment. *J Urban Health* 85(2): 206–216.

Moore L.V. 2007. Measuring the local food environment and its associations with diet quality. PhD Dissertation, Ann Arbor, MI: University of Michigan.

Moore, L.V. and A.V. Diez-Roux. 2006. Associations of neighborhood characteristics with the location and type of food stores. *Am J Public Health* 96(2): 325–331.

Morland, K., S. Wing, and A.V. Diez-Roux. 2002. The contextual effect of the local food environment on residents' diets: The atherosclerosis risk in communities study. *Am J Public Health* 92(11): 1761–1767.

Mujahid, M.S., A.V. Diez-Roux, J.D. Morenoff, and T. Raghunathan. 2007. Assessing the measurement properties of neighborhood scales: From psychometrics to ecometrics. *Am J Epidemiol* 165(8): 858–867.

Ohri-Vachaspati, P., D. Martinez, M.J. Yedidia, and N. Petlick. 2011. Improving data accuracy of commercial food outlet databases. *Am J Health Promot* 26(2): 116–122.

Ohri-Vachaspati, P. and L.C. Leviton. 2010. Measuring food environments: A guide to available instruments. *Am J Health Promot* 24(6): 410–426.

Paquet, C., M. Daniel, Y. Kestens, K. Leger, and L. Gauvin. 2008. Field validation of listings of food stores and commercial physical activity establishments from secondary data. *Int J Behav Nutr Phys Act* 5: 58.

Powell, L.M., E. Han, S.N. Zenk, T. Khan, C.M. Quinn, K.P. Gibbs, O. Pugach, et al. 2011. Field validation of secondary commercial data sources on the retail food outlet environment in the U.S. *Health Place* 17(5): 1122–1131.

Raudenbush, S.W. and R.J. Sampson. 1999. Ecometrics: Toward a science of assessing ecological settings, with application to the systematic social observation of neighborhoods. *Sociol Methodol* 29: 1–41.

Reidpath, D.D., C. Burns, J. Garrard, M. Mahoney, and M. Townsend. 2002. An ecological study of the relationship between social and environmental determinants of obesity. *Health Place* 8(2): 141–145.

Robins, J.M., M.A. Hernan, and B. Brumback. 2000. Marginal structural models and causal inference in epidemiology. *Epidemiology* 11(5): 550–560.

Rose, D.J. 2011. Captive audience? Strategies for acquiring food in two Detroit neighborhoods. *Qual Health Res* 21(5): 642–651.

Rose, D. and R. Richards. 2004. Food store access and household fruit and vegetable use among participants in the U.S. food stamp program. *Public Health Nutr* 7(8): 1081–1088.

Rubin, D.B. 1997. Estimating causal effects from large data sets using propensity scores. *Ann Intern Med* 127(8): 757–763.

U.S. Department of Agriculture. 2013. Snap Retailer Locator. http://www.snapretailerlocator.com/ (Accessed October 08, 2013).

U.S. Department of Agriculture and U.S. Department of Health and Human Services. 2012. Dietary Guidelines for Americans, 2010. Washington, DC: U.S. Government Printing Office.

U.S. Department of Labor. 2012. National Longitudinal Survey of Youth 1979 (NLSY79), cohort user's guide. https://www.nlsinfo.org/content/cohorts/NLSY79 (Accessed October 27, 2013).

Wrigley, N., D. Warm, and B. Margetts. 2003. Deprivation, diet, and food-retail access: Findings from the Leeds 'food deserts' study. *Environ Plann A* 35(1): 151–188.

Yang, Y., A.V. Diez-Roux, A.H. Auchincloss, D.A. Rodriguez, and D.G. Brown. 2011. A spatial agent-based model for the simulation of adults' daily walking within a city. *Am J Prev Med* 40(3): 353–361.

Zenk, S.N., L.L. Lachance, A.J. Schulz, G. Mentz, S. Kannan, and W. Ridella. 2009. Neighborhood retail food environment and fruit and vegetable intake in a multiethnic urban population. *Am J Health Promot* 23(4): 255–264.

8 Local Food Environments Outside of the United States

A Look to the North: Examining Food Environments in Canada

Jennifer Black

Canada stands committed to the United Nations Covenant on Social, Economic and Cultural Rights specifying the right of everyone to adequate food, and endorses a food security action plan stating "the fundamental right of everyone to be free from hunger" and "food security exists when all people at all times have physical and economic access to sufficient, safe and nutritious food to meet their dietary needs and food preferences for an active and healthy life."

Canada's Action Plan for Food Security (1998)

INTRODUCTION TO LOCAL FOOD ENVIRONMENTS IN CANADA

A swell of international interest is growing among health practitioners, researchers, and urban planners regarding potential strategies for redesigning local food environments (LFEs) to maximize human health and social justice and to reduce long-term environmental impacts. As highlighted throughout this book, emerging evidence from the United States has demonstrated that both the availability of nutritious food and the prevalence of diet-related health outcomes such as obesity and diabetes vary across neighborhoods and among geographic regions. Outside the United States, a growing knowledge base about LFEs is also emerging, but little systematic attention has examined the food environment literature in other affluent countries such as America's nearest neighbor, Canada.

Many of the research questions and policy debates related to U.S. food environments described throughout this book are also topics of interest in the Canadian context. Although Canada faces many similar food system challenges, Canadian history, geography, healthcare system design and food-related policies, programs and funding differ in meaningful ways. Moreover, findings from Canadian research regarding the distribution and potential implications of LFEs on dietary practices have diverged in some ways from U.S. findings. As such, lessons can be learned from successes and challenges on both sides of the border to inform international research, policies, and program planning related to LFEs.

Brief Overview of Canadian Geography, Agriculture, and Food System Issues

While Canada's vast land mass spans nearly nine million square kilometers (or over three million square miles), its estimated total 2011 population of approximately 33 million residents is still but a fraction of the 312 million estimated residents living in the United States. (Statistics Canada 2011a; United States Census Bureau 2011). The Canadian map shown in Figure 8.1 depicts how Canada's population is spread across 10 provinces and three northern territories (Yukon, Northwest Territories, and Nunavut). Similar to estimates from the United States, approximately 81% of Canadians live in urban areas and roughly 70% of the population lives in one of Canada's 33 census metropolitan areas (Statistics Canada 2011b). Moreover, over one-third of residents (35%) live in one of Canada's three largest cities: Toronto, Montreal, or Vancouver (Statistics Canada 2011c).

The patterning of regions with darker orange or red shading in Figure 8.1 illustrates that the majority of the Canadian population lives in cities and towns along the southern edge of the country. Population density is highest proximate to the U.S. border where the winter climate is relatively more hospitable compared to the extreme low temperatures common in northern regions where population density is far more sparse, shown in yellow. Although the clustering of primary agricultural production is not shown in Figure 8.1, farming remains an important economic sector in the Canadian economy, with diverse agricultural production taking place across the 10 provinces. The provinces of Manitoba, Saskatchewan, and Alberta (known as the Prairie Provinces) are home to over 80% of Canada's farmland, with the majority of the remaining farms housed in British Columbia, Ontario, and Quebec (Agriculture and Agri-Food Canada 2008).

Outputs from the food system (including revenues from farming, food and beverage processing, retailing and foodservice industries) have significant impacts on where Canadians live, work, and eat. Food-system-related jobs contributed to approximately 8% of Canada's gross domestic product and one in eight jobs in 2008 (Agriculture and Agri-Food Canada 2008). As a result, agricultural production and food systems issues are important drivers of (and are substantially impacted by) national and regional politics and related food policies. Canada's agricultural system is also highly dependent on international trade, particularly for exporting products such as oilseeds, beef, pork, poultry, and grain products. Compared to the United States and European Union, whose estimated exported agricultural production was 18% and 7%, respectively, Canada exported approximately 45% of its products in 2006 (Agriculture and Agri-Food Canada 2008). Canada also imports approximately 30% of its food supply from other countries, over half of which comes from the United States (Statistics Canada 2008). But farming practices have changed rapidly in Canada and the proportion of

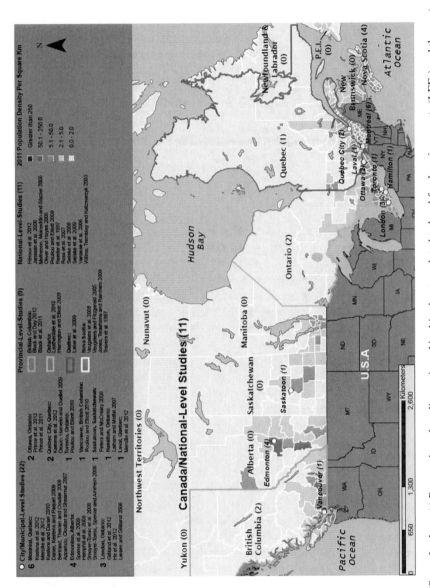

FIGURE 8.1 (See color insert.) Peer-reviewed studies reviewed in this chapter related to local food environments (LFEs) and the contextual determinants of obesity and dietary outcomes in Canada, published in 2012 or earlier.

small- and medium-sized farms has shrunk since the 1980s, although the number of farms with the highest gross revenues has increased dramatically. Farms grossing over $1 million accounted for just 2.5% of Canadian farms in 2006, but earned 40% of the country's gross farming revenue (Agriculture and Agri-Food Canada 2008).

Compared to countries outside of North America, Canadians spend a relatively low proportion of their household expenditures on groceries, estimated at approximately 10% in 2008. Still, low-income families spend a significantly higher proportion of their budget on food, and socioeconomic inequities in health- and nutrition-related outcomes persist in Canada (Agriculture and Agri-Food Canada 2008; Raphael et al. 2008; Tarasuk et al. 2010), warranting a closer examination of the social and contextual factors that shape diet-related outcomes in the Canadian context.

NUTRITION-RELATED HEALTH OUTCOMES IN CANADA

Estimated life expectancy in Canada in 2009 was approximately 81 years (slightly higher than the 2011 U.S. life expectancy of 78 years) and infant mortality rates fell below 5 deaths per 1000 births (slightly lower than the 2011 U.S. infant mortality of 6 deaths/1000) (National Vital Statistics Report 2012; Statistics Canada 2012a). Despite these promising outcomes, Canada's healthcare and public health systems are facing many of the same priority challenges as their U.S. neighbors, including growing rates of nutrition-related chronic disease. For example, the prevalence of both overweight ($25 \geq$ body mass index [BMI] > 29.9 kg/m^2) and obesity (BMI $\geq$ 30 kg/m^2) has increased significantly in Canada in recent decades, affecting all age and gender groups from coast to coast (Katzmarzyk 2002; Tremblay et al. 2002; Luo et al. 2007; Shields et al. 2011). Nearly one-quarter of Canadian adults now meet the BMI criteria for obesity based on measured height and weight, contributing to increased morbidity and mortality from cardiovascular disease, type 2 diabetes, and some cancers and an estimated 4.1% ($6 billion) of Canada's total healthcare costs (Katzmarzyk and Ardern 2004; Katzmarzyk and Janssen 2004; Katzmarzyk and Mason 2006; Anis et al. 2009; Lee et al. 2009).

Nationally representative estimates based on measured height and weight suggest that in 2007–2009, adult obesity prevalence in Canada was approximately 10 percentage points below national estimates from the United States (Shields et al. 2011). Still, BMI has increased in all provinces and the distribution of obesity and related outcomes is not uniform across Canada. For example, residents in Eastern Canada and remote northern communities are disproportionately affected (Willms et al. 2003; Katzmarzyk and Ardern 2004; Belanger-Ducharme and Tremblay 2005; Ross et al. 2007; Pouliou and Elliott 2009;). Individual-level explanations based on genetic predisposition, individual sociodemographic factors, cultural preferences, and health behaviors have been helpful in explaining why some individuals are more likely than others to consume a healthful diet and maintain a lower BMI. But individual-focused explanations have not adequately explained why people living in certain geographic regions have higher rates of chronic disease than would be expected based on individual-level characteristics (Power 2005; Raine 2005; Taylor et al. 2005), or how and why U.S. cities and neighborhoods differ from those of their neighbors to the north in Canada.

Neighborhood- and contextual-level factors such as area-level socioeconomic factors, limited access to retailers selling affordable, nutritious food, and persistent exposure to unhealthy foods in and around the school context have been proposed as potential explanations for geographic differences related to dietary choices and obesity outcomes. LFEs have further been proposed as a potential locus for intervention for improving community food security—that is aiming to ensure that community members can obtain a safe, personally acceptable, nutritious diet through a sustainable food system that maximizes healthy choices, community self-reliance, and socially just access to needed health resources (Dietitians of Canada 2007).

There is now a small but emerging literature evaluating the role of LFEs and neighborhood-level determinants of nutrition and health-related outcomes in the Canadian context that has received little systematic review. To that end, this chapter examines the literature on geographic variations in LFE exposures in Canada, the evidence regarding the associations between food environment characteristics with dietary outcomes and BMI, and remaining methodological and empirical gaps in the Canadian literature.

This chapter focuses on studies published in 2012 or earlier, identified using the search strategy described in Table 8.1. Studies were reviewed and abstracted if they (1) were conducted in Canada and (2) assessed at least one measure of body weight status (e.g., BMI, overweight, obesity, or waist circumferences) or dietary intake, in two or more geographic regions, and/or included at least one measure related to the LFE (e.g., number of food stores or restaurants, density by population or land area, or proximity to local food retailers). Only English-language articles were reviewed, potentially overlooking valuable contributions from French publications. This review was guided conceptually by the theoretical framework for understanding how neighborhoods influence body weight and obesity proposed by Black and Macinko (2008).

TABLE 8.1
Literature Search Strategy

Electronic Databases Searched	PubMed, PsychInfo, CINAHL, EMBASE, Social Services Abstract, Sociological Abstracts and ABI INFORM
Primary Search Terms	*food availability* OR *obesity* and *neighbourhood* OR *neighborhood*
Secondary Search Terms	*neighborhood$*[a], *neighborhood$, obes$, overweight, BMI, waist circumference, grocer$, supermarket, restaurants, food store, socioeconomic, deprived, food desert$, diet$, nutrition, deprivation, income, poverty, food$,* "available or availability or affordability or affordable or price or pricing or prices or cost or costs or retail$ or store or stores or market or markets or shop" in abstracts or titles

[a] The money sign ($) is a Boolean search function indicating truncation, allowing multiple forms of a given word (e.g., diet$ can identify diet, diets, dietary, dietetic, etc.).

LOCAL FOOD ENVIRONMENT RESEARCH IN CANADA

WHERE HAS LOCAL FOOD ENVIRONMENT RESEARCH BEEN CONDUCTED IN CANADA AND AT WHAT SCALE?

Figure 8.1 illustrates the main geographic areas where Canadian research related to LFEs and neighborhood-level determinants of diet and health outcomes have been focused. This map shows that at least 11 studies have used *national-level* data and have examined varied geographic scales including differences between provinces, urban/rural areas, health regions, school food environments, or various definitions of neighborhood geographies. At least nine studies from four provinces (British Columbia, Ontario, Quebec, and Nova Scotia) have applied data from several regions within a *single province*, but the majority of studies have focused on variations *within municipal areas*.

The largest cluster of research has emerged in the urban areas of Quebec and Ontario, in cities relatively proximate to the U.S. border, neighboring states such as New York and Vermont. Only a small handful of LFE-related studies have focused on other cities, including Edmonton, Alberta (4), Saskatoon, Saskatchewan (1), or Vancouver, British Columbia (1). Although not highlighted explicitly in Figure 8.1, barriers to accessing nutritious food are also an ongoing area of study and concern among some of Canada's northern and Aboriginal communities. Many remote northern areas face issues related to extreme cold climates, reliance on food transport by plane, high food costs, diminished access to traditional foods such as wild fish and game, and local food sources, resulting in unique food security challenges that are distinct from those faced in Canada's urban centers (Wein 1994; Chan et al. 2006; Lambden et al. 2006; Kuhnlein et al. 2008).

A brief description of the main administrative and geographic boundaries used in the Canadian LFE literature is also provided for reference in the table in the Appendix. Like the geographic boundaries used in the U.S. literature described in depth by Morland in Chapter 4, Canadian studies vary widely in their definitions of *neighborhoods* and LFE exposures. Small- and medium-sized geographic boundaries including dissemination areas (e.g., Oliver and Hayes 2005) or census tracts (e.g., Daniel et al. 2009; Black et al. 2011) have commonly been used, particularly among studies drawing on census data to examine demographic or socioeconomic characteristics of given regions. Studies comparing regions within a single city such as Ottawa (Prince et al. 2012), Edmonton (Hemphill et al. 2008), or Saskatoon (Peters and McCreary 2008) have also commonly relied on the municipally defined neighborhood boundaries or definitions constructed for specific research purposes. It is therefore difficult to directly compare neighborhood boundaries between cities as they can differ widely in terms of total area, population density, and level of demographic heterogeneity.

Food environment exposures have frequently been measured in terms of relative access within an area surrounding a specific geographic location such as a school or residential address, often defined by specific buffer zones (circular distances surrounding a point) or the nearest distance a person would theoretically travel to reach the closest food retailer. There remains no consensus regarding how best to measure the appropriate distance for assessing *good* or *poor* access to food resources or how best to account for transportation routes (i.e., whether people walk, cycle, drive, or rely on public transit) to reach amenities. Resources that are walkable within an approximately 10–15 minute commute by foot or within 500–1000 m have been proposed in recent studies (Apparicio et al. 2007; Smoyer-Tomic et al. 2008; Seliske et al. 2009a; Spence et al. 2009; Pouliou and Elliott 2010). However, larger buffer sizes have also been considered, particularly for residential contexts where the majority of residents conduct food shopping with a private vehicle. Several researchers have therefore recommended using multiple, varied measures of food environment amenities to more comprehensively assess nuanced aspects of LFE variety, proximity, and the concentration of exposures instead of a single crude measure of access such as number of nearby food retailers or the closest distance from home to a supermarket (Talen and Anselin 1998; Apparicio et al. 2007).

EVIDENCE OF GEOGRAPHIC VARIATION IN OBESITY

The findings from available studies assessing the distribution and/or area-level determinants of BMI outcomes in Canada are summarized in Table 8.2 and describe differences in the distribution of obesity between geographic regions, in urban versus rural contexts, and based on area-level socioeconomic and demographic conditions.

East versus West and Provincial Divides

Substantial variation has been reported across Canada's provinces and health regions (administrative units used to organize the provision of health services). In 2005, the vage-standardized rates of self-reported overweight or obesity (BMI $\geq$ 25 kg/m^2) for adult women ranged from a low of 17% in the Vancouver health region to nearly double that (37%) in Interlake, Manitoba (Pouliou and Elliott 2009). For men, rates ranged from a low of 32% in Richmond to 52% in the Zone 5 health region in Nova Scotia (Pouliou and Elliott 2009).

There is evidence that the prevalence of obesity rises in a gradient from Western to Eastern Canada among adults and children (Reeder et al. 1997; Willms et al. 2003; Pouliou and Elliott 2009). Population clusters with elevated BMI have been identified in the northern regions of Alberta, Saskatchewan, and Manitoba (Pouliou and Elliott 2009) and in remote northern Aboriginal communities (Belanger-Ducharme and Tremblay 2005). Findings further indicate that residing in Quebec versus all other Canadian provinces predicts a significantly lower BMI for women (but not men) even after controlling for individual factors and neighborhood socioeconomic status (SES) (Ross et al. 2007).

Obesity is also an important public health issue for Canadian children and youth for whom prevalence of elevated BMI is rising faster than for adults (Tremblay et al. 2002; Willms et al. 2003). Data on 2- to 11-year-old children from the 1998–99 National Longitudinal Survey of Children and Youth (NLSCY) suggest that 35% of girls and 38% of boys are overweight and 17% of girls and 19% of boys are obese as defined by age- and sex-specific cutoffs (Belanger-Ducharme and Tremblay 2005). From 1981 to 1996, the prevalence of overweight among 7- to 13-year olds rose significantly in every province; although rates of change varied by province (Willms et al. 2003). Willms et al. (2003) reported that the rates of increase and 1996 prevalence rates of overweight were generally higher among Canada's four Atlantic (eastern) provinces (Newfoundland, Nova Scotia, Prince Edward Island, and New

TABLE 8.2

Studies of Neighborhood, Area-Level, and School-Level Socioeconomic Resources, Contextual Factors, and Obesity

	Study Description			Area-Level Measure and Association with BMI/Weight Status				Measure(s) of Weight Status
Reference	Study Population	Sample Size (Area Metric)	Study Design	Area-Level SES	Area-Level Demographics	Spatial Location	Built Environment and/or Food Environment	Body Weight/ BMI Outcome(s)
(Gilliland et al. 2012)	London, Ontario (10- to 14-year olds)	891 (28 Schools)	Cross-sectional, multilevel	N/A	N/A	N/A	(−) Recreation facilities within 500 m from home (+) Fast-food availability within school *walkshed* Ø Fast food or convenience store availability around home environment	BMI z-scores Self-reported
(Kestens et al. 2012)	Montreal and Quebec City, Quebec (adults)	5,578 (29 Montreal health service units and 38 Quebec City neighborhoods from 2 municipalities)	Cross-sectional, Multilevel	N/A	N/A	N/A	(−) Living in NH with highest quartile of food store density (+) Living in NH with higher proportion of fast-food restaurants	Overweight = BMI ≥ 25 Self-reported
(Prince et al. 2012)	Ottawa, Ontario (adults)	4,727 (86 neighborhoods)	Cross-sectional	Ø SES index	N/A	N/A	(+) Density of convenience stores and fast-food outlets among women; Ø among men	Overweight/ obesity = BMI ≥ 25 Self-reported

(Prince et al. 2011)	Ottawa, Ontario (adults)	3,883 (85 neighborhoods)	Cross-sectional, Multilevel	(+) SES scores (for men) Ø SES scores (for women)	N/A	N/A	Ø Density of convenience stores, FFOs, grocery stores (−) Density of restaurants (+) Density of specialty stores for women (+) Green space for women (−) Green space for men	Overweight/ obesity = BMI ≥ 25 Self-reported
(Leatherdale et al. 2010)	Ontario (students in grades 5–8)	2,449 (30 elementary schools)	Cross-sectional, Multilevel	N/A	N/A	N/A	Ø Number of gas stations, bakeries, variety stores, recreation facilities within 1 km of school	Overweight/ obesity = BMI ≥ 85 percentile, self-reported
(Pouliou and Elliott 2010)	Toronto, Ontario and Vancouver, British Columbia (adults)	115,548 (1 km buffers around residential locations)	Cross-sectional, Multilevel	N/A	N/A	N/A	Ø Density of fast food, convenience stores, grocery stores, recreation activities	BMI Self-reported
(Harrington and Elliott 2009)	Ontario (adults)	2,039 (163 forward sortation areas)	Cross-sectional, Multilevel	(−) (For women) Ø (for men), dwelling value and % high-school educated[a] Ø average household income, % LICO families, unemployment	N/A	N/A	Ø Rural, older homes, homes in need of repair, rental homes	BMI, waist circumferences measured

(Continued)

TABLE 8.2 (Continued)
Studies of Neighborhood, Area-Level, and School-Level Socioeconomic Resources, Contextual Factors, and Obesity

	Study Description			Area-Level Measure and Association with BMI/Weight Status				Measure(s) of Weight Status
Reference	Study Population	Sample Size (Area Metric)	Study Design	Area-Level SES	Area-Level Demographics	Spatial Location	Built Environment and/or Food Environment	Body Weight/ BMI Outcome(s)
(Lebel et al. 2009)	Quebec (adults)	20,449 (51 Spatial units)	Cross-sectional, Multilevel	Ø NH material and social deprivation	N/A	N/A	(+) Rural w/BMI ≥ 25 for men	Overweight/ obesity = BMI ≥ 25 Self-reported
(Pouliou and Elliott 2009)	National (adults)	115,915 (101 Health regions)	ecologic	N/A	N/A	(+) North & Atlantic (−) South and West	N/A	Overweight/ obesity = BMI ≥ 25 Self-reported
(Spence et al. 2009)	Edmonton, Alberta (adults)	2,900 (800 m and 1600 m buffers around residential locations)	Cross-sectional	N/A	N/A	N/A	(+) Retail Food Environment Index within 800 m from residence Ø Retail Food Environment Index within 1,600 m from residence	Obesity = BMI ≥ 30 Self-reported
(Matheson et al. 2008)	National (urban adults)	267,108 (3,522 census tracts from 25 urban areas)	Cross-sectional, multilevel	(+) For women (−) For men NH material deprivation	N/A	N/A	N/A	BMI Self-reported

Reference	Setting	Sample	Design					Outcome
(Seliske et al. 2009a)	National (grades 6–10 students)	9,672 (178 schools with 1 and 5-km radius around schools)	Cross-sectional, Multilevel	N/A	N/A	N/A	Ø Individual food retailers (+) Food retail index (w/overweight)	Overweight and obesity, age and sex specific
(Veugelers et al. 2008)	Nova Scotia (grade 5 students)	5,471 (282 school catchment areas)	Cross-sectional, multilevel	N/A	N/A	N/A	(−) Perceived access to shops (+) Rural school location	Overweight and obesity, age and sex specific; Measured
(Ross et al. 2007)	National (urban adults)	15,686 Men, 17,278 women (2,615 census tracts from 27 CMAs)	Cross-sectional, Multilevel	(+)% Without high-school diploma Ø Median household income	(−)% Immigrants (for men)	(−) For Quebec	Ø Dwelling density (+) Sprawl (for men)	BMI; Self-reported
(Janssen et al. 2006)	National (grade 6–10 students)	6,684 (169 Schools with 5 km radius around school)	Cross-sectional, Multilevel	(+) %Unemployed, low income[b], % without high-school diploma	N/A	N/A	N/A	Obesity = BMI ≥ 30; Self-reported
(Vanasse et al. 2006)	National (adults)	106 Health regions	Ecologic	N/A	(+)% Aboriginal	(−) Vancouver, Toronto, Montreal	N/A	Obesity, age, and sex specific; Self-reported
(Oliver and Hayes 2005)	National (5- to 17-year olds)	11,455 (5,531 Dissemination Areas)	Cross-sectional, Multilevel	(−) Composite SES	N/A	N/A	N/A	Overweight, age, and sex specific; Self-reported
(Veugelers and Fitzgerald 2005)	Nova Scotia (grade 5 students)	4,298 (242 catchment areas)	Cross-sectional, Multilevel	(−) Mean household income	N/A	N/A	(−) Urban	Overweight and obesity, age and sex specific; Measured

(Continued)

TABLE 8.2 (Continued)
Studies of Neighborhood, Area-Level, and School-Level Socioeconomic Resources, Contextual Factors, and Obesity

	Study Description				Area-Level Measure and Association with BMI/Weight Status				Measure(s) of Weight Status
Reference	Study Population	Sample Size (Area Metric)	Study Design	Area-Level SES	Area-Level Demographics	Spatial Location	Built Environment and/or Food Environment	Body Weight/BMI Outcome(s)
(Willms et al. 2003)	National (7- to 13-year olds in 1981 and 1996)	3,036 Boys 3,024 girls (by province)	Cross-sectional, Multilevel	N/A	N/A	(+) Gradient from western to eastern provinces	N/A	Overweight and obesity, age and sex specific Measured
(Reeder et al. 1997)	National (adults in 1986–1992)	27,120 Adults (9 provinces excluding Nova Scotia)	Cross-sectional	N/A	N/A	(+) Atlantic Canada	(−) Urban (in Western Canada)	Mean BMI and BMI ≥ 27 kg/m² Measured

[a] %High-school educated only significantly associated with waist circumference for women (not BMI).

[b] Results not statistically significant after controlling for individual-level covariates.

Note: BMI, body mass index; SES, socioeconomic status; N/A, not applicable; (−), negative association; (+), positive association; Ø, no significant association; NH, neighborhood; LICO, low-income cutoff; CMA, census metropolitan area.

Brunswick) and lower for the three Prairie provinces (Manitoba, Saskatchewan, and Alberta). Compared to the rest of Canada, children in the province of Newfoundland had the highest increase in the odds of overweight (odds ratio = 1.40; 95% confidence interval = 1.13–1.73) from 1981 to 1996.

Urban–Rural Differences

Prevalence of overweight or obesity is lower in the three largest metropolitan areas, Toronto, Montreal, and Vancouver than the rest of the country (Pouliou and Elliott 2009) and there is evidence that residents in rural communities have significantly higher odds of obesity compared to urban-dwelling Canadians. Lebel et al. (2009) estimated that men living in rural communities in Quebec are 17% more likely to be overweight or obese versus those in urban areas. Reeder et al. (1997) also reported significantly higher obesity prevalence in rural- versus urban-dwelling residents in western Canada, but not in a national sample. In addition, grade 5 students in Nova Scotia who attended rural schools were more likely to be overweight or obese than children in urban schools, potentially the result of lower participation rates in coached sports and increased time playing video games, using the computer, or watching television (Veugelers and Fitzgerald 2005; Veugelers et al. 2008).

Residing in a sprawling area where walking is inconvenient or where individuals spend more time in cars may further contribute to obesity (Frank et al. 2004; Lopez-Zetina et al. 2006; Joshu et al. 2008). To date, most evidence on the associations between metropolitan sprawl and obesity come from the United States. However, significant positive associations between sprawl and BMI have been reported for Canadians as well (Ross et al. 2007).

Role of Area-Level Socioeconomic and Demographic Composition

There is substantial evidence from U.S. studies that living in an economically deprived neighborhood is associated with increased likelihood of obesity, even after controlling for individual-level SES (see Chapter 6 of this book and publications such as: Papas et al. [2007]; Black and Macinko [2008]; Beaulac et al. [2009]; USDA [2009]). In Canada, the role of area-level SES is inconsistent and varies between studies and by gender, for children versus adults and in different parts of the country.

There is some evidence that decreased area-level SES including lower composite SES, mean household income, educational attainment and higher unemployment rates is associated with higher BMI, particularly for children (Oliver and Hayes 2005; Veugelers and Fitzgerald 2005; Janssen et al. 2006; Ross et al. 2007; Harrington and Elliott 2009). However, other studies find no associations between BMI with median area income, percent earning below the low-income cutoff, neighborhood deprivation or income inequality (Ross et al. 2007; Harrington and Elliott 2009; Lebel et al. 2009; Prince et al. 2012). There is additional evidence that neighborhood poverty is associated with obesity for women, while living in a more affluent neighborhood may promote higher BMI for men (Matheson et al. 2008; Lebel et al. 2009; Prince et al. 2011).

Three studies of Canadian youth reported significantly lower odds of overweight or obesity for children in wealthier neighborhoods (Oliver and Hayes 2005; Veugelers and Fitzgerald 2005; Janssen et al. 2006). Analysis of the 2000/2001 NLSCY indicates that after controlling for individual characteristics, living in a low- versus high-SES neighborhood is associated with a 29% increase in the odds of overweight for 5- to 17-year olds (Oliver and Hayes 2005). Furthermore, Veugelers and Fitzgerald (2005) reported half the odds of obesity for children in Nova Scotia living in high-versus low-income neighborhoods and Janssen et al. (2006) found reduced odds of self-reported obesity for youth in grades 6–10 associated with multiple measures of area SES.

A dearth of studies has assessed the associations between neighborhood demographic characteristics such as ethnic/racial composition, percent immigrants or newcomers, residential stability or age composition (e.g., percent elderly or youth) with BMI or dietary outcomes in Canada. Preliminary evidence from one study found that the percent of recent immigrants living in urban census tracts was associated with lower BMI for men, even after controlling for individual-level immigrant status and sociodemographic factors (Ross et al. 2007); but it is otherwise difficult to compare Canada to U.S. findings in regards to the role of disparities in obesity or food environment outcomes associated with area-demographic composition.

In summary, at least 17 studies have explored the geographic distribution and area-level determinants of BMI in Canada. This preliminary evidence indicates that rates of obesity are higher in eastern versus western and in rural versus urban areas of the country. Unlike studies from the United States that have suggested a relatively consistent negative association between neighborhood-level SES and BMI, Canadian studies report mixed findings regarding the relations between area-level SES and obesity outcomes, and Canadian analyses of the role of area-demographic composition are virtually nonexistent (Table 8.3).

GEOGRAPHIC VARIATION AND LOCAL FOOD ENVIRONMENTS CHARACTERISTICS

The pathways through which area sociodemographics influence weight remain contested. U.S. evidence suggests that marginalized neighborhoods characterized by higher proportions of low-income and minority residents may have significantly higher exposure to amenities that promote weight gain and decreased access to resources that promote healthy body weight. For example, there is evidence that access to stores that sell healthful food at affordable prices is associated with improved dietary quality (Morland et al. 2002a; Laraia et al. 2004; Rose and Richards 2004; Moore et al. 2008), and in the United States, there is strong evidence that neighborhoods characterized by lower area-level income and more minority residents experience reduced access to stores that sell nutritious food, particularly large supermarkets. Underserved neighborhoods may subsequently face reduced access to affordable healthful foods such as fresh fruits and vegetables, whole grains and lean meats, and increased reliance on convenience stores and small local vendors (Morland et al. 2002a; Horowitz et al. 2004; Zenk et al. 2005; Gallagher 2006; Moore and DiezRoux 2006; Papas et al. 2007; Black and Macinko 2008; Beaulac et al. 2009; USDA 2009).

TABLE 8.3

Studies Assessing Neighborhood- and School-Level Built Environment and Food Environment Characteristics and Associations with Dietary Outcomes

Reference	Study Population	Sample Size (Area Metric)	Study Design	Built Environment and/or Food Environment Variables and Association with Dietary Outcomes	Dietary Outcome
(He et al. 2012)	London, Ontario (grades 7 and 8 students)	810 Students (21 elementary schools)	Cross-sectional	(−) Increased density of and closer proximity to fast-food outlets near school and closer proximity to convenience stores near home associated with diet quality	Dietary quality (modified Healthy Eating Index)
(Héroux et al. 2012)	Canada, Scotland, United States (13- to 15-year olds)	26,778 (687 schools)	Cross-sectional, multilevel	(+) Density of chain food retailers (convenience stores, fast food, chain cafes) within 1 km of school with eating lunch at a food retailer (in Canada only) ∅ School food retail environment and self-reported BMI (in Canada, Scotland or United States)	Location where students usually consume mid-day meal
(Mercille et al. 2012)	Montreal and Laval, Quebec (older adults age 68–84)	751 (500 m buffer distances around residential locations)	Cross-sectional	(−) Proportion of fast-food outlets relative to all restaurants within 500 m buffer with prudent diet, but ∅ with western diet (−) Proportion of healthful food stores with western diet scores but ∅ with prudent diet scores	*Prudent* and *Western*-style diet scores derived from categorical principal components analysis of semi-quantitative food frequency questions

Note: (−), negative association; (+), positive association; ∅, no significant association; BMI, body mass index.

FOOD RETAILING IN CANADA

In recent decades, major shifts have taken place in regard to where, what and how much food Canadians prepare, purchase and consume, as well as the types and locations of food retailers and foodservice outlets available in many communities (Garriguet 2007; Agriculture and Agri-Food Canada 2008). Although 67% of Canadian meals were consumed at home and purchased from a retail outlet selling groceries in 2007, Canadian spending on foods purchased from restaurants and fast-food outlets has increased dramatically, contributing to $37 billion in sales in 2004 (Statistics Canada 2006a; Agriculture and Agri-Food Canada 2008). Canada currently houses approximately 35,000 fast-food outlets and both the number of outlets and national sales figures are forecast by industry analysts to rise further in coming years (Euromonitor International 2012).

Although the availability of fast-food outlets has risen, there is evidence that access to grocery stores has declined in Canadian cities in recent decades. Canadian food retailing has changed from a system characterized mainly by small-scale, local neighborhood grocers to a centralized, consolidated, *scaled up* system dominated by a few large food retailers (Agriculture and Agri-Food Canada 2008; Bedore 2012). In 2008, Canadian grocery stores brought in approximately $78 billion in sales (Condon 2009). Yet, just a handful of Canada's largest retailers including Loblaw, Sobeys, Metro, Canada Safeway, Costco, and Wal-Mart soaked up nearly three quarters of the market share in 2007, whereas the number of smaller, independent grocers and their market share has substantially declined (Agriculture and Agri-Food Canada 2008; Bedore 2012). The following sections will examine literature assessing if and how the resulting distribution of food retailer availability has contributed to systematic disparities in access to nutritious foods, exposure to *obesogenic* foods or varied health outcomes among or between Canadian communities.

AVAILABILITY OF SUPERMARKETS, GROCERY STORES, AND ACCESS TO NUTRITIOUS FOOD IN CANADA

In total, over 50 studies from high-income countries including the United States, the United Kingdom, Canada, Australia, and New Zealand have examined differences in access to nutritious food and retail stores across sociodemographically diverse geographic areas (Beaulac et al. 2009; Larson et al. 2009). U.S. studies have found that residents of lower income and higher ethnic minority concentration neighborhoods experience reduced access to stores selling healthy foods, but higher exposure to vendors of poor quality foods, particularly fast-food outlets (Morland et al. 2002a; Powell et al. 2007; Beaulac et al. 2009). However, few studies yielding mixed results have assessed the distribution of supermarkets, grocers, fruit and vegetable stores, and vendors of nutritious food in Canada (described in Table 8.4).

Although preliminary findings do reveal that access to food retailers differs within cities and between regions of the country, results are inconclusive about whether area-level or sociodemographic factors systematically shape food availability. Several researchers have hypothesized that wealthier neighborhoods are likely to have improved access to healthful food and supermarkets, as is commonly

TABLE 8.4
Studies Documenting Geographic Differences in Food Availability

Reference	Setting	Area Metric	Main Area Characteristics	Main Measures of Food Availability	Main Findings
(Black and Day 2012)	British Columbia	800 m distance around and closest distance to 1392 public schools	School type, school size, median income, population density	Number of FFOs, beverage and snack stores, delis and convenience stores within 800 m buffer and closest distance to schools	(+) bw population density and availability of all food outlets (−) bw median area income and availability of all food outlets (+) bw larger school size and availability of FFOs, snack/beverage stores, and convenience stores
(Black et al. 2011)	British Columbia	630 Census tracts from eight metropolitan regions	Median household income, % visible minorities, % detached houses, % using public transit, population density, presence of a highway exit	Number of large supermarkets and fresh food stores (grocers, markets, stores selling fresh ingredients) within 1 km buffers and closest distance to stores	(−) bw median income and access to food stores (+) bw minority composition and availability of fresh food stores (−) bw % detached housing and fresh food stores
(Kestens and Daniel 2010)	Montreal, Quebec	750 m buffers around and closest distance to 1168 schools	Median household income, commercial density	Number of FFOs, restaurants, fruit and vegetable stores within 750 m buffer and closest distance to schools	(−) bw median income and availability of all food outlets (+) bw median commercial density and availability of all food outlets
(Daniel et al. 2009)	Montreal, Quebec	862 Census tracts	Household income, age structure, language spoken at home, marital status, household type, educational attainment	FFOs and fruit and vegetable stores within 1 km buffers	(+) bw FFOs and % full-time students, non-English or French speakers, fewer % married, children and older adults and more high-traffic roads (+) bw fruit and vegetable stores with higher % single residents, university educated, non-French or English, more local roads

(Continued)

TABLE 8.4 (Continued)
Studies Documenting Geographic Differences in Food Availability

Reference	Setting	Area Metric	Main Area Characteristics	Main Measures of Food Availability	Main Findings
(Drouin et al. 2009)	Quebec City, Quebec	4 Urban and rural areas	Rural/urban, material deprivation index (low, medium, high)	Food prices at a sample of 56 food stores (convenience, grocery, large grocery and green grocers) and number of stores per 100 km²	(−) bw food costs and food stores categorized as large grocery or greengrocers compared to convenience stores (+) bw availability of all store types in urban versus rural settings (+) bw number of convenience stores and increased material deprivation ØØ bw food costs with level of urbanization or material deprivation index
(Jones et al. 2009)	Nova Scotia	266 Communities	Material deprivation, psychosocial deprivation	FFOs per 1000	(−) bw material deprivation and mean number of FFOs per 1000 (+) bw psychosocial deprivation and mean number of FFOs per 1000
(Seliske et al. 2009b)	National	1 km and 5 km distance around 188 schools	Average household income, unemployment, % with less than high-school education	Number of full-service restaurants, fast-food restaurants, sub/sandwich shops, donut/coffee shops, convenience stores, and grocery stores	(+) bw full-service restaurants and low-SES schools within 1 km Ø bw other food retailers and area SES at 1 km (−) bw all food retailers combined and area SES at 5 km Overall, access to food retailers not generally associated with area SES in immediate school proximity

	Location	Unit of analysis	SES measure	Food access measure	Findings
(Bertrand et al. 2008)	Montreal, Quebec	3158 Dissemination Area	Median income	Fruit and vegetable supply, *accessibility index* with 3 km buffer (for motorized households) and 0.5 km buffer (without car)	Ø bw median income and food supply; (−) Access for consumers without a car
(Hemphill et al. 2008)	Edmonton, Alberta	218 Municipally defined units	% Low income, unemployment, renters, no high-school diploma, recent immigrants	Low, medium, high access to FFOs	(+) bw FFO access with higher % low income, unemployment, renters
(Larsen and Gilliland 2008)	London, Ontario in 1961 and 2005	76 Census tracts	% Lone-parent families, low income, low-educational attainment, unemployment, distress level	Supermarket accessibility by walking and public transit	(−) Access to supermarkets for inner-city neighborhood residents with low SES; Increasing inequalities between 1961 to 2005
(Peters and McCreary 2008)	Saskatoon, Saskatchewan	All neighborhoods defined by the City of Saskatoon	% Below low income cutoff	Grocery and convenience store locations and food pricing (1984–2004)	Over time, access to grocery stores changed resulting in reduced access to affordable healthful foods among areas with highest levels of poverty
(Smoyer-Tomic et al. 2008)	Edmonton, Alberta	215 Residential neighborhoods with populations > 275	Race/ethnicity composition, SES, age and family status, housing tenure, urbanization	Supermarkets within 800 m and FFOs within 500 m	Ø bw supermarkets and area SES; (+) bw FFOs and % Aboriginal, renters, lone parents, low-income households, public transportation commuters; (−) bw FFOs and higher median income and dwelling value
(Apparicio et al. 2007)	Montreal, Quebec	506 Census tracts	Low-income population and social deprivation index	Chain supermarkets: proximity to nearest, number within 1000 m and variety of food items and prices	(−) bw access to nearest supermarket and average distance to three closest chains with social deprivation; (+) bw number of supermarkets within 1000 m and social deprivation; Supermarket accessibility decreases from central city to peripheral areas

(Continued)

TABLE 8.4 (*Continued*)
Studies Documenting Geographic Differences in Food Availability

Reference	Setting	Area Metric	Main Area Characteristics	Main Measures of Food Availability	Main Findings
(Latham and Moffat 2007)	Hamilton, Ontario	Uptown (high SES) versus downtown (lower SES) neighborhoods	Higher versus lower SES neighborhoods	Cost of Ontario Nutritious Food Basket from supermarkets, grocery stores, and variety stores	Ø For food cost bw two varied SES neighborhoods (+) For food costs and (−) for availability of produce in variety stores
(Smoyer-Tomic et al. 2006)	Edmonton, Alberta	212 Neighborhoods	High-need areas (% low-income, elderly, lacking a vehicle)	Supermarkets within 1 km buffer and minimum distance	(+) Supermarket availability in inner city, along major roads and intersections (+) bw supermarket accessibility and high-need neighborhoods, higher percent without a vehicle, rates of low-income households and % elderly (−) 6 High-need neighborhoods had poor supermarket accessibility
(Travers et al. 1997)	Nova Scotia	8 Counties	Population density and income	Price of consumption food basket and alternate food basket	(−) Food costs in urban areas and larger stores, and in Central regions that include Halifax Ø and food costs and neighborhood income within urban Halifax

Note: FFOs, fast-food outlets; (+), positive association; bw, between; (−), negative association; Ø, no significant association.

reported in the U.S. literature. However, three studies in Montreal, Quebec (using multiple measures of food store availability and access) found that socioeconomically deprived neighborhoods did not have reduced access to supermarkets or fruit and vegetable vendors compared to wealthier areas (Apparicio et al. 2007; Bertrand et al. 2008; Daniel et al. 2009).

Furthermore, there is preliminary evidence that some economically disadvantaged Canadian neighborhoods, particularly in urban areas, have *better* access to supermarkets than wealthier and suburban areas (Apparicio et al. 2007; Black et al. 2011). For example, Smoyer-Tomic et al. (2006, 2008) reported that in Edmonton, the capital of Alberta, neighborhoods housing at least one supermarket had lower median income than those without any supermarkets, but overall, SES was not a consistent indicator of supermarket distribution. Inner-city and high-need neighborhoods had better access to supermarkets than elsewhere in Edmonton, where food stores appear to cluster in the city center along major roads and intersections (Smoyer-Tomic et al. 2006). Metropolitan Edmonton is North America's most northern city with over one million residents (Statistics Canada 2012b).

In urban regions of British Columbia, Canada's westernmost province, more affluent neighborhoods seem to house fewer food retailers within walking distance from residential areas and are located farther from the nearest supermarket or fresh food store compared to lower income areas (Black et al. 2011). Recent analyses by Black et al. (2011) suggest that, at least in the province of British Columbia, urban planning factors, particularly zoning and transportation considerations, are likely to have a greater impact on the distribution of food stores than area sociodemographic characteristics. For example, the percent of detached housing was found to explain an estimated 52% of the variation in models predicting the distance to the nearest fresh food store from home.

Health practitioners may view neighborhoods with limited access to healthful, affordable foods, and grocers as a problem, particularly in disadvantaged neighborhoods (USDA 2009; White House Task Force 2010). However, there is evidence that North American urban planning practices value neighborhoods dominated by detached, single-family dwellings above other possible uses including commercial uses for food retailers and restaurants (Perrin 1979; Flanagan 2006; Levine 2006). These practices consequently act to restrict commercial venues from residential areas mainly used for single-family housing to preserve home values in these neighborhoods (Shlay and Rossi 1981). This sort of planning clearly has the potential to create communities with limited access to local food stores. However, this would seem more likely to undermine food access for more stable, residential neighborhoods than for poorer, more marginalized neighborhoods.

Studies conducted in high-income countries outside of Canada have similarly yielded mixed and sometimes contrary findings about the area-level predictors of food store availability. For example, studies from the United Kingdom and New Zealand have found that socioeconomically deprived areas housed more food stores overall, more large independent food stores and are closer in proximity to supermarkets in the most versus least deprived areas (Cummins and Macintyre 1999, 2002; White et al. 2004; Pearce et al. 2007). Moreover, in Australia, few differences in food store availability were reported among demographically varied urban areas (Winkler et al. 2006).

Still, vulnerable neighborhoods with relatively poor supermarket access have been identified in Canada and warrant consideration from health researchers and urban planners (Bertrand et al. 2008; Larsen and Gilliland 2008; Bedore 2012). For example, spatial inequalities were reported in access to supermarkets in London, Ontario particularly for low-income inner-city residents; although, no significant associations were identified between supermarket access and percent low-income residents, area educational attainment or employment rates. The most distressed city neighborhoods had the lowest access by foot, but had relatively higher public transit access. London is a mid-sized city, with a population close to 500,000 residents, ranking it as Canada's eleventh most populous metropolitan area in 2011 (Statistics Canada 2012b).

Supermarket closures over time may further exacerbate barriers to accessing nutritious food in some communities in London where the average proportion of the population with easy access to a supermarket fell from 45.2% to 18.3% between 1961 and 2005 (Larsen and Gilliland 2008). Further evidence from a case study in Saskatoon, Saskatchewan, suggests that store closures between 1984 and 2004 resulted in reduced access to affordable, nutritious foods in the most economically vulnerable neighborhoods of the city (Peters and McCreary 2008).

A recent study by Bedore (2012) argues that changes in the centralization of the retail food industry in Canada have contributed to reduced access to food retailers in the small city of Kingston, located less than 300 km from each of Montreal, Ottawa, and Toronto in southeastern Ontario. Using a historical perspective and qualitative data from a low-income area of Kingston, this study suggests that the food economy has shifted over time. The preindustrial foodscape was characterized by a diverse set of decentralized independent food retailers with close community ties and connections. Bedore's findings suggest that changing land-use policies, the move toward a centralized chain store model, and need for economies of scale in food retailing in Kingston, like other Canadian cities, have resulted in a dramatic decline in the number of food stores. This has resulted in a scaling up of the average store size and sales volume and consolidation of market share by a few large food retailers, which is consistent with national trends in food retailing (Agriculture and Agri-Food Canada 2008).

Findings in British Columbia, Kingston, London, Edmonton, Saskatoon, and Montreal therefore illustrate that important gaps in access still exist for some vulnerable communities. Even though the literature does not consistently show reduced access to healthful food and supermarkets among lower-SES neighborhoods in Canada, there is evidence that increased centralization among Canada's food retailers have resulted in a food landscape where increasingly large stores are located near main roads, aimed at providing convenient access for residents with private vehicles.

Exposure to Fast-Food Outlets and *Obesogenic* Food Environments

Fast-food retailers have been another recent area of focus for food environment researchers. Foods sold at fast-food restaurants are often higher in calories, fat, and sodium than home-prepared foods and a growing body of evidence suggests that more frequent visits to fast-food outlets are associated with higher energy intake, reduced dietary quality and increased obesity risk (Paeratakul et al. 2003; Bowman and Vinyard 2004; Larson et al. 2011). Consequently, fast-food outlets have served as a central (albeit still rather crude) measure of potential exposure to *obesogenic* or obesity promoting food vendors.

Studies from the United States and Britain have suggested that low-SES and minority neighborhoods have higher exposure to fast-food chains (Morland et al. 2002b; Cummins et al. 2005; Powell et al. 2007), however findings from at least five studies in Canada are mixed. Two studies reported that fast-food outlets were more prevalent in Edmonton, Alberta neighborhoods with higher proportions of low-income residents, unemployment rates, and renter-occupied housing (Hemphill et al. 2008; Smoyer-Tomic et al. 2008). However, in Nova Scotia, Jones et al. (2009) reported that significantly more fast-food outlets were available in communities with more affluence. In Montreal, Daniel et al. found no significant association between fast-food availability and median income, but reported significantly higher availability of fast food in areas with more full-time students, households speaking neither French nor English, lower proportions of children, older adults and married residents and more high-traffic roads. These limited studies only speak to a small selection of Canadian locations but show that area-level SES is not a clear unidirectional correlate of fast-food exposure.

Food Availability Surrounding Schools

Recent concern has been raised about the possibility that the food environment surrounding schools may act as a barrier to healthful dietary choices for children. As a result, policy recommendations in British Columbia, Quebec, and outside of Canada have now called for the development of guidelines to restrict the sale of minimally nutritious food and beverages and fast-food outlets immediately surrounding schools (Institute of Medicine 2009; Frieden et al. 2010; Association Pour La Sante Publique Du Qubec 2011). Moreover, regulations restricting the number of new fast-food restaurants have recently been implemented in some communities in the United States (Mair et al. 2005; Sturm and Cohen 2009; Eisenberg et al. 2011). Still, large gaps remain in knowledge and research regarding the distribution of food outlets surrounding Canadian schools and the net impact on students' food purchases and dietary choices.

In the United States, approximately one-third of schools are within walking distance of a fast-food outlet or convenience store (Zenk and Powell 2008). National estimates from Canada are similar, estimating that 31% of schools are located within 1 km of a fast-food restaurant, but vary between and within provinces and geographic regions (Zenk and Powell 2008; Seliske et al. 2009b; Insitut National De Sante Publique Du Quebec 2010; Black and Day 2012).

U.S. studies have found that secondary schools serving older students and schools in commercially dense urban areas and in neighborhoods characterized by lower SES are more likely to have access to a nearby fast-food vendor (Austin et al. 2005; Kipke et al. 2007; Simon et al. 2008; Zenk and Powell 2008; Neckerman et al. 2010). Table 8.4 similarly describes two Canadian studies conducted in Montreal (Kestens and Daniel 2010) and the province of British Columbia (Black and Day 2012), which found higher availability of limited service food outlets near schools located in neighborhoods with higher commercial and population densities and in areas characterized by lower SES. In Montreal, schools in the lowest income neighborhoods have 10 times more food stores within 750 m compared to schools in the highest income areas (Kestens and Daniel 2010). However, a national study found that schools in higher SES neighborhoods have higher exposure to food retailers including fast-food restaurants, donut/coffee shops, convenience stores, full-service restaurants, sub/sandwich shops, and grocery stores within 5 km than lower SES areas (Seliske et al. 2009b).

Overall, little empirical work in Canada (or elsewhere) has clearly elucidated the impact of food environment characteristics surrounding schools on students' dietary practices or related health outcomes. However, two recent Canadian studies described in Table 8.3 have pointed toward a possible connection (He et al. 2012; Héroux et al. 2012). First, Héroux et al.'s (2012) findings suggest that even though a sample of Canadian schools were less likely to have nearby exposure to fast-food outlets compared to a sample of U.S. schools, Canadian students were more likely than American students to report eating lunch on school days at a fast-food restaurant, café, or snack bar. Canadian students attending schools with a higher density of chain food retailers including convenience stores, fast-food outlets, and chain cafes within 1 km were also more likely to report regularly eating lunch at an off-campus chain food retailer compared to students at schools with no nearby chain retailers. Interestingly, no significant associations were found between the school neighborhood food retail environment and lunchtime eating behaviors among the U.S. students in this study.

Unlike the United States, there is no federal school lunch program in Canada. Canadian provinces, school boards and individual schools vary widely in the types of food sold within and surrounding schools. In Vancouver, for example, public elementary school students commonly bring bagged lunches from home because most elementary schools do not provide or sell lunches on a regular basis. It could be hypothesized that in Canadian schools (particularly where meal programs and on-campus food vending is limited), students could be more heavily influenced by the retail environment within walking distance around school grounds.

Moreover, several Canadian provinces, including British Columbia, have implemented school food and beverage guidelines to limit the sales of foods with poor nutritional quality in cafeterias, vending machines, fundraising efforts, and school events aiming to improve access to nutritious foods *within schools* that align with Canada's Food Guide's recommendations (BC Ministry of Education and Ministry of Health 2007). However, little research has examined whether reduced access to *junk food* on campus has unintentionally resulted in increased food purchases from nearby retailers. He et al. (2012) however, recently reported that increased density and closer proximity to fast-food outlets near schools was associated with slightly lower total diet quality (quantified using a modified version of the Healthy Eating Index) among grades 7 and 8 students in London, Ontario. In the United States, evidence from California similarly suggests that increased access to fast-food restaurants near schools predicts increased soda intake, lower fruit and vegetable consumption, and higher BMI (Davis and Carpenter 2009).

However, few other studies have showed a significant association between food availability surrounding schools with obesity outcomes. Data from 11 high schools in Maine found no significant associations between food store access surrounding schools with student-level BMI (Harris et al. 2011). The authors suggested that students, at least in the Maine context, have access to sugar-sweetened beverages and fast food at a plethora of locations near school and home; thus, reduced access near school alone is unlikely sufficient to elicit substantive dietary improvements. Moreover, students attending schools with the highest exposure to limited service food retailers in a national sample of Canadian schools were estimated to have significantly *lower* odds of being overweight (Seliske et al. 2009a). Further evidence is therefore needed to explain how food availability and contextual factors near school and home contribute to differences in health behaviors and BMI among youth.

Do the Poor Pay More for Food?

In addition to physical availability of food vendors and the types of products available at school, work, or in local retailers, price is an important factor shaping dietary choice. Despite the relative affluence enjoyed by many Canadians, nearly one in ten households reports experiencing food insecurity, characterized by insufficient financial resources to meet the nutritional needs of themselves and their families (Health Canada 2007). In particular, Canadians relying on social assistance, seniors' pension, employment insurance, or worker's compensation are more likely to report food insecurity. In British Columbia, it is estimated that families on income assistance would need to spend between 34% and 39% of their disposable income to afford an adequate amount of nutritious food, thus leaving insufficient resources to cover the costs of housing, clothing, and other necessities (Dietitians of Canada 2012). Consequently, food bank use is at an all-time high in Canada and in this province, nearly one-third of food bank users are children and youth (Food Banks Canada 2011).

Evidence from the Canadian Heart and Stroke Foundation (2009) suggests that residents in some Canadian regions may experience additional barriers to consuming a nutritionally adequate diet owing to inequitably higher food costs. Striking differences were identified regarding the prices of fresh foods including fruits and vegetables, grain products, dairy, and meat across Canada. For example, the average price of six medium-sized apples among five communities with the lowest prices was $1.51 compared to $5.71 in the five communities with the highest prices. As a result, low-income residents living in areas with higher prices likely face large barriers to accessing healthful food, even when living near large grocers that offer nutritious choices. It remains to be seen whether food costs are systematically higher in low-SES neighborhoods or stores serving marginalized communities in Canada. Food costs (and availability) are also a particularly salient issue among many remote northern communities (Wein 1994; Lawn et al. 1998).

Only three studies were identified that explicitly compared food prices and availability in diverse Canadian neighborhoods. One study compared the cost of an *Ontario Nutritious Food Basket* in Hamilton, Ontario, reporting no significant differences in food costs between a low- and a high-income neighborhood (Latham and Moffat 2007). However, variety stores tended to offer more expensive food items and were more common in the lower income neighborhood, which also had lower availability of fresh produce. Similarly in Quebec City, area-level material deprivation was not associated with varied food prices. However, convenience stores were more prevalent than all other food stores in deprived urban areas where food prices (particularly for fruits and vegetables) were significantly more expensive than comparable items sold at large grocers or green grocers (Drouin et al. 2009). In Nova Scotia, lower food costs were reported in the Central province (including Halifax), but not between neighborhoods with varied SES in urban Halifax (Travers 1996).

SUMMARY OF INSIGHTS FROM THE CANADIAN LITERATURE

This chapter adds to the burgeoning international knowledge base about regional variations in LFE characteristics and highlights a growing interest in social and contextual explanations for disparities in health and diet-related outcomes in Canada. This chapter offers one of the first syntheses of this young literature, from which main conclusions and suggestions for strengthening the literature are presented later.

First, there is evidence that diet-related health outcomes and obesity rates vary across Canada and disparities are not fully explained by differences in individual-level demographics, SES, or lifestyle choices. Substantial differences exist between Canadian cities and health regions, with a rising gradient in obesity from west to east and clusters of high prevalence in the north, particularly in Aboriginal communities (Pouliou and Elliott 2009). Rural-living Canadians are more likely than urbanites to have increased BMI, warranting the need for better understanding of the causal pathways and potentially modifiable loci for intervention in rural Canada.

Second, the role of macro-level social factors such as area-level SES and material deprivation remains unclear in Canada. There is certainly some indication that area-level SES is relevant, particularly for women and children in low-income neighborhoods. Neighborhood context is estimated to explain from as little as 1% to as much as 5%–8% of variation in obesity outcomes in Canadian cities (Matheson et al. 2008; Harrington and Elliott 2009; Prince et al. 2011). However, several studies identified no significant associations between neighborhood SES and BMI, and there is some indication of a detrimental effect of living in an affluent neighborhood for men, leaving many remaining questions about the intermediary processes that structure obesity and the intersecting effects of gender, place, and health.

At least two theoretical pathways could explain how neighborhood SES could influence behavioral risk factors that shape BMI including dietary choices and physical activity (Black and Macinko 2008). The first explanation suggests that neighborhood living conditions such as the percent of affluent or low-income residents shapes health behaviors by impacting the availability of amenities and exposures in a given neighborhood. For example, if there were systemic barriers that prevent retailers from selling healthy food in lower income neighborhoods (e.g., through zoning restrictions, higher operating costs, or a perceived lower demand for fresh food detracting local vendors), it is feasible that a direct lack of access to health-promoting resources could impede the purchase and consumption of foods that are not locally accessible. Given that food environment variables, particularly grocery store availability, do not appear to be consistently patterned based on area-level SES in Canada, it is also not surprising to find that the associations between area-level SES and diet-related outcomes are similarly inconsistent.

The second theoretical explanation suggests that neighborhood context could impact health outcomes by influencing attitudes, perceived norms, and the level of commitment that an individual feels about undertaking a given behavior. For example, students attending schools where a variety of fast-food restaurants are conveniently located nearby, may have increased interest in spending time there if peers commonly meet and socialize and consider such venues as desirable locations to hang out, eat, and spend money. However, few studies have empirically examined the pathways and psychosocial factors that mediate the associations between school and neighborhood food environment exposures and behavioral outcomes.

In the United States, a wider body of literature has explored other potential area-level social conditions that impact health, and there is evidence that neighborhoods with fewer visible minority residents have better access to nutritious food and health-related amenities (Morland et al. 2002b; Galvez et al. 2008; Beaulac et al. 2009). However, few studies in Canada have explicitly examined the associations between obesity and area-level racial or ethnic composition. There is evidence that a higher proportion of new immigrants may serve a protective function for weight gain, but the mechanisms are unresolved. This may be explained by an underlying *healthy immigrant effect*, as new immigrants have lower odds of being obese than native Canadians, whereas obesity risk increases gradually with years of residence (McDonald and Kennedy 2005). Newcomers also potentially shape the norms and health amenities in neighborhoods and influence the demand for and supply of foods. Still, little work has described the role of immigrant composition on the neighborhood food environment or BMI in Canada.

Several neighborhood-level barriers to accessing healthy food have been identified that may reduce the opportunities for some Canadians to adhere to the dietary recommendations from Canada's Food Guide. There is evidence that some residential neighborhoods lack convenient access to stores that sell healthy and affordable foods. This is particularly a concern for low-income persons, families without access to a vehicle or reliable public transportation, elderly and disabled persons,

Aboriginals, and residents in rural areas, many of whom have to make difficult trad-eoffs to access nutritious food.

Moreover, studies from the United States, Britain, Australia, and New Zealand have provided important insights about how neighborhood-context and food ameni-ties are patterned and shape dietary choices and obesity, but Canadian findings dif-fer meaningfully. Compelling evidence shows that U.S. neighborhoods with higher proportions of minority and low-income residents have poorer access to healthy food (Beaulac et al. 2009). The term *food desert* is now commonly used to describe eco-nomically disadvantaged areas with poor access to healthful, affordable foods and grocers. However, the food desert paradigm appears to be insufficient for character-izing areas with barriers to access in the Canadian context, where food vending does not appear to cluster systematically in wealthier or suburban neighborhoods. In several U.S. cities, there is evidence that many large food retailers have abandoned inner-city neighborhoods, whereas the Canadian literature suggests that central city, urban neighborhoods often have better food access than their suburban or more affluent counterparts.

Although neighborhood-level poverty may not confer systematic disadvantage to accessing food in Canada, individual and family-level poverty surely still does. There is evidence that low-income families, those on social assistance and workers earn-ing the minimum wage have inadequate income to afford a nutritious diet in Canada and subsequently consume lower intakes of health-promoting foods such as fruits and vegetables (Kirkpatrick and Tarasuk 2003; Power 2005; Williams et al. 2006; Tarasuk et al. 2010). A low-income family living in an affluent urban neighborhood or advantaged suburb may still face disproportionate barriers acquiring nutritious food, owing to further travel distances to food stores, reduced public transit or lack of access to a private vehicle. Therefore, in the Canadian context, the notion of *food insecurity* may be more relevant than that of the food desert. Food insecurity has been characterized as the insufficient availability of safe and nutritionally adequate foods or the inability to acquire sufficient and acceptable foods in socially acceptable ways (Nord et al. 2005; Casey et al. 2006), capturing both individual and contextual barriers to food.

KEY REMAINING GAPS IN THE CANADIAN LITERATURE

Several important gaps remain in Canadian literature, which is prone to the same widely acknowledged critiques challenging studies of neighborhood determinants of health and obesity internationally. Such limitations are described in depth in previ-ous publications and elsewhere in this book (e.g., Macintyre et al. 2002; Diez Roux 2004; Oakes 2004; Papas et al. 2007; Larson et al. 2009) but briefly include: reliance on cross-sectional data; a lack of reliable, valid, comprehensive, and consistent mea-sures of food access and availability; the challenges inherent to defining an appro-priate neighborhood (and comparing studies that use different metrics); differences between researcher-defined versus perceived neighborhood characteristics; failure of most studies to account for exposures outside of a single context of exposure (e.g., measuring only home or school exposure but seldom jointly assessing exposures at work and/or when eating or shopping outside of a residential neighborhood); limited use of detailed or meaningful measures of dietary practices or nutritional adequacy and quality; and the shortage of well-developed theory to explain neighborhood determinants of dietary choice and obesity.

In addition to these shared limitations, there are specific gaps in the Canadian literature that deserve mention and future research attention. First, as shown in Figure 8.1, many parts of the country have received little systematic study. Much of the national-level analysis of the distribution of obesity has assessed large regions defined by provincial or health region boundaries. These large units of analysis combine areas with varied composition and context, potentially occluding meaningful differences. Analyses of food availability have clustered mainly in Quebec, Alberta, Nova Scotia, and some parts of Ontario, but little is known about access in other metropolitan and rural areas, provinces, or the northern territories.

Second, several key area-level variables and food resources have been overlooked. Virtually no published work has assessed the role of area-level ethnic or racial composition and associations with obesity or food availability. There is early evidence that immigrant and Aboriginal composition is meaningful, but little is known about how residential composition and heterogeneity structures opportunities for healthful food or how it may intersect with social class, gender, and other experiences of discrimination or disability to shape health outcomes. McNeill et al. (2006) laid out several key dimensions of the social environment with potential effects on health behaviors that influence obesity including social support and social networks, socioeconomic position and income inequality, racial discrimination, social cohesion and social capital and neighborhood factors, but few of these social dimensions have been explored in Canada.

Food environment research in Canada has mainly focused narrowly on the food *retailing* environment, concentrating on a limited set of food stores, predominantly supermarkets and fast-food outlets. Little discussion has assessed the role of alternative food sources such as community supported agriculture programs, farmers markets, community, school or backyard gardens, or emergency and charitable food organizations. In addition, mobile vendors such as food trucks and produce stands and online food purchasing, potentially relevant sources of food as well as potential intervention strategies for bolstering access to nutritious food, have received little attention.

However, a small but growing area of scholarship suggests that broader conceptions of the food environment should consider the extent to which school, home and community gardens (Wakefield et al. 2007), emergency, charitable and community-based food programs (Kirkpatrick and Tarasuk 2009) and alternative food procurement strategies and traditional foodways (e.g., food sharing, gleaning, hunting, and fishing) contribute to dietary practices and health outcomes. The role of traditional food procurement strategies and their contribution to food security are particularly salient in Canada's northern and arctic communities, where challenges related to nutritional adequacy, food availability, and cost have been documented (Campbell et al. 1997; Chan et al. 2006; Kuhnlein et al. 2008; Ford 2009;). Also, little work has described how experiences of food insecurity and inadequate money or transportation additionally hinder food access, or how the distribution of commercial food retailers are shaped by local land-use policies such as zoning restrictions.

The totality of the evidence in Canada demonstrating that the food environment directly shapes dietary choices or BMI is in the early stages of development. There has been much progress in the literature over the past five years, but little is known about exactly for whom, by how much, or why food availability matters for shaping diet, BMI, or health in Canada. Future efforts from prospective and quasi-experimental intervention studies are needed to determine the feasibility and efficacy of modifying the food environment to improve health. Ultimately, improved conceptual and empirical work is needed to understand the underlying historical, economic, social, and political context that buffers some and exacerbates poor outcomes for others. This would help explain the differences within Canada, as well as between Canada and its southern neighbor and other high-income countries.

CONCLUSIONS

The importance of a nutritious diet and maintaining a healthy body weight for good health and longevity has long been recognized in Canada. Canada's first food guide, the Official Food Rules, was released in 1942 (Health Canada 2009) and myriad governmental agencies including Health Canada, the Public Health Agency of Canada, and the Canadian Food Inspection Agency now work to promote improved nutrition and access to a healthy food supply. Still, many Canadian children and adults do not meet the well-known dietary recommendations suggested by Canada's Food Guide (Garriguet 2007) and rates of obesity and nutrition-related chronic diseases have risen steeply.

Several Canadian stakeholders have already begun efforts to measure (and improve) food availability and geographic disparities in BMI and nutrition-related outcomes. For example, several Canadian cities, including Toronto, Vancouver, and Calgary, have developed Food Policy Councils and Food Charters to address the need for improved policy and intervention to ensure equitable access to adequate nutritious, affordable and culturally appropriate foods. Cities are also taking on leadership roles in articulating goals and new policy frameworks for improving urban food systems. For example, in January 2013, Vancouver's City Council approved the city's first Food Strategy that aims to: (1) support food-friendly neighborhoods; (2) empower residents to take action; (3) improve access to healthy, affordable, culturally diverse food for all residents; (4) make food a centerpiece of Vancouver's green economy; and (5) advocate for a just and sustainable food system (City of Vancouver 2013). The research community is now charged with the task of providing well-designed research and evaluation tools to guide effective and timely strategies to achieve these ends.

APPENDIX

Description of Common Area-Level Metrics Used in the Canadian Literature

Area Metric	Description	Examples from Literature
Provinces	Canada's land area is divided into 10 provinces and 3 territories governed by a political authority (Statistics Canada 2006b)	(Willms et al. 2003)
Health Regions	Defined by the provinces to represent administrative areas or regions of interest to health authorities. (Statistics Canada 2007)	(Pouliou and Elliott 2009)
Census Metropolitan Area (CMA)	Consists of one or more adjacent municipalities located around a major urban core with a population of at least 100,000 (Statistics Canada 2006c)	(Ross et al. 2007)
Census Tracts	Usually have a population of 2,500 to 8,000 and are located in large urban areas with population of 50,000 or more if urban core (Statistics Canada 2006c)	(Daniel et al. 2009)
Dissemination Areas	Small area of 400 to 700 persons with one or more neighboring blocks. All of Canada is divided into dissemination areas. (Statistics Canada 2006c)	(Oliver and Hayes 2005)
Forward Sortation Areas (FSA)	The area represented by the first 3 digits of a Canadian postal code. Over 1,600 across Canada. (Canada Post 2009)	(Harrington and Elliott 2009)

REFERENCES

Agriculture and Agri-Food Canada. 2008. An Overview of the Canadian Agriculture and Agri-Food System Publication 10770E. Available at http://www.agr.gc.ca/eng/about-us/publications/economic-publications/alphabetical-listing/overview-of-the-canadian-agriculture-and-agri-food-system-2008/?id=1228246364385. Edited by Strategic Policy Branch, Research and Analysis Directorate.

Anis, A. H., W. Zhang, N. Bansback, D. P. Guh, Z. Amarsi, and C. L. Birmingham. 2009. Obesity and overweight in Canada: An updated cost-of-illness study. *Obes Rev* 11:31–40.

Apparicio, P., M. S. Cloutier, and R. Shearmur. 2007. The case of Montreal's missing food deserts: Evaluation of accessibility to food supermarkets. *Int J Health Geogr* 6:4.

Association Pour La Sante Publique Du Qubec. 2011. The School Zone and Nutrition: Courses of Action for the Municipal Sector ISBN: 978-2-920202-53-5. Available at http://www .aspq .org/documents/file/guide-zonage-version-finale-anglaise.pdf. Accessed: April 16, 2014.

Austin, S. B., S. J. Melly, B. N. Sanchez, A. Patel, S. Buka, and S. L. Gortmaker. 2005. Clustering of fast-food restaurants around schools: A novel application of spatial statistics to the study of food environments. *Am J Public Health* 95 (9):1575–81.

BC Ministry of Education and Ministry of Health. 2007. Guidelines for Food and Beverage Sales in BC Schools Ministry of Education and Ministry of Health.

Beaulac, J., E. Kristjansson, and S. Cummins. 2009. A systematic review of food deserts, 1966–2007. *Prev Chronic Dis* 6 (3):A105.

Bedore, M. 2012. Geographies of capital formation and rescaling: A historical-geographical approach to the food desert problem. *Can Geogr* 57:133–53.

Belanger-Ducharme, F. and A. Tremblay. 2005. Prevalence of obesity in Canada. *Obes Rev* 6 (3):183–6.

Bertrand, L., F. Therien, and M. S. Cloutier. 2008. Measuring and mapping disparities in access to fresh fruits and vegetables in Montreal. *Can J Public Health* 99 (1):6–11.

Black, J. L. and J. Macinko. 2008. Neighborhoods and obesity. *Nutr Rev* 66 (1):2–20.

Black, J. L. and M. Day. 2012. Availability of limited service food outlets surrounding schools in British Columbia. *Can J Public Health* 103 (4):255–9.

Black, J. L., R. M. Carpiano, S. Fleming, and N. Lauster. 2011. Exploring the distribution of food stores in British Columbia: associations with neighbourhood socio-demographic factors and urban form. *Health Place* 17:961–70.

Bowman, S. A. and B. T. Vinyard. 2004. Fast food consumption of U.S. adults: impact on energy and nutrient intakes and overweight status. *J Am Coll Nutr* 23 (2):163–8.

Campbell, M. L., R. M. Diamant, B. D. Macpherson, and J. L. Halladay. 1997. The contemporary food supply of three northern Manitoba Cree communities. *Can J Public Health* 88 (2):105–8.

Canadian Food Security Summit. 1998. available at: http://www.agr.gc.ca/misb/fsec-seca /pdf/action_e.pdf. Accessed May 5, 2014.

Casey, P. H., P. M. Simpson, J. M. Gossett, M. L. Bogle, C. M. Champagne, C. Connell, D. Harsha, B. McCabe-Sellers, J. M. Robbins, J. E. Stuff, and J. Weber. 2006. The association of child and household food insecurity with childhood overweight status. *Pediatrics* 118 (5):e1406–13.

Chan, H. M., K. Fediuk, S. Hamilton, L. Rostas, A. Caughey, H. Kuhnlein, G. Egeland, and E. Loring. 2006. Food security in Nunavut, Canada: Barriers and recommendations. *Int J Circumpolar Health* 65 (5):416–31.

City of Vancouver. 2013. Vancouver Food City Strategy. Available at http://vancouver.ca/files /cov/vancouver-food-strategy-final.PDF, accessed February 7, 2013.

Condon, G. 2009. Market Survey 2008. *Canadian Grocer* 123 (1):25–29,31.

Cummins, S. and S. Macintyre. 1999. The location of food stores in urban areas: A case study in Glasgow. *Br Food J* 101 (7):545–53.

Cummins, S. C., L. McKay, and S. Macintyre. 2005. McDonald's restaurants and neighborhood dDeprivation in Scotland and England. *Am J Prev Med* 29:308–10.

Cummins, S. C. and S. Macintyre. 2002. A systematic study of an urban foodscape: The price and availability of food in great Glasgow. *Urban Stud* 39:2115.

Daniel, M., Y. Kestens, and C. Paquet. 2009. Demographic and urban form correlates of healthful and unhealthful food availability in Montreal, Canada. *Can J Public Health* 100 (3):189–93.

Davis, B. and C. Carpenter. 2009. Proximity of fast-food restaurants to schools and adolescent obesity. *Am J Public Health* 99 (3):505–10.

Dietitians of Canada. 2007. Community Food Security. Position of Dietitians of Canada. *Public Policy Statement*:1–13.

Dietitians of Canada. 2012. Cost of Eating in British Columbia, 2011. Available at http://www.dietitians.ca/Downloadable-Content/Public/CostofEatingBC2011_FINAL.aspx, accessed april 16, 2014.

Diez Roux, A. V. 2004. Estimating neighborhood health effects: The challenges of causal inference in a complex world. *Soc Sci Med* 58 (10):1953–60.

Drouin, S., A. M. Hamelin, and D. Ouellet. 2009. Economic access to fruits and vegetables in the greater Quebec City: do disparities exist? *Can J Public Health* 100(5):361–4.

Eisenberg, M. J., R. Atallah, S. M. Grandi, S. B. Windle, and E. M. Berry. 2011. Legislative approaches to tackling the obesity epidemic. *Can Med Assoc J* 183 (13):1496–500.

Euromonitor International. 2012. Fast Food in Canada. Available at http://www.euromonitor.com/fast-food-in-canada/report, accessed January 10, 2013.

Flanagan, M. 2006. The Workshop or the Home? Gender Visions in the History of Urban Built Environments: Canada and the United States. *London J Can Stud* 22:58–83.

Food Banks Canada. 2011. Hunger Count: A comprehensive report on hunger and food bank use in Canada, and recommendations for change. Available at http://foodbankscanada.ca/getmedia/dc2aa860-4c33-4929-ac36-fb5d40f0b7e7/HungerCount-2011.pdf.aspx, accessed april 16, 2014.

Ford, J. D. 2009. Vulnerability of Inuit food systems to food insecurity as a consequence of climate change: A case study from Igloolik, Nunavut. *Reg Environ Change* 9:83–100.

Frank, L. D., M. A. Andresen, and T. L. Schmid. 2004. Obesity relationships with community design, physical activity, and time spent in cars. *Am J Prev Med* 27 (2):87–96.

Frieden, T. R., W. Dietz, and J. Collins. 2010. Reducing childhood obesity through policy change: Acting now to prevent obesity. *Health Affairs* 29 (3):357–63.

Gallagher, M. 2006. *Examining the Impact of Food Deserts on Public Health in Chicago.* Chicago, IL: LaSalle Bank.

Galvez, M. P., K. Morland, C. Raines, J. Kobil, J. Siskind, J. Godbold, and B. Brenner. 2008. Race and food store availability in an inner-city neighbourhood. *Public Health Nutr* 11 (6):624–31.

Garriguet, D. 2007. Canadians' eating habits. *Health Rep* 18 (2):17–32.

Gilliland, J. A., C. Y. Rangel, M. A. Healy, P. Tucker, J. E. Loebach, P. M. Hess, M. He, J. D. Irwin, and P. Wilk. 2012. Linking childhood obesity to the built environment: A multi-level analysis of home and school neighbourhood factors associated with body mass index. *Can J Public Health* 103 (9):S15–21.

Harrington, D. W. and S. J. Elliott. 2009. Weighing the importance of neighbourhood: A multilevel exploration of the determinants of overweight and obesity. *Soc Sci Med* 68 (4):593–600.

Harris, D. E., J. W. Blum, M. Bampton, L. M. O'Brien, C. M. Beaudoin, M. Polacsek, and K. A. O'Rourke. 2011. Location of food stores near schools does not predict the weight status of Maine high school students. *J Nutr Educ Behav* 43 (4):274–8.

He, M., P. Tucker, J. D. Irwin, J. Gilliland, K. Larsen, and P. Hess. 2012. Obesogenic neighbourhoods: The impact of neighbourhood restaurants and convenience stores on adolescents' food consumption behaviours. *Public Health Nutr* 15:2331–9.

Health Canada. 2007. Health Canada. Canadian Community Health Survey Cycle 2.2, Nutrition (2004). Income-related Household Food Security in Canada. Available at http://www.hc-sc.gc.ca/fn-an/surveill/nutrition/commun/income_food_sec-sec_alimeng.php#fg34. Ottawa, ON: Health Canada, accessed April 16, 2014.

Health Canada. 2009. Canada's Food Guides from 1942 to 1992. Available at http://www.hc-sc.gc.ca/fn-an/food-guide-aliment/context/hist/fg_history-histoire_ga-eng.php [cited July 12, 2009].

Heart and Stroke should be on a new line (it's a different reference than Health Canada 2009) Heart and Stroke Foundation. 2009. 2009 Report Card—What's in Store for Canada's Heart Health? Available at http://www.heartandstroke.ab.ca/site/lookup.asp?c=lqIRL1PJJtH&b=4969983, accessed April 16, 2014.

Hemphill, E., K. Raine, J. C. Spence, and K. E. Smoyer-Tomic. 2008. Exploring obesogenic food environments in Edmonton, Canada: The association between socioeconomic factors and fast-food outlet access. *Am J Health Promot* 22 (6):426–32.

Héroux, M., R. J. Iannotti, D. Currie, W. Pickett, and I. Janssen. 2012. The food retail environment in school neighborhoods and its relation to lunchtime eating behaviors in youth from three countries. *Health Place* 18 (6):1240–7.

Horowitz, C. R., K. A. Colson, P. L. Hebert, and K. Lancaster. 2004. Barriers to buying healthy foods for people with diabetes: Evidence of environmental disparities. *Am J Public Health* 94 (9):1549–54.

Insitut National De Sante Publique Du Quebec. 2010. Geographical analysis of the accessibility of fast-food restaurants and convenience stores around public schools in Quebec. Report.

Institute of Medicine. 2009. *Local Government Actions to Prevent Childhood Obesity.* Washington, DC: The National Academies Press.

Janssen, I., W. F. Boyce, K. Simpson, and W. Pickett. 2006. Influence of individual- and area-level measures of socioeconomic status on obesity, unhealthy eating, and physical inactivity in Canadian adolescents. *Am J Clin Nutr* 83 (1):139–45.

Jones, J., M. Terashima, and D. Rainham. 2009. Fast food and deprivation in Nova Scotia. *Can J Public Health* 100 (1):32–5.

Joshu, C. E., T. K. Boehmer, R. C. Brownson, and R. Ewing. 2008. Personal, neighbourhood and urban factors associated with obesity in the United States. *J Epidemiol Community Health* 62 (3):202–8.

Katzmarzyk, P. T. 2002. The Canadian obesity epidemic: An historical perspective. *Obes Res* 10 (7):666–74.

Katzmarzyk, P. T. and C. Mason. 2006. Prevalence of class I, II and III obesity in Canada. *Can Med Assoc J* 174:156–7.

Katzmarzyk, P. T. and C. I. Ardern. 2004. Overweight and obesity mortality trends in Canada, 1985–2000. *Can J Public Health* 95 (1):16–20.

Katzmarzyk, P. T. and I. Janssen. 2004. The economic costs associated with physical inactivity and obesity in Canada: An update. *Can J Appl Physiol* 29 (1):90–115.

Kestens, Y., A. Lebel, B. Chaix, C. Clary, M. Daniel, R. Pampalon, M. Theriault, and P. Subramanian SV. 2012. Association between activity space exposure to food establishments and individual risk of overweight. *PloS One* 7 (8):e41418.

Kestens, Y. and M. Daniel. 2010. Social inequalities in food exposure around schools in an urban area. *Am J Prev Med* 39:33–40.

Kipke, M. D., E. Iverson, D. Moore, C. Booker, V. Ruelas, A. L. Peters, and F. Kaufman. 2007. Food and park environments: Neighborhood-level risks for childhood obesity in east Los Angeles. *J Adolesc Health* 40 (4):325–33.

Kirkpatrick, S. and V. Tarasuk. 2003. The relationship between low income and household food expenditure patterns in Canada. *Public Health Nutr* 6:589–97.

Kirkpatrick, S. I. and V. Tarasuk. 2009. Food insecurity and participation in community food programs among low-income Toronto families. *Can J Public Health* 100 (2):135–9.

Kuhnlein, H. V., O. Receveur, R. Soueida, and P. R. Berti. 2008. Unique patterns of dietary adequacy in three cultures of Canadian Arctic indigenous peoples. *Public Health Nutr* 11 (4):349–60.

Lambden, J., O. Receveur, J. Marshall, and H. V. Kuhnlein. 2006. Traditional and market food access in Arctic Canada is affected by economic factors. *Int J Circumpol Health* 65:331–40.

Laraia, B. A., A. M. Siega-Riz, J. S. Kaufman, and S. J. Jones. 2004. Proximity of supermarkets is positively associated with diet quality index for pregnancy. *Prev Med* 39 (5):869–75.

Larsen, K., and J. Gilliland. 2008. Mapping the evolution of 'food deserts' in a Canadian city: Supermarket accessibility in London, Ontario, 1961–2005. *Int J Health Geogr* 7 (1):16.

Larson, N., D. Neumark-Sztainer, M. N. Laska, and M. Story. 2011. Young adults and eating away from home: Associations with dietary intake patterns and weight status differ by choice of restaurant. *J Am Diet Assoc* 111 (11):1696–703.

Larson, N. I., M. T. Story, and M. C. Nelson. 2009. Neighborhood environments: Disparities in access to healthy foods in the U.S. *Am J Prev Med* 36:74–81.

Latham, J. and T. Moffat. 2007. Determinants of variation in food cost and availability in two socioeconomically contrasting neighbourhoods of Hamilton, Ontario, Canada. *Health Place* 13 (1):273–87.

Lawn, J., H. Robbins, and F. Hill. 1998. Food affordability in air stage communities. *Int J Circumpolar Health* 57 (Suppl 1):182–8.

Lebel, A., R. Pampalon, D. Hamel, and M. Theriault. 2009. The geography of overweight in Quebec: A multilevel perspective. *Can J Public Health* 100 (1):18–23.

Lee, D. S., M. Chiu, D. G. Manuel, K. Tu, X. Wang, P. C. Austin, M. Y. Mattern, T. F. Mitiku, L. W. Svenson, W. Putnam, W. M. Flanagan, and J. V. Tu. 2009. Trends in risk factors for cardiovascular disease in Canada: Temporal, socio-demographic and geographic factors. *Can Med Assoc J* 181:E55–66.

Levine, J. 2006. *Zoned Out: Regulation, Markets, and Choices in Transportation and Metropolitan Land-Use.* Washington, DC: RFF Press.

Lopez-Zetina, J., H. Lee, and R. Friis. 2006. The link between obesity and the built environment. Evidence from an ecological analysis of obesity and vehicle miles of travel in California. *Health Place* 12 (4):656–64.

Luo, W., H. Morrison, M. de Groh, C. Waters, M. DesMeules, E. Jones-McLean, A. M. Ugnat, S. Desjardins, M. Lim, and Y. Mao. 2007. The burden of adult obesity in Canada. *Chronic Dis Can* 27 (4):135–44.

Macintyre, S. and A. Ellaway. 2003. Neighborhoods and health: An overview. In: *Neighborhoods and Health*, edited by Kawachi, I. and L. F. Berkman. New York: Oxford University Press, p. 24.

Mair, J. S., M. W. Pierce, and S. P. Teret. 2005. The Use of Zoning to Restrict Fast Food Outlets: A Potential Strategy to Combat Obesity. Available at http://www.publichealthlaw.net/Zoning%20Fast%20Food%20Outlets.pdf, accessed January 5, 2012.

Matheson, F. I., R. Moineddin, and R. H. Glazier. 2008. The weight of place: A multilevel analysis of gender, neighborhood material deprivation, and body mass index among Canadian adults. *Soc Sci Med* 66 (3):675–90.

McDonald, J. T., and S. Kennedy. 2005. Is migration to Canada associated with unhealthy weight gain? Overweight and obesity among Canada's immigrants. *Soc Sci Med* 61 (12):2469–81.

McNeill, L. H., M. W. Kreuter, and S. V. Subramanian. 2006. Social environment and physical activity: A review of concepts and evidence. *Soc Sci Med* 63 (4):1011–22.

Mercille, G., L. Richard, L. Gauvin, Y. Kestens, B. Shatenstein, M. Daniel, and H. Payette. 2012. Associations between residential food environment and dietary patterns in urban-dwelling older adults: Results from the VoisiNuAge study. *Public Health Nutr* 15:2029–39.

Moore, L. V. and A. V. Diez Roux. 2006. Associations of neighborhood characteristics with the location and type of food stores. *Am J Public Health* 96 (2):325–31.

Moore, L. V., A. V. Diez Roux, J. A. Nettleton, and D. R. Jacobs, Jr. 2008. Associations of the local food environment with diet quality—A comparison of assessments based on surveys and geographic information systems: The multi-ethnic study of atherosclerosis. *Am J Epidemiol* 167:917–24.

Morland, K., S. Wing, and A. Diez Roux. 2002a. The contextual effect of the local food environment on residents' diets: The atherosclerosis risk in communities study. *Am J Public Health* 92 (11):1761–7.

Morland, K., S. Wing, A. Diez Roux, and C. Poole. 2002b. Neighborhood characteristics associated with the location of food stores and food service places. *Am J Prev Med* 22 (1):23–9.

National Vital Statistics Report. 2012. Deaths: Preliminary Data for 2011. Available at http://www.cdc.gov/nchs/data/nvsr/nvsr61/nvsr61_06.pdf. 61 (6):1–65.

Neckerman, K. M., M. D. Bader, C. A. Richards, M. Purciel, J. W. Quinn, J. S. Thomas, C. Warbelow, C. C. Weiss, G. S. Lovasi, and A. Rundle. 2010. Disparities in the food environments of New York City public schools. *Am J Prev Med* 39 (3):195–202.

Nord, M., M. Andrews, and S. Carlson. 2005. *Household Food Security in the United States, 2004 Food Assistance and Nutrition Research Program Report 11*. Washington, DC: US Department of Agriculture, Economic Research Service.

Oakes, J. M. 2004. The (mis)estimation of neighborhood effects: Causal inference for a practicable social epidemiology. *Soc Sci Med* 58 (10):1929–52.

Oliver, L. N., and M. V. Hayes. 2005. Neighbourhood socioeconomic status and the prevalence of overweight Canadian children and youth. *Can J Public Health* 96 (6):415–20.

Paeratakul, S., D. P. Ferdinand, C. M. Champagne, D. H. Ryan, and G. A. Bray. 2003. Fast-food consumption among U.S. adults and children: Dietary and nutrient intake profile. *J Am Diet Assoc* 103 (10):1332–8.

Papas, M. A., A. J. Alberg, R. Ewing, K. J. Helzlsouer, T. L. Gary, and A. C. Klassen. 2007. The built environment and obesity. *Epidemiol Rev* 29 (1):129–43.

Pearce, J., K. Witten, R. Hiscock, and T. Blakely. 2007. Are socially disadvantaged neighbourhoods deprived of health-related community resources? *Int J Epidemiol* 36 (2):348–55.

Perrin, C. 1979. *Everything In Its Place: Social Order and Land Use in America*. Princeton, NJ: Princeton University Press.

Peters, E. J. and T. A. McCreary. 2008. Poor neighbourhoods and the changing geography of food retailing in Saskatoon, Saskatchewan, 1984–2004. *Can J Urban Res* 17 (1):78–106.

Pouliou, T. and S. Elliott. 2010. Individual and socio-environmental determinants of overweight and obesity in Urban Canada. *Health Place* 16 (2):389–98.

Pouliou, T. and S. J. Elliott. 2009. An exploratory spatial analysis of overweight and obesity in Canada. *Prev Med* 18:362–7.

Powell, L. M., F. J. Chaloupka, and Y. Bao. 2007. The availability of fast-food and full-service restaurants in the United States: associations with neighborhood characteristics. *Am J Prev Med* 33 (4 Suppl):S240–5.

Power, E. M. 2005. Determinants of healthy eating among low-income Canadians. *Can J Public Health* 96 (Suppl 3):S37–48.

Prince, S. A., E. A. Kristjansson, K. Russell, J. M. Billette, M. Sawada, A. Ali, M. S. Tremblay, and D. Prud'homme. 2011. A multilevel analysis of neighbourhood built and social environments and adult self-reported physical activity and body mass index in Ottawa, Canada. *IntJ Environl Res Public Health* 8 (10):3953–78.

Prince, S. A., E. A. Kristjansson, K. Russell, J. M. Billette, M. C. Sawada, A. Ali, M. S. Tremblay, and D. Prud'homme. 2012. Relationships between neighborhoods, physical activity, and obesity: A multilevel analysis of a large Canadian city. *Obesity* 20:2093–100.

Raine, K. D. 2005. Determinants of healthy eating in Canada: An overview and synthesis. *Can J Public Health* 96 (Suppl 3):S8-14, S8-15.

Raphael, D., A. Curry-Stevens, and T. Bryant. 2008. Barriers to addressing the social determinants of health: Insights from the Canadian experience. *Health Policy* 88 (2–3):222–35.

Reeder, B. A., Y. Chen, S. M. Macdonald, A. Angel, and L. Sweet. 1997. Regional and rural-urban differences in obesity in Canada. Canadian Heart Health Surveys Research Group. *Can Med Assoc J* 157 (Suppl 1):S10–6.

Rose, D. and R. Richards. 2004. Food store access and household fruit and vegetable use among participants in the US Food Stamp Program. *Public Health Nutr* 7 (8):1081–8.

Ross, N. A., S. Tremblay, S. Khan, D. Crouse, M. Tremblay, and J. M. Berthelot. 2007. Body mass index in urban Canada: Neighborhood and metropolitan area effects. *Am J Public Health* 97 (3):500–8.

Seliske, L. M., W. Pickett, W. F. Boyce, and I. Janssen. 2009a. Association between the food retail environment surrounding schools and overweight in Canadian youth. *Public Health Nutr* 12:1384–91.

Seliske, L. M., W. Pickett, W. F. Boyce, and I. Janssen. 2009b. Density and type of food retailers surrounding Canadian schools: Variations across socioeconomic status. *Health Place* 15 (3):903–7.

Shields, M., M. D. Carroll, and C. L. Ogden. 2011. Adult Obesity Prevalence in Canada and the United States. NCHS Data Brief no. 56. Hyattsville, MD: National Center for Health Statistics, pp. 1–8.

Shlay, A. and P. Rossi. 1981. Keeping up the neighborhood: Estimating net effects of zoning. *Am Sociol Rev* 46 (6):703–19.

Simon, P. A., D. Kwan, A. Angelescu, M. Shih, and J. E. Fielding. 2008. Proximity of fast food restaurants to schools: Do neighborhood income and type of school matter? *Prev Med* 47 (3):284–8.

Smoyer-Tomic, K. E., J. C. Spence, and C. Amrhein. 2006. Food deserts in the prairies? Supermarket accessibility and neighbourhood need in Edmonton, Canada. *Prof Geogr* 58 (3):307–26.

Smoyer-Tomic, K. E., J. C. Spence, K. D. Raine, C. Amrhein, N. Cameron, V. Yasenovskiy, N. Cutumisu, E. Hemphill, and J. Healy. 2008. The association between neighborhood socioeconomic status and exposure to supermarkets and fast food outlets. *Health Place* 14:740–54.

Spence, J. C., N. Cutumisu, J. Edwards, K. D. Raine, and K. Smoyer-Tomic. 2009. Relation between local food environments and obesity among adults. *BMC Public Health* 9:192.

Statistics Canada. 2006a. Canadians Spending More on Eating Out. Available at http://www41 .statcan.ca/2006/0163/ceb0163_002-eng.htm, accessed November 24, 2012.

Statistics Canada. 2006b. Province/Territory. Available at http:// geodepot.statcan. ca /Diss/Reference/COGG/ShortDescription_e.cfm?GEO_LEVEL=2&TUTORIAL = 0&ABBRV=e [cited August 5, 2009].

Statistics Canada. 2006c. Illustrated Glossary of Census Geography. Available at http:// geodepot.statcan.ca/Diss/Reference/COGG/ShortDescription_e.cfm?GEO _LEVEL=2&TUTORIAL=0&ABBRV=e [cited August 5, 2009].

Statistics Canada. 2007. Health Regions: Boundaries and Correspondence with Census Geography Product main page; Available at http://www.statcan.gc.ca/bsolc/olc-cel/olc -cel?lang=eng&catno=82-402-X [cited August 5, 2009].

Statistics Canada. 2008. Imports of Food into Canada by Country, 2007. Available at http:// www.statcan.gc.ca/pub/16-201-x/2009000/t240-eng.htm, accessed Jan 31, 2013.

Statistics Canada. 2011a. Census Profile. Available at http://www12.statcan.gc.ca/census -recensement/2011/dp-pd/prof/details/page.cfm?Lang=E&Geo1=PR&Code1=01&Ge o2=PR&Code2=01&Data=Count&SearchText=Canada&SearchType=Begins&Searc hPR=01&B1=All&Custom=&TABID=1, accessed January 3, 2012.

Statistics Canada. 2011b. The Canadian Population in 2011: Population Counts and Growth http://www12.statcan.gc.ca/census-recensement/2011/as-sa/98-310-x/98-310 -x2011001-eng.cfm, accessed January 3, 2012.

Statistics Canada. 2011c. Population and Dwelling Count Highlight Tables, 2011 http://www12.statcan.gc.ca/census-recensement/2011/dp-pd/hlt-fst/pd-pl/Table-Tableau.cfm?LANG=Eng&T=201&S=3&O=D&RPP=150 Census, accessed January 3, 2013.

Statistics Canada. 2012a. Tables by Subject: Life Expectancy and Deaths. Available at http://www.statcan.gc.ca/tables-tableaux/sum-som/l01/ind01/l3_2966_2979-eng.htm?hili_health30, accessed January 3, 2013.

Statistics Canada. 2012b. Population and Dwelling Counts, for Census Metropolitan Areas, 2011 and 2006 Censuses. Available at http://www12.statcan.gc.ca/census-recensement/2011/dp-pd/hlt-fst/pd-pl/Table-Tableau.cfm?LANG=Eng&T=205&S=3&RPP=50, accessed January 10, 2013.

Sturm, R. and D. A. Cohen. 2009. Zoning for health? The year-old ban on new fast-food restaurants in South LA. *Health Affairs* 28 (6):w1088–97.

Talen, E. and L. Anselin. 1998. Assessing spatial equity: An evaluation of measures of accessibility to public playgrounds. *Environ Plann A* 30 (4):595–613.

Tarasuk, V., S. Fitzpatrick, and H. Ward. 2010. Nutrition inequities in Canada. *Appl Physiol Nutr Metab* 35 (2):172–9.

Taylor, J. P., S. Evers, and M. McKenna. 2005. Determinants of healthy eating in children and youth. *Can J Public Health* 96 (Suppl 3):S20–6, S22–9.

Travers, K. 1996. The social organization of nutritional inequities. *Soc Sci Med* 43 (4):543–53.

Travers, K. D., A. Cogdon, W. McDonald, C. Wright, B. Anderson, and D. R. Maclean. 1997. Availability and cost of heart healthy dietary changes in Nova Scotia. *J Can Diet Assoc* 58:176–83.

Tremblay, M. S., P. T. Katzmarzyk, and J. D. Willms. 2002. Temporal trends in overweight and obesity in Canada, 1981–1996. *Int J Obes Relat Metab Disord* 26 (4):538–43.

United States Census Bureau. 2011. State and County QuickFacts. Available at http://quickfacts.census.gov/qfd/states/00000.html [cited January 3, 2013].

USDA. 2009. Access to Affordable and Nutritious Food: Measuring and Understanding Food Deserts and Their Consequences. Report to Congress.

Vanasse, A., M. Demers, A. Hemiari, and J. Courteau. 2006. Obesity in Canada: Where and how many? *Int J Obes (Lond)* 30 (4):677–83.

Veugelers, P., F. Sithole, S. Zhang, and N. Muhajarine. 2008. Neighborhood characteristics in relation to diet, physical activity and overweight of Canadian children. *Int J Pediatr Obes* 3 (3):152–9.

Veugelers, P. J., and A. L. Fitzgerald. 2005. Prevalence of and risk factors for childhood overweight and obesity. *Can Med Assoc J* 173:607–13.

Wakefield, S., F. Yeudall, C. Taron, J. Reynolds, and A. Skinner. 2007. Growing urban health: community gardening in South-East Toronto. *Health Promot Int* 22 (2):92–101.

Wein, E. E. 1994. The high cost of a nutritionally adequate diet in four Yukon communities. *CanJ Public Health* 85 (5):310–2.

White, M., E. Williams, S. Raybould, A. Adamson, J. Bunting, and J. Mathers. 2004. Do 'Food Deserts' Exist? A Multi-level Geographical Analysis of the Relationship between Retail Food Access, Socio-economic Position and Dietary Intake (Final report to Food Standards Agency). Newcastle, School of Population and Health Sciences, University of Newcastle upon Tyne. Available at http://www.ncl.ac.uk/biomedicine/research/groups/publication/55124, accessed September 28, 2013.

White House Task Force. 2010. White House Task Force on Childhood Obesity Report to the President. Available at http://www.letsmove.gov/sites/letsmove.gov/files/TaskForce_on_Childhood_Obesity_May2010_FullReport.pdf Accessed april 16, 2014

Williams, P. L., C. P. Johnson, M. L. Kratzmann, C. S. Johnson, B. J. Anderson, and C. Chenhall. 2006. Can households earning minimum wage in Nova Scotia afford a nutritious diet? *Can J Public Health* 97 (6):430–4.

Willms, J. D., M. S. Tremblay, and P. T. Katzmarzyk. 2003. Geographic and demographic variation in the prevalence of overweight Canadian children. *Obes Res* 11 (5):668–73.

Winkler, E., G. Turrell, and C. Patterson. 2006. Does living in a disadvantaged area mean fewer opportunities to purchase fresh fruit and vegetables in the area? Findings from the Brisbane food study. *Health Place* 12 (3):306–19.

Zenk, S., A. Schultz, B. Israel, S. James, S. Bao, and M. Wilson. 2005. Neighbourhood racial composition, neighborhood poverty, and the spatial accessibility of supermarkets in metropolitan Detroit. *Am J Public Health* 95 (4):660–7.

Zenk, S. N. and L. M. Powell. 2008. US secondary schools and food outlets. *Health Place* 14 (2):336–46.

Section III

Moving Forward
Local Food Environment Now and in the Future

9 State-Level Interventions
Pennsylvania's Fresh Food Financing Initiative

*Yael Lehmann, April White, Jordan Tucker, and
Allison Karpyn*

This is not just happening here in Chicago on the South Side, in so many neighborhoods, if people want to buy a head of lettuce or salad or some fruit for their kid's lunch, they have to take two or three buses, maybe pay for a taxicab, in order to do it.

First Lady Michelle Obama (Yaccino 2011)

On a crisp October day in 1968, 10,000 people gathered to mark the opening of Progress Plaza, the country's first African-American-owned shopping center, in the Yorktown neighborhood on Broad Street in North Philadelphia. The crowd was celebrating the shopping center, anchored by a big, beautiful A&P Supermarket, which brought much-needed services and jobs to the community—and they were celebrating the strong community partnerships that made Progress Plaza possible.

This was not a typical shopping center development, financed by developers, businessmen, and bankers and motivated mainly by profit. This was a true community development, financed by residents and motivated by the understanding that access to affordable, nutritious food was essential to the health of their neighbors and the health of their neighborhood. Reverend Leon Sullivan of the nearby Zion Baptist Church led the effort; 650 members of his congregation financed the project, contributing $10 a month, every month, for 3 years to bring a supermarket stocking fresh produce and 16 other stores to their neighborhood.

For three decades, that supermarket was a vital part of the Yorktown community. When it abruptly shut its doors in 1998, the community took the company to court in hopes of delaying the closure. When efforts to keep the supermarket failed, the plaza tried unsuccessfully to woo another supermarket. With its anchor market gone, the once-proud plaza fell into decline and Yorktown residents were forced to travel 19 blocks—via two buses—to the nearest supermarket for fresh fruits and vegetables and other healthy foods for their dinner tables.

It would take another decade—and another innovative community effort—to bring a supermarket back to the neighborhood.

IMPORTANCE OF SUPERMARKETS

While the closure of the supermarket was devastating for residents of Yorktown, the neighborhood's situation was not unique. A 1995 report found that Philadelphia had the second lowest number of supermarkets per capita of the country's major cities, but everywhere, supermarkets were leaving the urban and rural neighborhoods they had nourished for the spacious shopping centers and higher income levels of suburban residents (Cotterill 1995). Ultimately, their departure created communities that lacked food access.

The term *food access* describes a community's level of access to the high-quality, healthy, affordable food necessary to live a healthy life. It means a community that has numerous fast-food restaurants and convenience stores selling highly priced and highly processed foods but does not have a supermarket selling fresh produce at an affordable price is a community that lacks food access. These communities, colloquially called *food deserts*, are said to be *underserved* by supermarkets. The phenomenon is also referred to as the *grocery gap* because the afflicted communities are most often lower-income neighborhoods, communities of color, and rural areas.

As an increasing number of people living in urban and rural neighborhoods were lacking food access, rates of food insecurity and obesity started to climb.

ORIGINS OF THE GROCERY GAP

For much of the nation's history, grocery shopping was a neighborhood activity. It meant visiting a host of independent local vendors—butchers, fish markets, produce stands—or a nearby public market where these vendors gathered. Later, small *mom and pop* stores developed, offering a selection of groceries. It was not until the end of World War I that the country saw a growth of larger markets and regional grocery chains. The 1920s brought a shift from full-service grocery stores, in which a clerk collected goods from the shelves, to the self-service model prevalent today. In 1930, the first modern supermarket, King Kullen, opened in Queens, New York (Sarkar 2005). King Kullen introduced the supermarket business model that reigns today: a self-service model based on the volume of sales instead of the price of goods. By the 1960s, supermarkets commanded 70% of food retail sales (Food Marketing Institute 2005). With this successful business model came larger and larger stores and larger and larger parking lots, two changes well suited to the newly thriving suburbs where land was cheap and car ownership was common.

The same postwar period had marked the beginning of a population shift from the city and rural communities to the suburbs. In rural settings, advances in technology led to the increased mechanization and industrialization of agriculture. These changes meant a shrinking need for farm labor and declines in the number of farms and rural population losses (Dimitri et al. 2005; Johnson 2006; Johns Hopkins Center for a Livable Future 2012). At the same time, manufacturing in cities began to decline, leading to population shifts away from these areas (Larson 2003).

Between 1960 and 1970, 70% of the population's growth occurred in the suburbs, in part because of a phenomenon known as *white flight*, whereby large numbers of whites began moving out of cities and into the suburbs (Fernandez et al. 1982; The Association for Convenience & Fuel Retailing 2011). Increasingly, the bulk of the population in cities was comprised of minorities and lower income residents, and the trend of supermarket divestment in cities that started in the first decades of the twentieth century accelerated into its last decades. Between 1968 and 1984, the supermarket chain Safeway closed 600 of its inner-city stores, and many urban minority communities fell victim to *redlining*, a banking practice, though outlawed in 1970, that restricted investment in businesses locating in those neighborhoods (Kane 1984; Hillier 2003). Between 1970 and 1990, 34 of 50 chain supermarket locations in Boston closed, while in Los Angeles County, the number of supermarkets plummeted from 1068 to 694 (Blay-Palmer 2010).

IMPACTS OF THE GROCERY GAP

As communities lost supermarkets—the primary source of nutritious, affordable food for many Americans—the country's obesity rates soared. Today, nearly 10% of Americans live in lower-income communities that lack access to supermarkets and other retailers stocking affordable, nutritious foods and more than one-third of adults are obese, twice as many as just 30 years ago (Ogden et al. 2012a; Ver Ploeg et al. 2012). One out of every six children—12.5 million kids—is obese, more than triple the number who suffered from obesity in 1980 (Ogden et al. 2012b).

In 2010, The Food Trust, a nationally recognized food access nonprofit, and PolicyLink, a research and advocacy organization, published *The Grocery Gap: Who Has Access to Healthy Food and Why It Matters* (Treuhaft and Karpyn 2010). This literature review was the most comprehensive bibliography to date of studies of healthy food access and its impacts—132 studies conducted in the United States in the previous 20 years, including three nationwide analyses and geographically focused reports covering 22 states. Notably, *The Grocery Gap* included both peer-reviewed journal articles and gray literature, an important body of information produced by practitioners and community members working in communities underserved by supermarkets and other retailer stocking affordable, nutritious food.

Individually, these studies reveal communities in great need of improved food access:

- In Albany, New York, 80% of nonwhite residents cannot find low-fat milk or high-fiber bread in their neighborhoods (Hosler et al. 2006).
- In Mississippi, over 70% of Supplemental Nutrition Assistance Program (SNAP)-eligible (food stamp-eligible) households travel more than 30 miles to reach a supermarket (Kaufman 1998).
- In Washington, DC, the city's lowest-income communities have just one supermarket for every 70,000 people, while the highest income communities have one for every 12,000 people (D.C. Hunger Solutions 2006).

Taken together, these studies overwhelmingly showed disparities in food access. They found that millions of Americans—especially families in lower-income neighborhoods, communities of color, and rural areas—lack access to healthy food.

Distressingly, these studies also overwhelmingly found that disparities in food access lead to disparities in health equity. Lack of access to healthy food is a pressing public health issue. The studies showed that lack of access to healthy food is associated with a higher risk of obesity and other diet-related diseases. One study of more than 10,000 adults found that those living in a neighborhood with supermarkets had the lowest rate of obesity and those living in neighborhoods with no supermarkets had the highest (Morland et al. 2006). Another study of 70,000 teens found that increased availability of supermarkets was associated with lower rates of overweight (Powell et al. 2007).

But the literature review also found that the balance of the research showed that improved healthy food access can lead to better health. One study found that African-Americans living in a census tract with a supermarket were more likely to meet dietary guidelines for fruits and vegetables; for each additional supermarket in the community, produce consumption increased 32% (Morland et al. 2002). Another study, conducted in New Orleans, found that each additional meter of space for fresh vegetables in a community was associated with an additional 0.35 servings of vegetables eaten per day (Bodor et al. 2008).

Intriguingly, *The Grocery Gap* showed that improving food access through new and improved healthy food retail in an underserved community could also improve its economic health, creating job opportunities and serving as an anchor for neighborhood revitalization (Treuhaft and Karpyn 2010).

The Grocery Gap's findings presented a clear picture of the public health and social justice concerns associated with lack of food access and suggested encouraging the development of supermarkets and other healthy food retail as an economically viable solution.

This chapter will describe The Food Trust Framework, a local advocacy model that led to state and national financing efforts to address the lack of access to supermarkets. The Food Trust Framework has its roots in The Food Trust's on-the-ground activities in North Philly's Yorktown community and throughout Philadelphia and the state of Pennsylvania. As part of a comprehensive approach to preventing obesity and other diet-related diseases, the organization raised awareness of and consensus around the issue of food access in Philadelphia. The efforts led to the establishment of Pennsylvania's Fresh Food Financing Initiative (FFFI), an innovative public–private partnership to encourage supermarket development in underserved communities.

Recognized by Harvard University's Ash Center as one of the Top 15 Innovations in American Government and by the Centers for Disease Control and Prevention in its Showcase of Innovative Policy and Environmental Strategies for Obesity Prevention and Control, FFFI has approved funding for nearly 90 fresh-food retail projects across Pennsylvania, creating or retaining 5000 jobs and developing 1.67 million square feet of retail space (Ash Center for Democratic Governance and Innovation 2008; CDC Division of Media Relations 2009; The Reinvestment Fund 2013). These projects will improve access to healthy food and a healthier lifestyle for an estimated half-million Pennsylvanians.

This chapter will also discuss how Pennsylvania's successes in addressing food access issues—disparities in access, public health concerns, and missed economic opportunities—inspired similar advocacy campaigns based on The Food Trust Framework and fresh food financing programs in dozens of states and at the federal level. In addition, The Food Trust Framework may have broader implications for approaches to policy development.

SUPERMARKET CAMPAIGN IN PENNSYLVANIA

City planner Duane Perry, then executive director of the merchant association of the Reading Terminal Market, Philadelphia's historic central market, was one of the first to raise the issue of food access in Philadelphia in the early 1990s. He saw residents from all over Philadelphia coming to Reading Terminal in Center City for fresh produce, often because it was not available in their communities. What if Reading Terminal Market expanded, bringing affordable, nutritious foods to more residents of those neighborhoods and providing a new outlet for the region's farmers?

ESTABLISHMENT OF THE FOOD TRUST

Perry founded The Farmers' Market Trust—the original name of The Food Trust—in 1992 with the mission of ensuring that everyone has access to affordable, nutritious food. One of the first agency efforts was a farmers' market in the lower-income community of Tasker Homes, a public housing development in South Philadelphia. Each week The Food Trust, with the help of the Tasker Homes tenant council, set up one long table with an array of fresh vegetables and fruits for residents to purchase. "People hadn't seen that kind of quality produce in their neighborhood before," Perry recalled. Residents told the market staff about traveling long distances to buy healthy food for families and often complained of the prices and lack of quality or variety in small neighborhood corner stores.

The market was a tremendous success, confirming Perry's hypothesis that there was demand for healthy foods in neighborhoods underserved by supermarkets and other fresh food retailers. The Tasker Homes market and each new market The Food Trust opened showed that lower-income families, just like middle- and upper-income families, wanted to eat nutritiously.

But farmers' markets have their limitations. Most markets operate only a few hours a week and, particularly in Northeastern cities like Philadelphia, only seasonally, approximately June through October when the farmers' harvest is most abundant. Today, The Food Trust operates more than 25 markets in lower-income communities throughout the city, accepting SNAP and other benefits and serving 400,000 customers—but farmers' markets could be only one part of the food access solution in Philadelphia.

It was again the customers, buying healthy food for their families, who steered Perry to the next solution. As they shopped, they told market staff of the stores that used to sell fresh produce and other healthy foods in their neighborhood. They were frustrated that those supermarkets had closed—many moving to the suburbs—and that nothing had replaced them. As Perry surveyed the city, these comments seemed like more than isolated observations. A 1995 study found that the Greater Philadelphia region had a low ratio of supermarkets to population (Cotterill 1995) and needed about 70 stores to meet national standards. The farmers' markets had shown there were customers in the city's lower-income communities, so where were all the supermarkets?

In the late 1990s, with a staff of just four, The Food Trust set out to answer that question.

ADVOCATING FOR SUPERMARKETS

With the help of Dr. Amy Hillier of the University of Pennsylvania, then a student, The Food Trust used Geographic Information System software to map the locations of supermarkets in Philadelphia and discover the extent of the city's food access problem (Figure 9.1). The maps layered income data from the 1990 U.S. Census, supermarket sales data from commercial data firm Trade Dimensions, and diet-related mortality data (including deaths due to neoplasms or tumors; endocrine, nutritional, and immunity disorders such as diabetes; and diseases of the circulatory system) provided by the Philadelphia Department of Public Health.

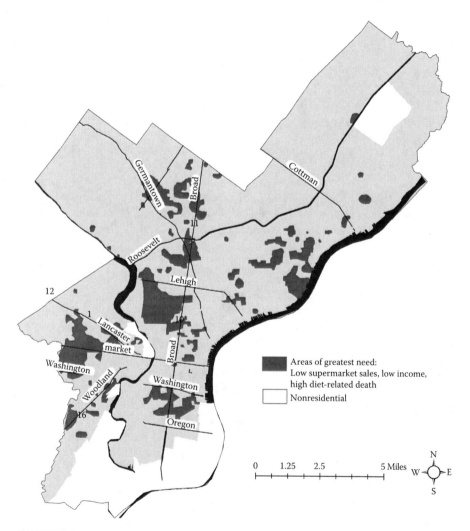

FIGURE 9.1 Map of Philadelphia: Areas with greatest need, based on supermarket sales, income, and diet-related deaths.

This last element offered a new perspective on the issue of food access. Early conversations with city officials about the Philadelphia's lack of supermarkets had not been encouraging. The social justice aspects of food access were a tough sell in a city mired in a bad economy. And talk of supermarkets as an economic development strategy was not initially popular in a city that saw its future, as it had its past, in manufacturing. But these maps showed something more compelling to city officials: the city's lower-income communities also had some of the lowest supermarket access and these lower-income, low-access communities had the highest rates of diet-related deaths. The maps, published in the 2001 report *Food For Every Child: The Need for More Supermarkets in Philadelphia*, showed that food access was not simply a social justice issue, nor simply an economic development issue; it was an urgent and expensive public health concern for Philadelphia (Perry 2001).

This data collection and dissemination was the first step in The Food Trust's fledgling supermarket campaign. The process, which would later be named The Food Trust Framework, and would be replicated across the country, grew out of the on-the-ground education and coalition building work the organization had been conducting in Philadelphia for a decade.

In 2002, the Philadelphia City Council, spurred by The Food Trust's report, called for hearings on the issue of supermarket access in Philadelphia. The hearings, which included testimony from dozens of concerned community members and leaders, generated wider awareness of the issue. One leader in particular became increasingly engaged.

State Representative Dwight Evans grew up in the Germantown and West Oak Lane neighborhoods of Philadelphia, a part of the community he now represented. He knew what it was like growing up without convenient access to a supermarket; the Oak Lane neighborhoods were among the lowest-income, lowest-access communities identified by The Food Trust's maps. Now Evans saw that the problem was not unique to Oak Lane and nearby Olney; it affected communities throughout the city, including large portions of North Philadelphia, the near Northeast, South Philadelphia west of Broad Street, and West Philadelphia.

"I already knew that there was a problem," Evans said. "The map just made it real. It put a face on it. It was like an exhibit in a courtroom."

As he continued to research the issue of food access, it became clear that the problem was not unique to Philadelphia either. It plagued other Pennsylvanian cities such as Pittsburgh, and rural towns such as Apollo and Gettysburg.

The Food Trust and key city and state leaders now knew the extent of the problem, but it was not clear how to solve the issue. What would it take to bring supermarkets back to these underserved communities?

In 2003, at the request of the Philadelphia City Council, The Food Trust organized the Food Marketing Task Force. Notably, this task force included high-level representatives from the public health, economic development and grocery retailing sectors, groups that did not often work together. To some public health advocates, in fact, the grocers had long been the enemy, given the sector's difficult history in lower income communities and communities of color. The co-chairs were representative of diverse perspectives: Walt Rubel was an executive of the ACME/Albertsons, Inc. grocery chain and Christine James-Brown was the president and chief executive officer (CEO) of the United Way International. The 30-member task force met four times to identify the challenges to operating a supermarket in an underserved area and to propose recommendations that could address these challenges (Giang et al. 2008).

At the conclusion of the task force process in 2004, The Food Trust published *Stimulating Supermarket Development: A New Day for Philadelphia*, which laid out the task force's 10 recommendations for encouraging supermarket development in Philadelphia and throughout Pennsylvania (Burton and Perry 2004):

1. The city should adopt food retailing as a priority for comprehensive neighborhood development.
2. The city should employ innovative, data-driven market assessment techniques to highlight unmet market demand in urban neighborhoods.
3. The city should identify targeted areas for supermarket development and promote them to real estate developers and the supermarket industry.
4. The city should give priority to assembling land for supermarket development.
5. The city should reduce regulatory barriers to supermarket investment.
6. The city should market available public incentives to maximize impact on supermarket site location decisions.
7. City and state economic development programs should be made available to the supermarket industry.
8. The Commonwealth of Pennsylvania should develop a business-financing program to support local supermarket development projects.
9. The appropriate city, regional, and state transportation agencies should develop safe, cheap, and convenient transportation services for shoppers who do not have access to a full-service supermarket.
10. The city should convene an advisory group of leaders from the supermarket industry and the civic sector to guide the implementation of these recommendations.

Key among these recommendations was the development of a business-financing program at the state level to encourage supermarket development in underserved communities. This recommendation addressed the number one issue identified through the task force process: the central barrier for grocery retailers interested in opening supermarkets in underserved communities, which often required higher development investment to address issues like land assembly and workforce development, was lack of access to capital (Figure 9.2).

"During that first task force meeting in Philadelphia, I was completely convinced that this was an opportunity to grow my business profitably and serve society in a profound way," recalled grocer Jeffery Brown. "One of the key elements was the platform to discuss the challenges and how government, nonprofits and businesses were willing to work together to mitigate some of these challenges. If we could find a way to address the financial gap created by the low profit margins typical of the supermarket industry and the higher expenses associated with opening in an underserved community, I knew we could bring supermarkets back to these neighborhoods."

Problem statement: A healthy diet contributes to obesity prevention. Limited access to healthier food choices in terms of availability and/or quality is a major barrier to maintaining a healthier diet among children in families with low incomes.

Pre-Program Inputs

Community need

Political will and leadership (program champion)

Establishment of evidence with background data collection
- Educating decision makers on findings

Task force representing a diversity of interests and committed to process
- Health interests
- University researchers
- Dept. of Public Health (to offer evidence)
- Industry operators
- Dept. of Planning

- Non-profit civic groups

Advocate at state and local levels for funding, building relationships among community sectors

Financing and selective grant-making to reduce structural barriers

Community buy-in

Tax credits for economic development

Financing Legislation Passed

Inputs

Community need

Political will and leadership

Public-private partnerships
- The Reinvestment Fund
- The Food Trust

- The Greater Philadelphia Urban Affairs Coalition
- Commonweath of Pennsylvania

Process for funding grants and loans
- Funding leveraged (New Market Tax Credits)

Financing or distribution mechanism to help establish or assist supermarkets in underserved areas
- Grants
- Debt financing

Activities/Process

Ongoing response to constituent need

Provision of technical assistance and human resources assistance to qualifying grantees and borrowers

- The Food Trust
- The Reinvestment Fund
- Others

Outreach to promote programs to communities and operators/locations

Determine eligible operators/locations

Match communities to willing operators

Land assembly (obtain space for construction of new supermarkets)

Community commitment to deal with hurdles

Outputs

Amount of funding to resource program

Number of applications for grants or loans

Number of grants and loans made

Number of stores constructed or renovated

Number of operators matched to communities

Number of new options for produce/healthier food

Number of jobs created

Short-Term Outcomes

Increase in number of supermarkets opening and operating in underserved areas

Revitalization of old stores and construction of new stores

Increased access to (and increased variety

of) affordable fresh produce and/or other healthier food options

Cost savings for community members
- Lower food prices
- Reduced transportation costs

Jobs for community members

Supermarkets both meeting needs of consumers and meeting probability objectives

Greater food diversity

Intermediate Outcomes

Increased purchase and consumption of fresh produce and/or healthier food options

Increased selection of fresh produce at markets in underserved areas

Increased workforce capacity

Increased safety due to improved lighting, access, and security

Increased development of other small enterprises
- Supermarkets anchor developments for other retail

Bundled health and social services in supermarkets
- Other positive community outcomes/spinoffs

Increased knowledge of new healthy foods

Long-Term Outcomes

Increased consumption of healthier food options

Ongoing construction of markets in underserved areas and maintenance of existing markets

Create jobs, revitalize commercial real estate, leverage private sector capital, and increase tax ratables

Provide lower cost, nutritious foods and savings on transportation

Promote a nutritionally balanced diet which leads to reduced rates of diet-related disease

Goals

Contribute to improving the access of fresh foods

Economic development

Improved health outcomes due to:
- Reduction in diet-related disease
- Increased social capital
- Improved well-being

FIGURE 9.2 **(See color insert.)** Pennsylvania's Fresh Food Financing Initiative logic model. (Copyright The Food Trust, 2009.)

CREATION AND IMPLEMENTATION OF PENNSYLVANIA'S FRESH FOOD FINANCING INITIATIVE

With strong support from all sectors represented on the task force and with Representative Evans as its champion, the recommendation for a business-financing program was realized in 2004 when the Pennsylvania state legislature established the FFFI. The fund was designed to encourage supermarket development through flexible grant and loan funding to expand or open supermarkets and other fresh food retail in underserved Pennsylvania communities.

The legislature seeded the fund with $30 million in three annual installments of $10 million. The seed money was leveraged by a Community Development Financial Institution (CDFI) that raised more than $117 million in private capital to match the state's $30 million grant.

Through FFFI, grocery retailers, and developers were eligible for loans of up to $5 million and grants of up to $250,000 per store. Projects that demonstrated both an extraordinary need and high potential for impact were eligible for up to $1 million in grant funding.

STRUCTURING THE INITIATIVE

The FFFI put Pennsylvania in the vanguard of states in addressing food access issues. Rarely had economic incentives, which exist for many other retail sectors, been targeted to the grocery industry. Two aspects of the fund's structure were keys to the pioneering program's success.

First, the fund was a public–private partnership, continuing the cross-sector partnerships established in the task force process. Pennsylvania provided initial funding for FFFI through the Pennsylvania Department of Community and Economic Development. The state also oversaw program management and tracked the economic impacts of the program. The Reinvestment Fund, a Philadelphia-based CDFI, leveraged the state's seed funding with additional investments from public and private sources and administered the fund, evaluating applicants' financial eligibility. The Food Trust, in its role as a food access advocate, conducted outreach and marketing to food retailers and community leaders and determined if a proposed project would improve food access in an underserved community. Another partner in FFFI, the Urban Affairs Coalition, oversaw outreach to women- and minority-owned businesses.

Second, recognizing that the barriers to food access are unique in each community, FFFI was designed to be flexible to best meet the needs of grocery retailers and developers and underserved neighborhoods. The program was flexible in terms of who was eligible for funding; full-size supermarkets were the primary focus, but smaller healthy food retailers, including corner stores and farmers' markets, were also eligible. And the program was flexible on how the funds could be used. FFFI funding could be used for costs associated with ground-up construction, as well as renovations to existing structures, equipment, employee training, and other needs.

The Food Trust's advocacy efforts did not end with the creation of the FFFI. The same network of cross-sector partnerships that led to the establishment of the initiative would be harnessed to implement the program. Marketing the new program to grocers and underserved communities and working with experienced partners to establish eligibility criteria and application processes would be essential to the success of the program.

RISE OF COMMUNITY DEVELOPMENT FINANCIAL INSTITUTIONS

Two major policy efforts are tied closely to the reinvestment of capital in lower- and moderate-income communities in the United States. One is the Community Reinvestment Act (CRA) of 1977, which mandated that banks respond to the credit needs of their entire service area. The act was a response to redlining practices where banks literally drew red lines on maps to isolate communities from investment. The second was the establishment of the 1994 Community Development Fund legislation (103rd Congress 1994), an important agenda item during President Bill Clinton's campaign and later in his administration. President Clinton was familiar with redlining and the lack of enforcement of CRA, and with the successful activities of the South Shore Bank of Chicago. As Arkansas governor, he worked to replicate the South Bank model with the Southern Development Bancorporation, a CDFI established for southwestern Arkansas, and wanted to see more such banks in the United States (Benjamin et al. 2004). Ultimately the CDFI Fund, established to increase economic opportunity and promote community development investments for underserved populations, was housed in the Treasury Department where today it continues to operate as a mechanism to provide loans, grants, and equity investments to CDFIs (Caskey and Hollister 2001). The CDFI Fund, and the subsequent rise in CDFIs, made programs like Pennsylvania's FFFI possible.

MARKETING THE INITIATIVE

Marketing the FFFI was central to cultivating qualified applicants for the program from across the state in both rural and urban areas.

The Food Trust did this by building relationships with the statewide grocery association and wholesalers and grocery operators across the state. The Food Trust connected with operators at industry tradeshows, through presentations at grocer board meetings, via one-on-one meetings at their stores and in the pages of trade publications. Referrals through trade associations or operators who had benefitted from the program proved to be the best method for attracting applicants to the program.

In addition to marketing the program to grocery operators throughout the state, The Food Trust also reached out to key community and economic development contacts in every county across the state. This outreach proved helpful in identifying regions of particular need.

DETERMINING ELIGIBILITY

There was a two-step process for applicants—developers or grocery operators—to the FFFI. First, the applicant completed a site eligibility application that was used to determine if the proposed site and store plan met FFFI eligibility guidelines. If the site eligibility application was approved, the applicant completed a financial application that was used to determine if the applicant was qualified to receive funding.

Step 1: Site Eligibility

The Food Trust evaluated the initial site eligibility application, which was designed to encourage applicants. It was just two pages long, required only basic information about site and store development plans and was evaluated within 10 business days.

The site eligibility application was judged based on three main criteria: Was the project located in a low- to moderate-income census tract? Was this community underserved by food retail, as determined by the food retail density of the area? And would the project be the right fit for the community, meeting its needs and expectations for improved access to healthy, affordable foods?

Developing a nuanced understanding of each community and each project was important to the evaluation process. In addition to using census tract information to determine a region's economic level, the organization consulted socioeconomic data at the borough and township level, especially in rural areas with large census tracts, and considered free- and reduced-lunch data as another indicator of poverty in an area.

To determine if a region was underserved, The Food Trust looked at the number of stores in the trade area. Trade areas were developed with industry partners and were based on the size of the store. Stores of less than 10,000 square feet were assigned a half-mile trade area; those of 10,000 to 25,000 square feet, a one-mile trade area; and those larger than 25,000 square feet, a two-mile trade area.

When evaluating the *community fit* of a project, the organization considered community support for the store quality, affordability, and site location; demonstrable potential for impact on the economy or well-being of the community where the project was located; demonstrated need for public funding; adherence to sound land-use principles; and coordination with community plan and other programs promoting community development. This part of the process involved interviews with local stakeholders, community meetings, and other ground testing of the data used to determine income level and retail density to ensure it reflected the actual experience of residents in each community.

Step 2: Financial Eligibility

If the criteria for site eligibility were met, applicants progressed to part two of the process, the financial application. At this stage, The Reinvestment Fund evaluated the applicant for financial strength, management and development team track record, budget integrity, appropriate collateral and the project's competitive advantage in the marketplace. Unlike traditional lenders, The Reinvestment Fund sought to work with applicants to strengthen their application and design an appropriate FFFI financing package—often including a combination of grants, loans, and New Markets Tax Credits—for the project.

> "We can attract the private capital to match public investment in healthy food choices in our communities," said Jeremy Nowak, then president and CEO of The Reinvestment Fund. "These investments can drive the health and economic vitality of these communities, particularly during difficult economic times."

IMPACTS OF PENNSYLVANIA'S FRESH FOOD FINANCING INITIATIVE

Since 2004, funding has been approved for 88 projects in more than half of Pennsylvania's counties. Approved stores have typically ranged from 12,000 to 65,000 square feet, with the larger, full-service supermarkets employing 150 to 200 full-time and part-time employees and having weekly sales of $200,000 to $300,000 (Karpyn and Treuhaft 2012). Projects approved for funding will create or retain over 5,000 jobs and improve access to healthy food for an estimated half-million Pennsylvania residents.

Research is underway to assess the health impacts of several of the stores opened with assistance from FFFI; studies of the immediate economic impact of the initiative found a positive influence on real estate values, job availability, tax revenue and food access, quality and prices in a neighborhood with an FFFI-funded supermarket (The Reinvestment Fund 2008). The results of the initiative can also been seen in communities throughout the state.

In Blossburg, Tioga County, funding from FFFI provided Melanie and Ryan Shaut, a young, local couple with entrepreneurial goals, with the financing they need to purchase the Bloss Holiday Market from its retiring owners. The Bloss Holiday Market is the only source of fresh produce for nearly eight miles in this north-central Pennsylvania town.

In south-central Adams County, Kennie's Market, a family- and employee-owned supermarket located in the heart of Gettysburg received FFFI funding for the construction of a new 32,000-square-foot store. The expanded store offers customers convenient, walkable access to an expanded selection of fresh food and created 50 new jobs for the city.

In Apollo, Armstrong County, and Vandergrift, Westmoreland County, near Pittsburgh, experienced supermarket operators Randy and Brenda Sprankle bought two stores on the verge of closure due to the previous owners' retirements with assistance from FFFI; both stores were the only supermarkets in their respective communities.

And on that vacant stretch of North Broad Street, the FFFI revitalized the fading Progress Plaza. In December 2009, more than a decade after the supermarket closed its doors and 40 years after Reverend Sullivan and his congregation built the center together, the public–private partnership of FFFI provided assistance to local chain Fresh Grocer to open a new 46,000-square-foot supermarket, an anchor for the rebuilt plaza and for the Yorktown community. The supermarket has improved food access and economic opportunities for the community and serves as a hub for nutrition education, offering supermarket tours, tastings and marketing materials to introduce customers to the market's healthy offerings.

"Reverend Leon Sullivan said we may not have much money but if a lot of us put a little bit together, maybe we can do something," Yorktown community member Anita Chappell recalled as the new Fresh Grocer prepared to open in Progress Plaza, filling a long empty hole in the community. "To see it come back to its strength and vibrancy the way he imagined it, it took years, it took money, it took patience, it took tears, a lot of prayers. So it's just marvelous to see it there. I'm just thrilled that I lived to see it."

SCALING UP: REPLICATION OF THE FOOD TRUST FRAMEWORK AND PENNSYLVANIA'S FRESH FOOD FINANCING INITIATIVE

The Food Trust Framework—a codification of the process that led to the country's first FFFI in Pennsylvania—has served as a model for addressing food access issues and the FFFI has been scaled up with the establishment of similar fresh food financing programs throughout the country.

Scaling up typically refers to the act of increasing a program's scope or impact while maintaining quality and is often the subject of conversations about sustainability. How scale-up is undertaken has been the source of academic articles since the mid-1990s (Uvin and Miller 1996). Diffusions of Innovations, a public health-oriented framework for explaining how programs move from small-scale reach to expansive reach, is another example of a model explaining approaches to program dissemination. An early requirement for scale-up is a common understanding of program elements. In the case of the supermarket campaign, an articulation of The Food Trust Framework was an important mechanism for accomplishing scale up and replication.

The Food Trust Framework, developed as a response to the lack of supermarkets in underserved areas, aligns closely with other theoretical models of policy development whereby the strategy begins with defining the problem or issue and moves to articulating an agenda for policy and ultimately settles on implementing components of the agenda. The Stages Model of the Policy Process, for example, outlines six stages for policy development (Issue Emergence, Agenda Setting, Alternative Selection, Enactment, Implementation, and Evaluation). Critics assert that the linear nature of the model may be flawed, in that it fails to recognize the dynamic nature of the practice of policy making. More recent models for policy development assert that a systems thinking approach, articulated first in the 1970s, is a better framework to understand policy. Systems thinking, when applied to policy making, recognizes that policy is dependent on inputs (media coverage, election results, personal experiences) interacting with feedback in a political system to create outputs (laws, regulations, or decisions). Put simply, activities, people, and demands are all intertwined in a system, which is not linear or one dimensional, which ultimately generates outputs. Systems thinking has also been emphasized by the Institute of Medicine and others as an important evaluation framework (Institute of Medicine 2010).

The advocacy portion of The Food Trust Framework consists of four phases: *Prepare and Inform*, during which data on a community's food-access issues are gathered, mapped, and disseminated to raise awareness; *Engage and Empower Stakeholders*, during which the task force is assembled, co-chairs are identified, and an agenda developed; *Strategize and Develop Recommendations*, during which the task force is convened to examine barriers to supermarket development in under-served communities and propose recommendations to promote food retail develop-ment; and *Change Policy*, during which these recommendations are released. The final fifth phase of The Food Trust Framework following a successful advocacy effort is *Implementation* (Figure 9.3).

In the 10 years after the first Food Marketing Task Force meeting in Pennsylvania, four additional states—Illinois, Louisiana, New Jersey, and New York—completed the advocacy portion of The Food Trust Framework and progressed to the implemen-tation phase, establishing fresh food financing programs based on Pennsylvania's FFFI. Another eight states—Colorado, Georgia, Massachusetts, Maryland, Minnesota, Mississippi, Tennessee, and Texas—were in the midst of the advocacy phases. In that time, Pennsylvania's FFFI also served as a model for the California FreshWorks Fund and the federal Healthy Food Financing Initiative.

With the growth of the PA FFFI model came momentum and interest to create a federal Healthy Food Financing Initiative. By working with key partners including The Reinvestment Fund and PolicyLink, an advocacy campaign for the federal pro-gram was developed and sought to replicate efforts to inform and convene stakehold-ers to address our nations need to improve food access for all Americans. Together the three organizations educated federal policymakers on how the Pennsylvania model could be adapted, forming a national program.

PHASE 1: PREPARE AND INFORM

The first phase of The Food Trust Framework includes gathering data to describe the nature and extent of the problem and identifying potential stakeholders for the creation of a task force.

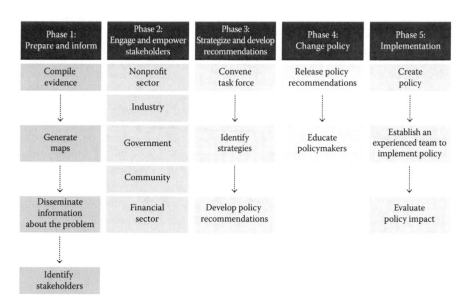

FIGURE 9.3   Food Trust framework.

In the case of the supermarket campaigns for which this framework was developed, this phase included reporting on the scientific evidence on the issue of food access and the development of maps that laid out the relationship between areas suffering from high rates of death due to diet-related disease, supermarket sales, and demographic information, such as income and population density.

These maps showed the location of supermarkets and supermarket sales volume along with layers of different data sets for income levels of residents and the rates of diet-related death. The final in the series of six maps illustrating the process and the problem showed the *areas of greatest need*, lower-income areas with low access to supermarkets and a high incidence of deaths due to diet-related disease (Figure 9.4).

These maps served as the basis for a mapping report highlighting specific neighborhoods of a metropolitan region or specific areas of a state in need of improved healthy food access. Additional data, including obesity and overweight levels of adults and children, the leading causes of death in the state and the overall wealth and well-being of the state, further illustrated the need for healthy food access in the state. Groups already addressing the issue of food access—such as organizations and agencies working on antiobesity and healthy food access efforts, CDFIs, foundations, grocers associations and government agencies, and staff dedicated to healthy food access—were resources and evidence of existing community support for a solution.

In these supermarket campaigns, potential stakeholders—many of whom were also important sources of information about the state of food access in their communities—included food access organizations, supermarket industry leaders, government and civic sector leaders, community leaders, financial sector representatives, economic development leaders, public health leaders, and children's health advocates.

PHASE 2: ENGAGE AND EMPOWER STAKEHOLDERS

The next phase in The Food Trust Framework is the recruitment of local partners to participate in a task force. To connect with potential task force members, the convening organization engages in extensive outreach efforts via phone, e-mail, and in-person meetings. Throughout the outreach, the conveners evaluate the level of knowledge and engagement potential stakeholders have around the advocacy issue, using the data collected in the first phase to engage stakeholders on the areas of greatest interest to each one. In the supermarket campaigns, stakeholders were invested in different aspects of issue—public health, social justice, community development. The knowledge of the issue gained in the first phase of the framework allows the convener to address stakeholders' specific interests. This diversity of perspectives on the issue at hand is essential to creating an effective task force, as is keeping the task force to a manageable size of 30 to 40 members. Co-chairs, who facilitate the task force process and, if identified early in the process, can assist in recruiting task force members, should represent different and vital perspectives. In the supermarket campaigns, one co-chair was always from the grocery industry and the other from the civic sector.

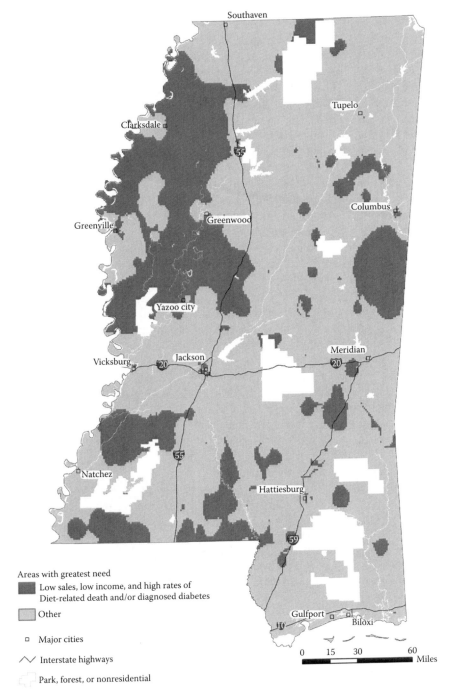

Areas with greatest need
▮ Low sales, low income, and high rates of
  Diet-related death and/or diagnosed diabetes
▯ Other

▫ Major cities

⋀⋁ Interstate highways

⬚ Park, forest, or nonresidential

0   15   30   60
                              Miles

FIGURE 9.4   Map of Mississippi: Areas with greatest need. (Data from Trade Dimensions Retail Database, 2009; Mississippi Department of Public Health, 2008; U.S. Centers for Disease Control and Prevention, 2008; U.S. Census Bureau, American Community Surveys, 2005–2009.)

PHASE 3: STRATEGIZE AND DEVELOP RECOMMENDATIONS

The third phase focuses on generating viable policy recommendations to address the issue through task force meetings. Once stakeholders have been identified, they are asked to join the task force and to commit to participating in four two-hour meetings held over the course of nine months to a year—with the ultimate goal of creating public policy solutions. Before the first meeting, the convener works with co-chairs to establish the agenda and clear goals for the process. The first meeting lays the groundwork for the task force process, articulating the collected evidence of the problem and fostering discussion between the represented sectors. In the second meeting the focus shifts toward problem solving, with presentations by stakeholders from different sectors. The task of the third meeting is crafting policy recommendations, which are approved at the fourth meeting. This final meeting is also an opportunity to discuss strategies for the next step of The Food Trust Framework. Between meetings the convener contacts task force members to encourage additional feedback on the process to best steer the subsequent meetings.

In the supermarket campaigns, the task forces were charged with developing policies to encourage supermarket and other fresh food retail investment in underserved communities. The first two meetings examined the challenges to the grocery industry that prevent or discourage investments in lower income, underserved communities and potential solutions. During these meetings, the conveners and select task force members provided presentations on specific geographic areas that were underserved by supermarkets and specific challenges for the grocery industry, often showcasing local examples. Among the challenges discussed by task forces were a lack of access to financing, higher costs for land assembly, the need for workforce training, and the need for improved security.

The final two task force meetings considered potential policy solutions to those challenges discussed in the first two meetings and focused on drafting and finalizing a set of policy recommendations. Presentations on local programs and policies, as well as those from other states that have addressed particular challenges for the grocery industry to improve access to healthy food, were typically a part of the agenda for the final two meetings. Policy recommendations in states that have undertaken supermarket campaigns include a variety of strategies for encouraging supermarket development, including the provision of tax credits and other incentives for the grocery industry, improvements to public transportation, and a flexible fresh-food-financing program of grants and loans. In every state, the task force issued their recommendations in a final report that was widely shared with lawmakers and the public.

PHASE 4: CHANGE POLICY

The *Change Policy* phase includes all the activities necessary to move the policy platform from a set of recommendations to enacted policy. Often this phase will include public hearings and briefings, meetings with individual lawmakers and media events, such as news conferences and press releases. Prioritizing and focusing efforts on recommendations that spark the most public interest can be helpful. Identifying a key proponent for those recommendations in government is often a critical step toward making recommended policy solutions a reality.

In Pennsylvania, the supermarket campaign from which The Food Trust Framework was developed, lobbying and educational efforts were undertaken by civic leaders, child health advocates, retailers and retail associations, and partners. In many states that have undertaken supermarket campaigns, the recommendation proposing a fresh-food-financing program was a high priority. Key proponent State Representative Dwight Evans, who was involved with the Pennsylvania efforts throughout the process, held an important seat as the chair of the state appropriations committee and was instrumental in achieving policy change: the establishment of Pennsylvania's FFFI, the first such program established in the nation.

PHASE 5: IMPLEMENTATION

Efforts do not end with policy change. Successfully implementing the changes is essential to enacting a long-term solution. In The Food Trust Framework, the implementation phase draws on the knowledge and cross-sector partnerships developed through the first four advocacy phases to create a team of experienced organizations that can work together to implement the resulting policy and evaluate its effectiveness.

In the supermarket campaigns, this policy has been a fresh-food-financing program modeled after the FFFI. In this model, a government entity or foundation provides the seed funding for the program and oversees implementation. A CDFI raises capital and administers the funds, determines the applicants' financial eligibility and underwrites projects for loans and grants. A food access organization conducts outreach and marketing to food retailers and community leaders, determines the applicants' site eligibility and advocates for community needs. These organizations are also charged with evaluating the economic and health impacts of the initiative. Together, this team of experienced organizations works toward the policy's ultimate goal: the opening of new and expanded supermarkets selling healthy, affordable food in previously underserved communities, thereby improving the health of residents and the neighborhood economy.

In New Orleans, the recommendations of the New Orleans Food Policy Advisory Committee—a cross-sector task force convened by Tulane University, Second Harvest Food Bank, the Louisiana Retailers Association, and The Food Trust—led to the creation of the New Orleans Fresh Food Retailer Initiative. To implement the program, the City of New Orleans partnered with Hope Enterprise Corporation and The Food Trust. The City of New Orleans seeded the fund with $7 million in Disaster Community Development Block Grant Funding. The investment was matched by Hope Enterprise Corporation, a CDFI. The Food Trust served as the food access organization for the initiative. The implemented program offers interest-bearing loans up to $1 million and forgivable loans up to $500,000 or 20% of the total financing need.

One of the first communities to benefit from the initiative was the seventh Ward, home to the iconic Circle Food Store. Incorporated in 1938, the sleek curved stucco market with the red-tile roof was the thriving epicenter of this working class neighborhood in the shadows of downtown. The city's first African-American-owned grocery over time became the place to buy school uniforms, get a dental checkup and pick up holiday candy. But the signature product at Circle Food Store was its famed, farm-fresh bell pepper, sold five for $1.

"People used to come from all over the city to get those bell peppers, especially at Easter and Christmas," recalled Dwayne Boudreaux, who has owned the grocery spot for more than two decades.

That was before Hurricane Katrina struck the Gulf Coast in 2005, burying Circle Food Store under five-and-a-half feet of water and silt that did not recede for nearly a month. It took far longer —nearly 8 years—for Boudreaux to round up the more than $9 million in capital necessary to restore the trashed historic building. He said the nonstop pleading of Mid-City residents begging him to reopen and the sight of his former customers lugging groceries on city buses encouraged him to keep fighting for aid.

It would never have happened, the entrepreneur said, without $1 million in financing from the New Orleans Fresh Food Retailer Initiative.

"This was the glue," said Boudreaux. Both the money and the seal of official approval that came with the loan helped Circle Food Store complete a financial package that also included historic renovation dollars and private capital.

On January 17th, 2014 Circle Food Store reopened its doors and its aisles were quickly packed with grateful community members. "I've had people calling me," Boudreaux said, "telling me it won't feel like the community is back until Circle Food Store is back."

COMPREHENSIVE APPROACH TO IMPROVING FOOD ACCESS

The gleaming Progress Plaza Fresh Grocer, one of 18 projects in Philadelphia approved for funding through the FFFI, is now a beacon of fresh food in North Philadelphia, but the anchor supermarket is not the only effort to improve food access in the once-underserved Yorktown community.

Encouraging supermarket development is one part of a comprehensive approach to increasing access to healthy, affordable foods and combating obesity, and other diet-related diseases in Philadelphia. Other efforts include nutrition education and strong healthy vending machine standards in schools, menu-labeling laws, active-commuting policies, more farmers' markets and healthier options in corner stores.

And in the same period these interventions were underway, the rate of obesity among Philadelphia school children decreased by 5%, documenting one of the first reversals in the country's obesity trends. The study also found an 8% decrease in the obesity rate among African-American boys and a 7% decrease in the obesity rate among Hispanic girls, the largest decline reported to date for these populations.

Although the study does not assess the causes of the decline in obesity rates, it cites Philadelphia's comprehensive approach to obesity prevention as a potential contributor, and other cities and states, such as New York City (Centers for Disease Control and Prevention 2011) and California (Babey et al. 2011) that have shown a similar commitment to supermarkets and a comprehensive approach to improving food access have also seen the early signs of a reversal of the obesity trend (Robbins et al. 2012).

Ten years ago, its only supermarket shuttered, the Yorktown community was part of an unhealthy trend of supermarket divestment occurring at the same time there was a rise in the number of underserved communities and obesity rates. Today, thanks to the combined efforts of the city's public, private, and civic sectors, Yorktown residents can find fresh produce and other healthy foods at the supermarket, at the neighborhood farmers' markets and even at their nearest corner store. Now Yorktown is part of a much healthier trend: communities investing in supermarkets as part of a comprehensive approach to improving food access through state-level programs like Pennsylvania's FFFI and through the federal Healthy Food Financing Initiative.

In 2010, the Obama Administration announced the creation of the national Healthy Food Financing Initiative, a grants and loan program to encourage supermarket development modeled on Pennsylvania's program. As a partnership between three agencies—the U.S. Department of Agriculture, U.S. Department of Treasury, and U.S. Department of Health and Human Services—the Healthy Food Financing Initiative provides funding to a variety of healthy food retailers, from grocery stores and coops, to farmers markets' and small retailers in underserved communities across the country.

In February 2010, First Lady Michelle Obama came to Philadelphia to kick off her signature Let's Move! Campaign and announce the Obama administration's commitment to the Healthy Fresh Food Financing, as well as other efforts to improve food access and decrease rates of diet-related disease. She toured the Progress Plaza Fresh Grocer, talking with and hugging employees and shoppers, and she visited Fairhill Elementary School in North Philadelphia, where she was introduced to the crowd by a sixth-grader active in her school's healthy eating efforts. Taking the stage, the First Lady challenged the nation to work together to solve the obesity crisis and offered Philadelphia's comprehensive, cross-sector efforts as an inspiration.

"You all have done extraordinary and some could say revolutionary work here in this city. And as you all have said consistently, you couldn't do it without each other. That has been the resonating message," Obama said. "It's really groundbreaking, and hopefully will set the tone for what we can do throughout the country."

REFERENCES

103rd Congress. 1994. H.R. 3474 (103rd): Riegle Community Development and Regulatory Improvement Act of 1994. H.R.3474.

Ash Center for Democratic Governance and Innovation. 2008. *Fresh Food Financing Initiative: 2008 Finalist Commonwealth of Pennsylvania*. Cambridge, MA: Harvard Kennedy School of Government.

Babey, S. H., J. Wolstein, A. L. Diamant, A. Bloom, and H. Gikdsteub. 2011. A patchwork of progress: Changes in overweight and obesity among California 5th, 7th, and 9th Graders, 2005–2010. UCLA Center for Health Policy Research and California Center for Public Health Advocacy.

Benjamin L, J. S. Rubin, and S. Zielenbach. 2004. Community development financial institutions: Current issues and future prospects. *J Urban Affairs* 26: 177–95.

Blay-Palmer, A. 2010. *Imagining Sustainable Food Systems: Theory and Practice*. Farnham, Surrey, England; Burlington, VT: Ashgate.

Bodor, J. N., D. Rose, T. A. Farley, C. Swalm, and S. K. Scott. 2008. Neighbourhood fruit and vegetable availability and consumption: The role of small food stores in an urban environment. *Public Health Nutr* 11: 413–20.

Burton, H and D. Perry. 2004. *Stimulating Supermarket Development: A New Day for Philadelphia*. Philadelphia, PA: The Food Trust.

Caskey, J. P. and R. Hollister. 2001. *Business Development Financial Institutions: Theory, Practice, and Impact*. Madison, WI: Institute for Research on Poverty.

CDC Division of Media Relations. 2009. *CDC Recognizes Innovative Obesity Prevention and Control Initiatives with Weight of the Nation Awards*. Atlanta, GA: Centers for Disease Control and Prevention.

Centers for Disease Control and Prevention. 2011. Obesity in K-8 students: New York City, 2006–07 to 2010–11 school years. *MMWR Morb Mortal Wkly Rep* 60: 1673–8.

Cotterill, R. W. 1995. The urban grocery store gap. edited by A. W. Franklin. Food Marketing Policy Center: University of Connecticut.

D.C. Hunger Solutions. 2006. *Healthy Food, Healthy Communities: An Assessment and Scorecard of Community Food Security in the District of Columbia*. Washington, DC: D.C. Hunger Solutions.

Dimitri, C., A. Effland, and N. Conklin. 2005. The 20th century transformation of U.S. agriculture and farm policy. Economic Information Bulletin No. 3, United States Department of Agriculture.

Fernandez, J. C., J. A. Pincus, J. Peterson, and United States Department of Housing and Urban Development. 1982. *Troubled Suburbs: An Exploratory Study, a Rand Note*. Santa Monica, CA: Rand Corporation.

Food Marketing Institute. 2005. Supermarket Anniversary Facts: 75 Facts for 75 Years. Available at http://www.fmi.org/research-resources/fmi-research-resources/supermarket-anniversary-facts#9 (accessed November 6, 2013).

Giang, T., A. Karpyn, H. B. Laurison, A. Hillier, and R. D. Perry. 2008. Closing the grocery gap in underserved communities: The creation of the Pennsylvania Fresh Food Financing Initiative. *J Public Health Manag Pract* 14: 272–9.

Hillier, A. E. 2003. Redlining and the Home Owners' Loan Corporation. *J Urban Hist* 29: 394–420.

Hosler, A. S., D. Varadarajulu, A. E. Ronsani, B. L. Fredrick, and B. D. Fisher. 2006. Low-fat milk and high-fiber bread availability in food stores in urban and rural communities. *J Public Health Manag Pract* 12: 556–62.

Institute of Medicine. 2010. Bridging the evidence gap in obesity prevention: A framework to inform decision making, edited by . S. K. Kumanyika, L. Parker, and L. J. Sim. Washington, DC: National Acadmies Press.

Johns Hopkins Center for a Livable Future. 2012. *History of Food in Teaching the Food System*. Available at http://www.jhsph.edu/research/centers-and-institutes/teaching-the-food-system/curriculum/_pdf/History_of_Food-Background.pdf (accessed November 6, 2013).

Johnson, K. 2006. Demographic trends in rural and small town America. *Reports on Rural America* 1 (1): 1–35. Durham, New Hampshire: Carsey Institute, University of New Hampshire.

Kane, J. 1984. "The Supermarket Shuffle." *Mother Jones*, July 1984.

Karpyn, A. and S. Treuhaft. 2012. The grocery gap: Finding healthy food in America. In *A Place at the Table*, edited by P. Pringle. New York, NY: Public Affairs.

Kaufman, P. 1998. Rural poor have less access to supermarkets, large grocery stores. *Rural De Perspect* 13: 19–26.

Larson, T. 2003. Why there will be no chain supermarkets in poor inner-city neighborhoods. *California Politics and Policy* 7: 22–45.

Morland, K., A. V. Diez Roux, and S. Wing. 2006. Supermarkets, other food stores, and obesity: The atherosclerosis risk in communities study. *Am J Prev Med* 30: 333–9.

Morland, K., S. Wing, and A. Diez Roux. 2002. The contextual effect of the local food environment on residents' diets: The atherosclerosis risk in communities study. *Am J Public Health* 92: 1761–7.

Ogden, C. L., M. D. Carroll, B. K. Kit, and K. M. Flegal. 2012a. Prevalence of obesity in the United States, 2009–2010. NCHS Data Brief no. 82. Hyattsville, MD: National Center for Health Statistics, pp. 1–8.

Ogden, C.L., M. D. Carroll, B. K. Kit, and K. M. Flegal. 2012b. Prevalence of obesity and trends in body mass index among us children and adolescents, 1999–2010. *JAMA* 307 (5): 483–90.

Perry, D. 2001. *Food for Every Child: The Need for More Supermarkets in Philadelphia.* Philadelphia, PA: The Food Trust.

Powell, L. M., M. C. Auld, F. J. Chaloupka, P. M. O'Malley, and L. D. Johnston. 2007. Associations between access to food stores and adolescent body mass index. *Am J Prev Med* 33: S301–7.

The Association for Convenience & Fuel Retailing. 2011. *Increased Business Costs and Growing Regulations Led to a Need for More Industry Education in the Early 1970s.* Available at http://www.nacs50.com/decades/70s/ (accessed November 6, 2013).

The Reinvestment Fund. 2008. The economic impacts of supermarkets on their surrounding communities. In *Reinvestment Brief.* Philadelphia, PA: The Reinvestment Fund.

The Reinvestment Fund. 2013. *Pennsylvania Fresh Food Financing Initiative.* Available at http://www.trfund.com/pennsylvania-fresh-food-financing-initiative/ (accessed November 6, 2013).

Robbins, J. M., G. Mallya, M. Polansky, and D. F. Schwarz. 2012. Prevalence, disparities, and trends in obesity and severe obesity among students in the Philadelphia, Pennsylvania school district, 2006–2010. *Prev Chronic Dis* 9: E145.

Sarkar, P. 2005. "Scrambling for Customers: The Supermarket Was Born 75 Years Ago; One-stop Shopping Has Come a Long Way." *San Francisco Chronicle*, August 4, 2005.

Treuhaft, S. and A. Karpyn. 2010. *The Grocery Gap: Who Has Access to Healthy Food and Why it Matters.* Oakland, CA: PolicyLink and The Food Trust.

Uvin, P. and D. Miller. 1996. Paths to scaling up: Alternative strategies for local nongovernmental organizations. *Hum Organ* 55: 344–54.

Ver Ploeg, M., V. Breneman, P. Dutko, R. Williams, S. Snyder, C. Dickens, and P. Kaufman. 2012. Access to affordable and nutritious food: Updated estimates of distance to supermarkets using 2010 data. Economic Research Service, USDA, Economic Research Report No. 143.

Yaccino, S. 2011. "In Chicago, Michelle Obama Takes on 'Food Deserts.'" *The New York Times*, October 25, 2011, The Caucus.

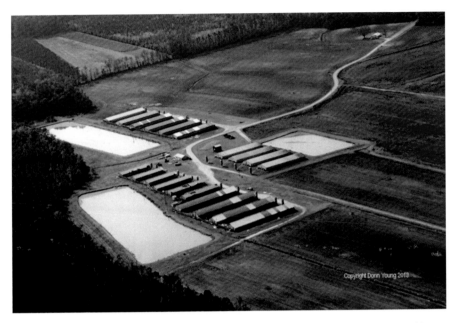

FIGURE 3.1 Industrial hog operation confinements, waste lagoons, spray fields, and home in the upper right. (Courtesy of Donn Young Photography, DSC no. 9566, Chapel Hill, North Carolina, 2013.)

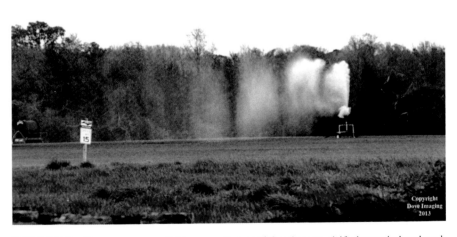

FIGURE 3.2 Hog waste spray fields aerosolize particles that can drift downwind and soak fields with fecal waste that can run off into surface waters and impact upper aquifers of ground water. (Courtesy of Dove, R., www.doveimaging.com, New Bern, North Carolina, 2013.)

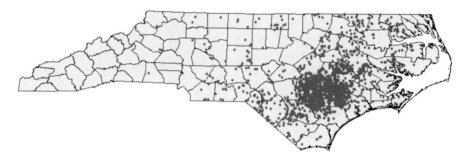

FIGURE 3.4 The 2407 industrial hog operations permitted by the North Carolina Division of Water Quality. (From Wing, S. et al., *American Journal of Public Health*, 98, 1390–1397, 2008.)

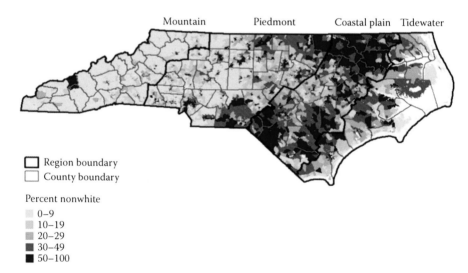

FIGURE 3.5 Nonwhite percentage of the population of census block groups, North Carolina, 2010. (Norton, J. et al., *Environmental Health Perspectives*, 115, 1344–1350, 2007.)

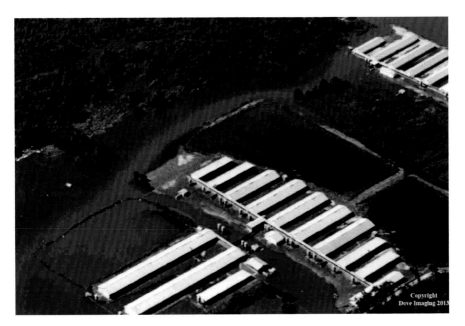

FIGURE 3.6 Fecal waste pits flooded following Hurricane Floyd. (Courtesy of Dove, R., www.doveimaging.com, New Bern, North Carolina, 2013.)

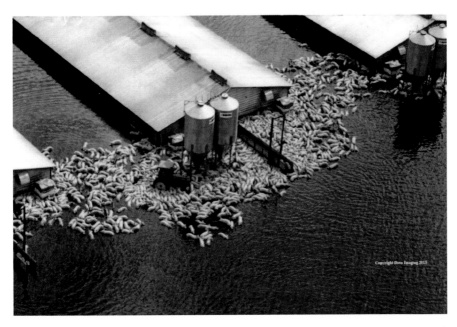

FIGURE 3.7 Tens of thousands of hogs drowned in the flooding from Hurricane Floyd. (Courtesy of Dove, R., www.doveimaging.com, New Bern, North Carolina, 2013.)

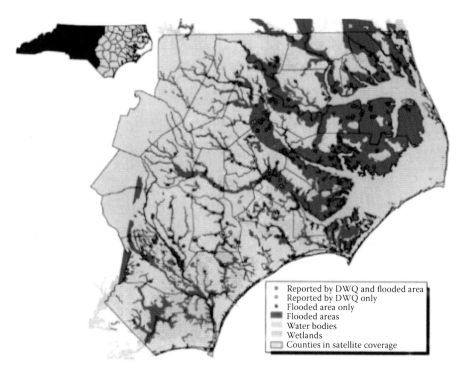

Reported by DWQ and flooded area
Reported by DWQ only
Flooded area only
Flooded areas
Water bodies
Wetlands
Counties in satellite coverage

FIGURE 3.8 Industrial animal production facilities with coordinates in the digital flood image or flooding reported by the North Carolina Division of Water Quality, September 1999. About 98% of these facilities were raising hogs. (From Wing, S. et al., *Environ. Health Perspect.*, 110, 387–391, 2002.)

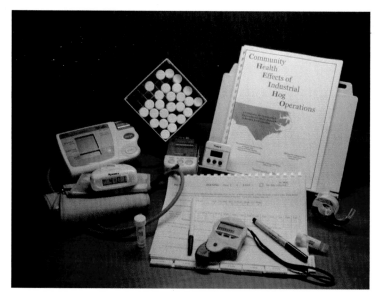

FIGURE 3.9 Instruments used for data collection by participants in the Community Health Effects of Industrial Hog Operations Study. (Courtesy of Denzler, B., University of North Carolina.)

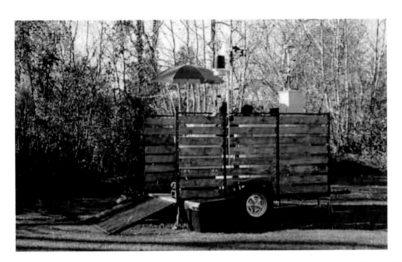

FIGURE 3.10 Monitoring trailer used to house equipment for measuring hourly pollution levels in 16 neighborhoods in eastern North Carolina. (Courtesy of Denzler, B., University of North Carolina.)

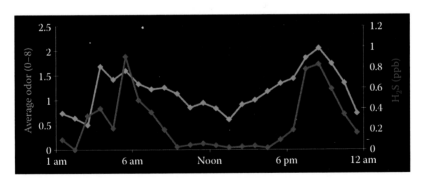

FIGURE 3.11 Average hourly odor levels (left vertical axis) and hydrogen sulfide (right vertical axis) in 16 eastern North Carolina communities located near industrial hog operations. (Based on Wing, S. et al., *American Journal of Public Health*, 98, 1390–1397, 2008.)

2010 Census: United States Profile

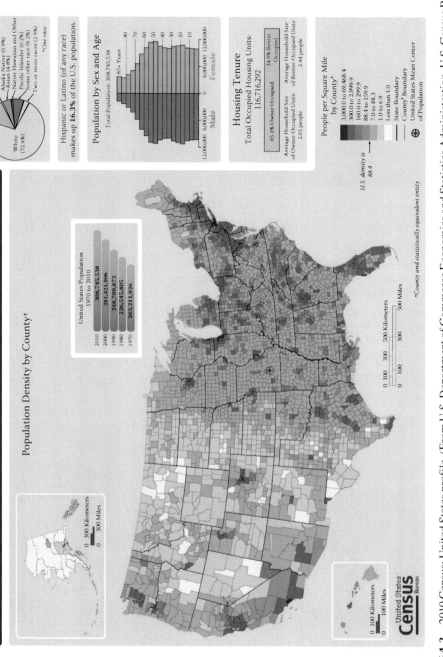

U.S. Race* Breakdown

- White (72.4%)
- Black or African American (12.6%)
- American Indian and Alaska Native (0.9%)
- Asian (4.8%)
- Native Hawaiian and Other Pacific Islander (0.2%)
- Some other race (6.2%)
- Two or more races (2.9%)

*One race

Hispanic or Latino (of any race) makes up **16.3%** of the U.S. population.

Population by Sex and Age
Total Population: 308,745,538

Male / Female
85+ Years, 80, 70, 60, 50, 40, 30, 20, 10
12,000,000 6,000,000 0 6,000,000 12,000,000

Housing Tenure
Total Occupied Housing Units: 116,716,292

65.1% Owner Occupied | 34.9% Renter Occupied

Average Household Size of Owner-Occupied Units: 2.65 people
Average Household Size of Renter-Occupied Units: 2.44 people

People per Square Mile by County†

- 3,000.0 to 69,468.4
- 300.0 to 2,999.9
- 160.0 to 299.9
- 88.4 to 159.9
- 7.0 to 88.3
- 1.0 to 6.9
- Less than 1.0

U.S. density is 88.4

— State Boundary
— County† Boundary
⊕ United States Mean Center of Population

†County and statistically equivalent entity

Population Density by County†

United States Population 1970 to 2010

- 2010: 308,745,538
- 2000: 281,421,906
- 1990: 248,709,873
- 1980: 226,545,805
- 1970: 203,211,926

0 100 300 500 Kilometers
0 100 300 500 Miles

0 300 Kilometers
0 300 Miles

0 100 Kilometers
0 100 Miles

United States Census Bureau

FIGURE 4.3 2010 Census: United States profile. (From U.S. Department of Commerce Economics and Statistics Administration, U.S. Census Bureau.)

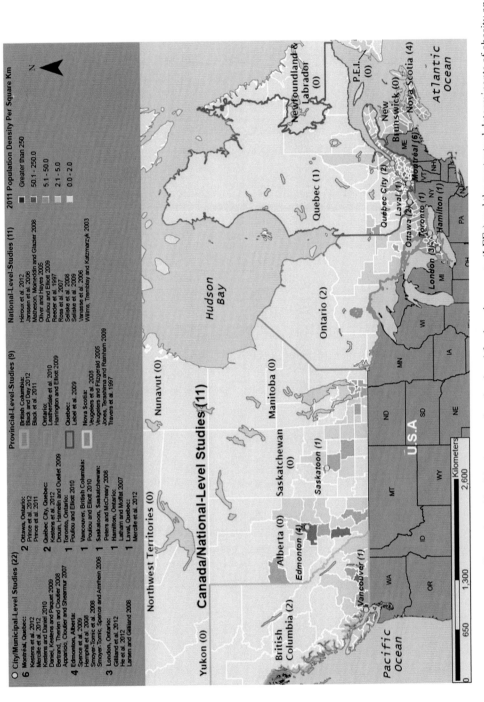

FIGURE 8.1 Peer-reviewed studies reviewed in this chapter related to local food environments (LFEs) and the contextual determinants of obesity and dietary outcomes in Canada, published in 2012 or earlier.

Problem statement: A healthy diet contributes to obesity prevention. Limited access to healthier food choices in terms of availability and/or quality is a major barrier to maintaining a healthier diet among children in families with low incomes.

Pre-Program Inputs

Community need

Political will and leadership (program champion)

Establishment of evidence with background data collection
- Educating decision makers on findings

Task force representing a diversity of interests and committed to process
- Health interests
  - University researchers
  - Dept. of Public Health (to offer evidence)
- Industry operators
- Dept. of Planning

- Non-profit civic groups

Advocate at state and local levels for funding, building relationships among community sectors

Financing and selective grant-making to reduce structural barriers

Community buy-in

Tax credits for economic development

Financing Legislation Passed

Inputs

Community need

Political will and leadership

Public-private partnerships
- The Reinvestment Fund
- The Food Trust

- The Greater Philadelphia Urban Affairs Coalition
- Commonweath of Pennsylvania

Process for funding grants and loans
- Funding leveraged (New Market Tax Credits)

Financing or distribution mechanism to help establish or assist supermarkets in underserved areas
- Grants
- Debt financing

Activities/Process

Ongoing response to constituent need

Provision of technical assistance and human resources assistance to qualifying grantees and borrowers

- The Food Trust
- The Reinvestment Fund
- Others

Outreach to promote programs to communities and operators/locations

Determine eligible operators/locations

Match communities to willing operators

Land assembly (obtain space for construction of new supermarkets)

Community commitment to deal with hurdles

Outputs

Amount of funding to resource program

Number of applications for grants or loans

Number of grants and loans made

Number of stores constructed or renovated

Number of operators matched to communities

Number of new options for produce/healthier food

Number of jobs created

Short-Term Outcomes

Increase in number of supermarkets opening and operating in underserved areas

Revitalization of old stores and construction of new stores

Increased access to (and increased variety

of) affordable fresh produce and/or other healthier food options

Cost savings for community members
- Lower food prices
- Reduced transportation costs

Jobs for community members

Supermarkets both meeting needs of consumers and meeting probability objectives

Greater food diversity

Intermediate Outcomes

Increased purchase and consumption of fresh produce and/or healthier food options

Increased selection of fresh produce at markets in underserved areas

Increased workforce capacity

Increased safety due to improved lighting, access, and security

Increased development of other small enterprises
- Supermarkets anchor developments for other retail

Bundled health and social services in supermarkets
- Other positive community outcomes/spinoffs

Increased knowledge of new healthy foods

Long-Term Outcomes

Increased consumption of healthier food options

Ongoing construction of markets in underserved areas and maintenance of existing markets

Create jobs, revitalize commercial real estate, leverage private sector capital, and increase tax ratables

Provide lower cost, nutritious foods and savings on transportation

Promote a nutritionally balanced diet which leads to reduced rates of diet-related disease

Goals

Contribute to improving the access of fresh foods

Economic development

Improved health outcomes due to:
- Reduction in diet-related disease
- Increased social capital
- Improved well-being

FIGURE 9.2 Pennsylvania's Fresh Food Financing Initiative logic model. (Copyright The Food Trust, 2009.)

10 Ecological Approaches to Creating Healthy Local Food Environments in the United States

Push and Pull Forces

Carol M. Devine and Jennifer L. Wilkins

If you wish to make an apple pie truly from scratch, you must first invent the universe.

(Carl Sagan (1980))

After more than a decade of research in the area of public health, there is evidence that, at least in the United States, disparities in access to food exist as a function of area wealth and racial composition. Although the measured impact of these disparities on dietary intake and health has limitations, some studies that have been conducted demonstrate the importance of equitable access to healthy foods. As we enter the next decade of research, investigators are challenged to conduct studies that will provide policy makers with evidence to support new legislation (e.g., city zoning requirement for food retailers, federal tax incentives for chain supermarkets to locate in restricted food environments, and/or policies that help small retailers carry perishable food products) that will improve public health nutrition and diet-related disease rates through the modification of local food environments. In spite of the limitation in current knowledge, many government, community-driven groups, and academics have used the precautionary principle to move forward and take action to improve many local food environments across the United States.

Overcoming substantial disparities in community local access to healthy food will require intentional transformations in local food environments. Limited access to nutritious foods, coincident with relatively easier access to calorie-dense foods, is increasingly seen as an important—and changeable—threat to public health. Creating sustainable change in local food environments in the United States will require ecological approaches that generate both push and pull forces at all levels.

This chapter describes existing and emerging approaches to increasing community access to healthy foods and decreasing disparities in local food environments, highlighting selected representative initiatives, programs, and interventions in the United States. It presents recommendations for research and evaluation of emerging changes to local food environments and their impact on nutrition and health.

In this chapter we first present objectives and definitions, describe an ecological push–pull model for framing interventions to change local food environments, and then provide examples of seven types of approaches originating at different levels of action. Finally, we will consider research and evaluation needs.

OBJECTIVES

By the end of this chapter readers will be able to

- Describe the ecological, multisectoral, push–pull, food systems-based nature of approaches to change local food environments to increase local access to healthy food.
- Identify approaches at multiple levels of action including individuals and families, civil society, local, state, and national levels and how food system sectors may be involved.
- Describe how efforts to increase local access to healthy food can take advantage of the push–pull nature of the food system.
- Discuss how changing local food environments may involve social, economic, physical, and policy inputs and outcomes.
- Identify surveillance, research, and program evaluation needs related to interventions to promote local access to healthy food.
- Identify several resources for those who wish to work in this area.

APPROACH AND DEFINITIONS

The approaches described in this chapter were shaped by a diverse set of available reports of efforts to increase access to healthy food in communities. These efforts include a few natural experiments (typically uncontrolled), a small number of research interventions, various public policy initiatives, and a large and increasing number of local community-driven efforts. Although research in this emerging field is on the rise, analyses in peer-reviewed publications are sparse, and the majority of local initiatives have not been formally evaluated. Thus, the chapter does not present a thorough review of existing evidence, but rather, describes and summarizes a number of promising approaches at a variety of levels that were initiated by actors in a food system context.

The focus of the approaches described in this chapter is on increasing access to healthy foods in communities or neighborhoods. Because of our focus on efforts to change these local food environments, we used the description of that environment, laid out in Chapter 1, to mean the places and distances consumers would routinely travel to acquire food for personal or family consumption. The distance, direction, and type of transportation differ by community context: a few blocks by foot or bus in an urban neighborhood and a few miles by car in a suburban or rural community.

As we considered approaches to increase healthy food access, we included initiatives aimed at three main related goals insuring that food in the environment was: (1) available or present, (2) affordable by all community residents, and (3) accessible in terms of proximity. Many of these initiatives also incorporated efforts to provide foods that were acceptable to community members in terms of quality, and consistent with their preferences, cultural practices, and desire for convenience. These considerations, however, were not the focus of the current discussion (for more see Caspi et al. [2012]).

Because of our focus on the community food environment, we did not review in depth interventions aimed primarily at individuals within institutional settings such as schools, worksites, or healthcare institutions, although the type and quality of food sold in these institutions is an important contributor to community health. The importance of the role these institutions play in community food access—especially for insufficiently resourced population groups—is without question. Interventions that were primarily educational or promotional in nature, such as those designed to change individual product purchasing behavior within supermarkets or grocery stores, were also not a focus. These latter types of interventions are also important contributors to overall consumption of healthy foods, but beyond the scope of this chapter.

The approaches discussed in this chapter aimed to increase access to healthy foods in the local food environment. The focus was on approaches designed to increase nutrient density and reduce current social and economic disparities in consumption. The largest number of interventions discussed in this chapter focused on increasing the availability of and access to vegetables and fruits. Other intervention targets include whole grains and lower-fat dairy products, and nutrient-dense snack foods. A few interventions aim to limit availability of or access to less healthy, energy-dense foods.

Approaches to changing local food environments to increase healthy food access were identified through a variety of means, including searches of the published research literature for the past 10 years; relevant reviews (Gittelsohn et al. 2012b); and government (CDC 2013), civil society (Wekerle 2004), and workshop (Whitacre et al. 2009) reports. Community-based initiatives were identified through Internet searches. References to specific programs in the citations of published reports were also investigated. Although the focus was primarily on community food access in the U.S. context, we also considered approaches used in other developed countries and historically important efforts. Because of the necessarily diverse and localized nature of these efforts, we include only a few examples that are representative of scores of local, regional, and state efforts to change local food environments.

ECOLOGICAL FRAMEWORK: MULTIPLE LEVELS OF ACTION

An ecological framework has been proposed as an effective way to portray the complex relationships between individual food choices, the food system, and the physical, social, economic, and policy environments in which food is acquired and consumed (Swinburn et al. 1999; Sallis et al. 2009). Interventions that focus solely on individual health behaviors (in the context of a fixed food environment) have had limited success in combating obesity and decreasing diet-related disease risk on a population scale (Hill and Peters 1998). The environmental and policy contexts of individual health behaviors have received increased attention (Story et al. 2008). An ecological approach engages multiple levels of action and multiple actors in efforts to create more comprehensive interventions. Dietary behavior change "is expected to be maximized when environments and policies support healthful choices, when social norms and social support for healthful choices are strong, and when individuals are motivated and educated to make those choices" (Glanz et al. 2008). Given the seemingly intractable nature of diet-related chronic diseases, obesity, and food insecurity, as well as the limited success of decades of investment in programs aimed at changing individual behavior, ecological approaches offer new possibilities for achieving and sustaining change in the public health landscape.

We emphasize three central themes in applying an ecological framework to changing local food environments (Figure 10.1): (1) multilevel embeddedness of local food access, (2) push–pull interactions within and between levels of the framework, and (3) multiple pathways to increasing access to healthy foods in the local

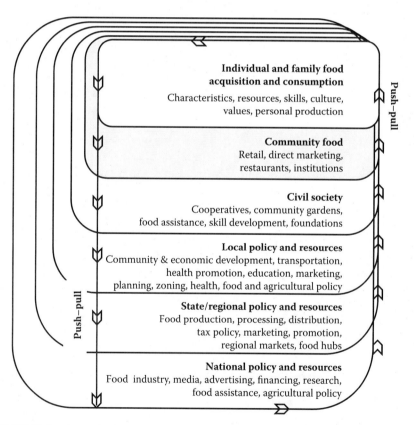

FIGURE 10.1   An ecological push–pull model for changing local food environments.

food environment. This framework also explicitly acknowledges the importance of engagement at all levels with public and private sectors of the food system from individual acquisition to national food and agricultural policy.

Multilevel Embeddedness of Local Food Access

Individual and family food choices are embedded within the physical, social, economic, and policy environments (Swinburn et al. 1999) in their local communities and, as shown in Figure 10.1, within a cascade of macrolevel environments that can both enhance and limit local access to food.

Ecological models bring into view how individuals and organizations interact with elements of the proximal and distal environments. These models propose that human behavior involves multiple levels of influence, including intrapersonal (biological, psychological), interpersonal (social, cultural), organizational, institutional, community, physical environmental, and policy. By applying such a framework, community actors may be able to better address multiple and interacting determinants of food access. Further, ecological models have become useful tools for developing intervention approaches for change at multiple levels of influence (Sallis et al. 2008).

Individual and family demand for food responds to and is shaped by many influences. These may include personal and household characteristics, acquisition and consumption preferences and patterns, knowledge, skills, values, and cultural preferences, as well as personal production (Sobal and Bisogni 2009).

Multiple community sites can provide food: retail grocery stores, corner stores, or supermarkets; direct marketing to consumers through farmers' markets (FMs) or green carts; restaurants of all types, institutions such as child care, schools, healthcare facilities, or workplaces; and food assistance outlets such as food pantries, soup kitchens, and food banks that are used by an increasing proportion of the population (Andrews 2010; Carson and Meub 2013). All of these settings are embedded within local, regional, and national food systems and are regulated and supported by government policies and available resources at all levels. Local food outlets serve simultaneously to provide food access to consumers and as markets and distribution outlets for the food production, processing, and distribution systems.

Increasingly, civil society plays active roles in improving food access at the community level. Nongovernmental organizations, groups, movements, and food-oriented campaigns may increase access by facilitating interactions between individuals and the food system or by fostering collective action to improve the local food environment. Food cooperatives and buying clubs and community gardens have long played active roles in the promotion of local food access. Civil society organizations are operating at community and regional levels to add to what had traditionally been a top–down model of the food system from production to consumption. In many communities they have led the charge to create pull forces in the form of increased consumer demand for improved healthy food access and policies at multiple levels to push for this access. By building social awareness, promotion, education, and community engagement, the involvement of these civil society organizations can often mean the difference between success and failure of a change in access that is built.

Perhaps the best-known example in this arena is The Food Trust (2012), founded in Philadelphia to ensure community access to healthy food.

Local health and agricultural policies and supporting regulations have long affected food access, but local policies seemingly tangential to food and health—such as transportation, city planning, and tax policy—can also affect food access in important structural ways. Increasingly, planning, economic development, and zoning efforts consider food access as important as traditional outcomes of local public policy. Local marketing efforts help to promote food access as a desirable community amenity.

State and regional policies can shape food production, processing, and distribution networks. State tax policies, transportation networks, marketing and promotion efforts, economic development initiatives, and comprehensive plans can provide incentives for healthy food access.

At the national level, federal food agricultural and food assistance policies have long affected the entire food system including what is grown, how it is processed, distributed, and labeled as well as how it is accessed by those with limited resources. For example, changes in the federal regulations governing the package of foods approved for purchase through the Special Supplemental Food Program for Women, Infants, and Children (WIC) to better reflect federal dietary guidelines are credited with creating local demand (or *pull*) for increased availability of a variety of fruits, vegetables, whole grain products, and lower-fat milk in WIC-authorized convenience and grocery stores (Andreyeva et al. 2011). A recent augmentation to the WIC benefit provides checks to be used specifically for the purchase of fruits and vegetables from retail outlets and, increasingly, from FMs with approved vendors (Connecticut Department of Agriculture 2010; NYS 2013). Federal financing initiatives, such as the Healthy Food Financing Initiative (HFFI), offer tools to help improve local healthy food access by promoting a range of community interventions such as developing and equipping grocery stores and other small businesses and retailers selling health food in areas lacking these options (HFFI 2011).

Local food access must be considered in the context of a global food system (Donald 2013). The multinational food, beverage, and restaurant corporations that make up the private sector are driven by the bottom line, but these food system actors are responding to the call to address public health issues in a variety of ways. Some are taking the lead with modest reformulations such as eliminating, reducing, and/or replacing caloric sweeteners, sodium, and trans fats (Sleator and Hill 2007), or signing onto high-level commitments (Partnership for a Healthier America) and/or promotions (Strom 2012). Although some of these actions may be taken in response to concerns about stiffer government regulations, their promise for improving public health has captivated the attention of national leaders and corporate investors alike. It remains to be seen, however, how effective these strategies will be in addressing local access to healthy foods, reducing diet-related chronic disease risk, and the reversal of obesity trends. In December 2012, the Federal Trade Commission issued an assessment of progress following its 2008 review of targeted food industry marketing activities to children and adolescents (Leibowitz et al. 2012). The findings of this report have relevance to local food access, given the preponderance of packaged and highly processed foods (with low nutrient density) in neighborhood stores located in underserved areas, thereby raising questions about whether food reformulations are likely to lead to meaningful differences in dietary quality and public health.

Push–Pull Interactions within and between Levels of an Ecological Framework

An ecological framework is not static; rather it should reflect dynamic interactions among its elements. Push and pull forces from the top down, from the bottom up, within and between layers create both a supply of food and a demand for healthy food in communities. Interactions at varying levels can focus on interpersonal actions, as well as organizational, environmental, and policy changes. Individuals and households, civil society organizations, or food assistance programs, such as WIC or the Farmer's Market Nutrition Program (FMNP), can help create demand for particular types of foods (e.g., fruits and vegetables) in underserved areas and thus a market for those who wish to sell those foods. Through purchases, individuals can *pull* on the system to signal demand for healthy foods when they are available. By supporting policies that incentivize healthy food access and voting for policy makers who author them, citizens and civil society can help *push* local food systems to change. City or town governments can develop zoning ordinances that encourage increased availability of nutritious foods—an effective push on the system. Citizens interested in improving access to healthy food in their communities can engage with city government through public hearing, building relationships with local officials, and providing input on proposed local zoning ordinances and incentives, such as tax abatement schemes.

Interactions between levels are an essential part of the ecological framework. Examples of such interactions include households with food cooperatives, grocery stores and restaurants with local farms or regional food hubs, and local planners with national financing initiatives for supermarkets in underserved areas. Interactions are also important between public and private sectors within levels of the ecological model. Examples include interactions between community civil society organizations and elected officials with planning and zoning responsibilities or state agricultural marketing efforts and food producers and processors.

Multiple Pathways to Local Food Access

The ecological model illustrates the importance of multiple partners and multiple pathways to change local food environments. No single action by a single actor is likely to result in success (Rose et al. 2009). The mere presence of a food store does not mean that it will succeed as a business. For example, failure to attract the confidence and purchases of local residents can challenge even a highly community-driven effort to increase local food access (Morland 2010). Nonetheless, increasing the number and variety of sources of healthy foods in the local environment and considering the needs of all interested parties—from consumer to producer—should lay the groundwork to increase the flow of healthy food to communities and, ultimately, to households and individuals.

Changing local food environments will result in and form changes in interactions among actors within each of the levels of influence portrayed in the model.

At the individual level, agency, self-efficacy, knowledge and skills, and awareness of proximal and distal opportunities, and influences are critical to increasing healthy food access. The interpersonal level involves social networks that can include family members, peers, and fellow nutrition assistance program recipients. At the organizational level, valuable skills include the ability to organize and work collaboratively toward common community food system/access goals.

FOOD SYSTEM INTERSECTIONS WITHIN AN ECOLOGICAL FRAMEWORK

Access to healthy food in communities requires shifts in proximal outlets with which individuals have direct contact and in which they express demand, as well as critical, more distal changes throughout the production, supply, and value chain. Although food purchases at the retail level are perhaps most accessible form of demand (pull), individuals and increasingly organizations, consumer groups, and other forms of civil society are also exerting pull toward healthier food access up the supply chain (i.e., distribution, processing, and production). For example, some grocery chains promote regionally grown vegetables and fruits, in large part because it is seen as something that is valued by customers (Guptill and Wilkins 2002; Ilbery and Maye 2006).

Likewise, local, state, and national policy is actively engaged in pushing the food system to increase the nutrient density of the food supply and close gaps in healthy food access within communities, city neighborhoods, and rural areas. Through nutrition and health promotion programs and nutrition assistance funding, policy exerts push influences at the individual consumer level with the aim of shifting demand (pull), but such policy efforts will only succeed if the various sectors of the local food access system are commercially healthy. As well, technology provides a push toward improved access to healthy food by enhancing capacity at production, processing, distribution, and marketing levels. So, we see interplay of push and pull forces on the entire food system at multiple levels within multiple sectors to achieve the desired outcome—increasing healthy food access.

APPROACHES TO INCREASING COMMUNITY FOOD ACCESS

The ecological model frames a variety of goals for and approaches to enhance local food access. Public health and nutrition goals may include midterm outcomes, such as enhancing the quality and nutrient density of food choices, as well as long-term outcomes of reduced diet-related chronic diseases incidence and lower obesity rates. At the same time, interventions to increase local food access may address related goals for community development and vitality, environmental health and sustainability, and other broad community issues (e.g., social cohesion).

Approaches to increase community food access can be divided into one of seven categories: (1) education and skill building, (2) social marketing, (3) direct-to-consumer, (4) healthy retail and direct-to-retail or institution, (5) economic, (6) transportation, and (7) development and planning approaches. We will describe examples of each and end by discussing surveillance and research activities that assist with needs assessment, targeting, and evaluation of several types of approaches. Keep in mind that the examples presented here represent only a very few of the scores of laudable initiatives underway in cities and towns across the country. As well, several initiatives can fit in more than one of the classifications presented here, but we offer this grouping as a way of highlighting key components or emphases.

EDUCATIONAL AND SKILL-BUILDING APPROACHES

Educational and skill-building approaches are typically aimed at enhancing food procurement and preparation skills, as well as gardening skills. These approaches occur primarily at the individual or household level, but they may also occur in neighborhoods. They are aimed at increasing access to healthy food at the household level and helping to develop sustained demand for community food by increasing individual and family capacity to use healthy foods. Broadly these types of efforts may also raise awareness of the need for local access to healthy foods and may increase demand for particular items such as low-fat dairy products (Reger et al. 1998). Such approaches have been traditionally carried out by local public health, Cooperative Extension, or civil society groups. Novel examples, from public–private partnerships, are Truck Farm mobile garden education projects in Tampa (Truck Farm Tampa 2012) and Chicago (Truck Farm Chicago 2013). With their truck beds planted with garden greens, peppers, tomatoes, and other vegetables, farmer/educators engage children and adults in neighborhoods, near schools, and along city streets in food education. The opportunity to taste fresh produce and see how plants grow gives consumers a direct connection to a novel local source of vegetables.

SOCIAL MARKETING APPROACHES

Social marketing approaches complement individual educational and skill-building approaches by drawing attention to healthy foods, often locally produced, through labeling and advertising through a variety of media (Curhan 1974). These efforts, although they do not directly increase healthy food access, do promote public conversation and create awareness of these foods that may be sold in grocery stores, FMs, and restaurants. In these ways, they change the social environment for food and eating and help to create demand or pull for healthy foods in local stores and other institutions. Examples of marketing approaches at federal, state, and local levels include the U.S. Department of Agriculture's Know Your Farmer, Know Your Food program (USDA 2013), NYS Department of Agriculture and Markets' Pride of New York program (2013), and Berkshire Grown (2013) in Massachusetts.

The use of locally produced food is neither necessary nor sufficient to increase local food access in underserved communities. Engagement of producers and encouraging FMs in efforts to increase sales of locally produced food may bring more push forces on community food availability. But success of this kind of effort will also rely on future directions in federal agricultural policy and in food consumption by consumers (Buzby et al. 2006). Community policies to encourage connections between producers and consumers can help to create a social and economic environment where food access becomes integrated into community development and planning on a broad scale (Kantor 2001).

DIRECT-TO-CONSUMER APPROACHES

Approaches that connect farmers directly to consumers, addressing availability and quality of healthy food in communities, abound. These approaches include Pick-Your-Own farm operations, farm stands, and Community Supported Agriculture (CSA) operations, but also the wide variety of FMs, including urban green markets, green carts featuring locally grown produce, and markets at workplaces, healthcare settings, schools, and transit points (e.g., highway rest stops, bus stations, or commuter routes). Although FMs may provide economic benefit to local communities and may even reduce the price of a healthy food basket in an underserved areas (Larsen and Gilliland 2009; Young et al. 2011), more evidence is needed to show their impact on food access and health, especially in the most underserved populations (Glanz and Yaroch 2004; Brown and Miller 2008; Martinez et al. 2010). More recently, FMs in fixed locations have been joined by mobile grocery stores that bring healthy foods to underserved neighborhoods. Examples include the People's Grocery in Oakland, California (2012). Although many direct markets may have originated in the private sector by producers themselves, efforts to bring these types of direct marketing to underserved areas often require partnerships between producers and civil society organizations or local governments to be successful. A recent report from the Centers for Disease Control and Prevention enumerated state-level efforts to increase local fruit and vegetable access and consumption through direct approaches including FMs, farm-to-school programs, voucher systems, and other policies (CDC 2013). States with more environmental supports such as these were noted as having higher consumption of fruits and vegetables.

HEALTHY RETAIL AND DIRECT-TO-RETAIL OR INSTITUTIONAL APPROACHES

Interventions designed to improve the local food environment through promotion of retail outlets carrying healthy foods typically focus on two approaches: (1) location of food retail outlets in underserved areas and (2) efforts to increase the proportion of healthy foods in existing stores.

Initiatives to attract the location of food retail outlets to underserved areas may be found in all parts of the United States. Over the past decade, there has been an explosion of initiatives emanating from city and regional planning that exercise local policy mechanisms to *zone* for better nutrition and healthy eating (Chen and Florax 2010). City planning can encourage or inhibit land use for community gardens. City regulations can encourage vending of fresh produce like the green carts that pepper New York City's (NYC) five boroughs with tiny oases for fresh fruits and vegetables, increasing healthy food access in areas regarded otherwise as food deserts (Lucan et al. 2011). Over 500 vendors participate in the NYC Green Cart program and help fill a void in low-income areas plagued with high rates of obesity and diet-related diseases.

Food Retail Expansion to Support Health (or FRESH) is an initiative of New York City's Mayoral Five-Borough Economic Opportunity Plan that promotes the establishment and retention of neighborhood grocery stores in underserved communities by providing zoning and financial incentives to eligible grocery store operators and developers (NYC Economic Development Corporation 2013). Like similar efforts in other cities, these community development strategies are aimed at improving healthy food access in areas where lack of nutritious, affordable fresh food has been linked to higher rates of diet-related diseases, including heart disease, diabetes, and obesity.

For more than 20 years, The Food Trust in Philadelphia has worked across the city and more recently throughout Pennsylvania to ensure that residents have access to affordable, nutritious food and to information to make healthy food decisions (Karpyn et al. 2010). Working with neighborhoods, schools, grocers, farmers, and policy makers, The Food Trust employs a comprehensive approach to improved food access combining nutrition education while tangibly increasing availability of affordable, healthy food. Work of The Food Trust (for more information see Chapter 9) is credited, in part, for the recent Philadelphia Department of Public Health finding that—for the first time in decades—the obesity rates among the city's school children decreased by 5% between 2006 and 2010. This is one of the first studies showing a reversal of the country's troubling obesity trends at the level of a large urban center, and suggests that comprehensive approaches that combine nutrition education and increased access to healthy foods are effective (Marks and Lavizzo-Mourey 2012).

Interventions to increase the number of healthy retail food outlets involve businesses of all scales and types from full-service supermarkets and independent grocery stores to corner stores, bodegas, and small box stores. Challenges to interventions in smaller stores may include the proportion of profits from snack items and beverages and competition for shelf space (Bodor et al. 2010), lack of funds to purchase healthy foods (Curran et al. 2005), high fixed costs of fruits and vegetables (Jetter and Cassady 2010), and lack of equipment for fresh foods needing refrigeration (Rose et al. 2009).

Among efforts to increase the proportion of healthy foods in neighborhood stores, the Baltimore Healthy Stores initiative is a well-known example (Gittelsohn et al. 2010a,b,c). The investigators recruited both small corner stores and some supermarkets in Baltimore to stock specific healthy foods. Although no difference in overall healthy food purchasing was found, the researchers reported a significant increase in preparation of healthy foods and purchasing of the marketed healthy foods in intervention areas, and in stocking and self-efficacy to stock healthy foods by owners (Song et al. 2009). Store owners reported increased customer flow and sales, illustrating the importance of assessing outcomes for customers and retailers (Gittelsohn et al. 2012a).

Related to these efforts to increase healthy foods in grocery stores are direct-to-retail approaches, which typically involve partnerships among producers, processors, grocery stores, and supermarkets. Similar relationships may also link producers with restaurants and institutional food service operations such as in public and private schools, universities, hospitals, and workplaces. Farm-to-school projects are a widespread example of the farm-to-institution model. Over the past decade, farm-to-school programs have emerged as a promising approach to improving the quality of school meals and thereby helping prevent childhood obesity. Farm-to-school projects are a response to demand or pull from parents, professional food and nutrition organizations, and health policy advocacy organizations for better quality school meals. At the same time, push is coming from agriculture marketing and community and economic development organizations to strengthen links between local agriculture producers and processor and area school districts (Allen and Guthman 2006). These programs are echoed in emerging programs linking producers to other institutions such as universities (Friedmann 2007) and worksites (Ross et al. 1999). Foundation grants have provided important support for these direct-to-retail efforts. For example, the National Farm-to-School Network receives support from the W.K. Kellogg Foundation that facilitates the involvement of school districts and states in farm-to-school, and the Robert Wood Johnson Foundation supports various farm-to-school initiatives (RWJF 2013). The USDA Food and Nutrition Service sponsors a grants program to support schools in their efforts to develop, sustain, and scale up farm-to-school programs (FNS 2013a).

Finally, regional food hubs, auctions, and markets, where large lots of regionally produced food is sold or auctioned off to local stores and institutions, simplify access to healthy foods by centralizing procurement of produce (Schmidt et al. 2011; Lerman et al. 2012). Information about these and many other projects is available on the Healthy Food Access Portal at http://www.healthyfoodaccessportal.org.

TRANSPORTATION APPROACHES

Transportation approaches to increasing local food access either bring food to the customer or the customer to the food. The lack of convenient and affordable transportation has been identified as a barrier to local food access, especially in rural areas (Dean and Sharkey 2011). While some city residents must rely on costly taxis, or infrequent buses, for grocery delivery, rural residents with limited transportation options may need to rely on relatives and friends to take them to grocery stores often as much as half an hour away to find affordable, high-quality produce (Maley 2007). Many interventions to improve local food access are aimed at bringing food to communities through location of supermarkets or mobile food stores in underserved areas, as described earlier. An alternative is to bring the shoppers to the food, by providing and/or subsidizing transportation to competitively priced retail food outlets that may be located on the outskirts of urban areas. Cities, such as Nashville, have set up shuttles or *grocery bus* routes to increase access to supermarkets (RWJF 2011).

ECONOMIC APPROACHES

Economic approaches to promote local healthy food access for consumers fall into two main categories: (1) vouchers to increase consumer purchasing power and (2) price subsidies to increase affordability of healthy foods. Vouchers for healthy foods do not promote local food access directly but they may have an indirect effect through the creation of demand for particular foods such as fruits and vegetables (Andreyeva et al. 2011). Economic approaches to increasing healthy food access at the consumer level center around increasing purchasing power for healthy foods, particularly fruits and vegetables, among low-income families. As described earlier, examples include the WIC and the FMNP, as well as the Senior Farmer's Market Nutrition Program targeting fruit and vegetable acquisition and consumption. There is evidence that these types of voucher programs are associated with increased fruit and vegetable consumption for seniors and WIC recipients (Balsam et al.

1994; Anderson et al. 2001; Kunkel et al. 2003). Installation of Electronic Benefits Terminals (EBT) for the federal Special Nutrition Assistance Program (SNAP) at FMs and supplying individual vendors with mobile card swipe devices also make it more convenient for SNAP recipients to purchase fruits and vegetables. To date, these terminals account for only a tiny fraction of the redemptions of SNAP benefits, but they have the potential to reach many more SNAP recipients as more FMs install EBT terminals (Young et al. 2011).

Civil society approaches to increasing local healthy food acquisition and consumption by low-income households include subsidized CSA shares or shares based on a sliding fee scale (Perez et al. 2003). For example, vouchers for fruits and vegetables and a novel fruit and vegetable prescription program are strategies used by Wholesome Wave as part of their mission to increase access and affordability of produce to historically underserved communities (2013).

A small number of experiments in laboratory or institutional settings such as workplaces, school cafeterias, and web-based simulations have assessed the effect of price reductions or subsidies on food purchasing behavior with modest short-term positive results (Jeffery et al. 1994; French et al. 2010; Waterlander et al. 2012). The effectiveness of so-called *fat taxes* on unhealthy foods has been much debated, but little real-world evidence is available to evaluate their effect (Thow et al. 2010). An exception was a fat tax on foods high in saturated fat in Denmark (Smed and Robertson 2012), which was repealed after about a year because people found substitutes or alternative sources for the taxed foods (Strom 2012).

Planning and Economic Development Approaches

Planning and economic development efforts to include food access as a broader goal of community development efforts have benefitted from recent financial incentives to promote local food retail businesses. Morgan (2009) points out that local food access is of interest to urban planners because it impinges on many other aspects of urban life such as public health, social justice, energy, economic development, and transportation, among others. Because of this, many cities and regions have begun to initiate coordinated efforts to increase food access that involve several sectors of the local community. These are often guided by community food policy or food systems councils or other types of local coalitions (Cyzman et al. 2009) and include examples such as the Chicago Metro Agency for Planning efforts to promote food access (CMAP 2013) and the Birmingham Urban Food Project (REV Birmingham 2013).

The National Healthy Food Financing Initiative (HFFI) aimed at promotion of retail food businesses in underserved areas through grants and loans to local communities, are an important entry into this arena. These types of programs provide community grants to promote food business development. The National HFFI, which operates through collaboration between the U.S. Treasury, and the U.S. Agriculture and Health and Human Service Departments, was first funded in 2012 to work with communities in several states to create and preserve grocery stores in underserved areas. The HFFI is modeled after the Pennsylvania Fresh Food Financing Initiative (FFFI), a public–private partnership that reported 83 new or improved grocery stores in underserved urban and rural neighborhoods as of 2009 (Reinvestment Fund

2006). An evaluation of the FFFI in an intervention and a comparison neighborhood (Flint et al. 2012) reported significant positive changes in neighborhood perceptions of the food environment but no changes in body mass index (BMI) or fruit and vegetable consumption. Other evaluations of this project will look at job creation and economic indicators, illustrating some of the close ties between community economic vitality and local food access (Fleischhacker et al. 2013). Similarly the New Market Tax Credits program provides tax credits to investors who provide capital for community development entities such as grocery stores in low-income communities (CDFI 2013).

Small business development efforts that support local food access also include job training and technical assistance for individuals, small businesses, and communities. The Detroit Grocery Incubator (Fair Food Network 2013) is an example of an approach to increasing local food access by providing training and experience to develop future *grocery entrepreneurs.*

Healthy food retailing legislation has been established in several states offering help such as tax incentives and grants and loans to help promote small business development in the food sector (CDC 2012). The Illinois Food, Farms, and Jobs program is an example (Food Farms Jobs 2013). In many states, cooperative extension county offices provide technical assistance to local producers to make their products available to local retail and direct market outlets, as well as through USDA's Farmers' Market Promotion Program, which offers a competitive grants program that funds expansion of direct-to-consumer marketing (FNS 2013b).

SURVEILLANCE AND RESEARCH NEEDS

Efforts to change local food environments have benefitted greatly from a number of surveillance activities ranging from multiple reports by the Economic Research Service of the U.S. Department of Agriculture on food deserts, on food prices, and on food insecurity and by the Centers for Disease Control and Prevention's report on fruit and vegetable consumption, FMs, and healthy food environments. These surveillance activities, together with state, regional, and local reports on food access and food supplies in local communities, have helped to raise alerts about food access issues, identify places in greatest need, and provide a critical baseline against which intervention efforts can be measured (Pothukuchi 2004).

Formal intervention research to increase local food access faces several barriers such as the difficulties inherent in measuring and controlling multiple sectors of the food system, the multiple influences on food access, the importance of local context to the outcomes of interventions, the relatively long time scale needed before behavioral or health outcomes are observable, and the small scale of much of the work in this area (Sallis et al. 2009). With the exception of some public policy initiatives, there has been little scaling up of interventions thus far, but growth in some entrepreneurial activities such as within the farmer's market and green cart sectors provides evidence of a secular change in retail food business models that may have an impact on community access to healthy foods. Another challenge is the need for interventions to increase food access in rural areas. With few exceptions (Gittelsohn et al. 2012b), the examples cited in this chapter originate primarily from urban areas.

The nature of this evolving work means that it is important to describe and evaluate promising approaches to support the development of this field, in spite of a limited evidence base.

The lack of formal research and the localized and uncontrolled nature of these interventions mean that there are serious limitations to interpretation of what works, how it works, and under what circumstances. Even the appropriate outcomes to measure and the best measures to use are unclear (Ver Ploeg et al. 2009). Some of the published reports and evaluations dealt specifically with healthy food availability, cost, and purchasing behavior. Others investigated dietary behavior and a few included health-related outcomes such as BMI. Further still, others examined community level and economic outcomes. Rose et al. (2010) point out the need to assess multiple dimensions of local food access including the effect on acquisition and consumption, as well as the effect on sales, prices, employment, economic vitality, and community cohesiveness. Because of the extremely localized nature of these types of interventions, research in this area will need to carefully assess contextual issues and processes at individual, household, neighborhood, community, and policy levels. Of necessity, this type of research will need to include investigators from multiple disciplines including public health and nutrition, as well as community development, planning, economics, and marketing, just to name a few.

GOING FURTHER

Helpful resources for further work in this area have been referenced throughout this chapter. We add a few general places to start for those who wish to investigate this area further:

CDC Healthy Food Access. Available at http://www.cdc.gov/healthyplaces /healthtopics/healthyfood_environment.htm.

USDA Food Access Research Atlas. Available at http://www.ers.usda.gov /data-products/food-access-research-atlas.aspx#.UcSpn8psuWE.

Healthy Food Access Portal—Policy Link, The Food Trust, The Reinvestment Fund. Available at http://www.healthyfoodaccess.org/home?destination =home.

REFERENCES

Allen, P. and J. Guthman. 2006. From "old school" to "farm-to-school": Neoliberalization from the ground up. *Agr Hum Values* 23: 401–15.

Anderson, J. V., D. I. Bybee, R. M. Brown et al. 2001. 5-a-day fruit and vegetable intervention improves consumption in a low income population. *J Am Diet Assoc* 101: 195–202.

Andrews, M. 2010. More Americans relied on food assistance during recession. Washington, DC: Economic Research Service, USDA. Available at http://www.ers.usda.gov /amber-waves/2010-december/more-americans-relied-on-food-assistance-during -recession.aspx (accessed November 9, 2013).

Andreyeva, T., J. Luedicke, A. Middleton, M. Long, and M. Schwartz. 2011. Changes in access to healthy foods after implementation of the WIC food package revisions. *J Acad Nutr Diet* 112: 850–8.

Balsam, A., D. Webber, and B. Oehlke. 1994. The farmers' market coupon program for low-income elders. *J Nutr Elder* 13: 35–42.

Berkshire Grown. 2013. Available at http://berkshiregrown.org (accessed June 26, 2013).

Bodor, J. N., V. M. Ulmer, L. F. Dunaway, T. A. Farley, and D. Rose. 2010. The rationale behind small food store interventions in low-income urban neighborhoods: Insights from New Orleans. *J Nutr* 140: 1185–8.

Brown, C. and S. Miller. 2008. The impacts of local markets: A review of research on farmers' markets and Community Supported Agriculture (CSA). *Am J Agr Econ* 90: 1298–302.

Buzby, J. C., H. F. Wells, and G. Vocke. 2006. Possible implications for U.S. agriculture from adoption of select dietary guidelines. Economic Research Service Report. Washington, DC: Economic Research Service, U.S. Department of Agriculture. Available at http://www.ers.usda.gov/publications/err-economic-research-report/err31.aspx (accessed November 9, 2013).

Carson, J. A. and W. W. Meub. 2013. Recent data show continued growth in Supplemental Nutrition Assistance Program use. Carsey Institute. The Carsey Institute at the scholars'repository. Paper 186. Issue Brief No. 58.

Caspi, C. E., G. Sorensen, S. V. Subramanian, and I. Kawachi. 2012. The local food environment and diet: A systematic review. *Health Place* 18: 1172–87.

CDC. 2012. State initiatives supporting healthier food retail: An overview of the national landscape. Available at http://www.cdc.gov/obesity/downloads/Healthier_Food_Retail.pdf (accessed June 26, 2013).

CDC. 2013. *State Indicator Report on Fruits and Vegetables.* Atlanta, GA: Centers for Disease Control and Prevention, U.S. Department of Health and Human Services.

CDFI. 2013. New Market Tax Credits Program. Available at http://www.cdfifund.gov/what_we_do/programs_id.asp?programid=5 (accessed June 26, 2013).

Chen, S. E. and R. J. G. M. Florax. 2010. Zoning for health: The obesity epidemic and opportunities for local policy intervention. *J Nutr* 140: 1181–4.

CMAP. 2013. Local food systems promote sustainable local food. Available at http://www.cmap.illinois.gov/2040/local-food-systems (accessed June 26, 2013).

Connecticut Department of Agriculture. 2010. WIC Fruit and Vegetable Check Program. Available at http://www.ct.gov/doag/lib/doag/marketing_files/05b__WIC_Fruit_and_Vegetable_Check_Program_3-24-2010.pdf (accessed June 26, 2013).

Curhan, R. C. 1974. The effects of merchandising and temporary promotional activities on sales of fresh fruits and vegetables in supermarkets. *J Market Res* 11: 286–94.

Curran, S., J. Gittlesohn, J. Anliker et al. 2005. Process evaluation of a store-based environmental obesity intervention on two American Indian reservations. *Health Educ Res* 20: 719–29.

Cyzman, D., J. Wierenga, and J. Sielawa. 2009. A community response to the food environment. *Health Promot Pract* 10: 146S–55S.

Dean, W. R. and J. R. Sharkey. 2011. Rural and urban differences in the associations between characteristics of the community food environment and fruit and vegetable intake. *J Nutr Educ Behav* 43: 426–33.

Donald, B. 2013. Food retail and access after the crash: Rethinking the food desert problem. *J Econ Geogr* 13: 231–7.

Dubofsky, J. E. 1969. Fair housing: A legislative history and a perspective. *Washburn Law J* 8:149–66.

Fair Food Network. 2013. Detroit Grocery Incubator. Available at http://www.fairfoodnetwork.org/detroitgroceryincubator (accessed November 9, 2013).

Fleischhacker, S. E., R. Flournoy, and L. V. Moore. 2013. Meaningful, measurable, and manageable approaches to evaluating healthy food financing initiatives: An overview of resources and approaches. *J Public Health Manag Pract* 19: 541–9.

Flint, E., S. Cummins, and S. A. Matthews. 2012. Do supermarket interventions improve food access, fruit and vegetable intake and BMI? Evaluation of the Philadelphia Fresh Food Financing Initiative. *J Epidemiol Community Health* 66: A33.

FNS. 2013a. Farm to school grant applications. Available at http://www.fns.usda.gov/cnd/f2s /f2_2013_grant_program.htm (accessed June 26, 2013).

FNS. 2013b. Farmers' markets and local food marketing. Available at http://www.ams.usda .gov/AMSv1.0/FMPP (accessed June 26, 2013).

Food Farms Jobs. 2013. Local food, farms, and jobs: Growing the Illinois economy. Available at http://foodfarmsjobs.org/ (accessed June 26, 2013).

French, S. A., L. J. Harnack, P. J. Hannan, N. R. Mitchell, A. F. Gerlach, and T. L. Toomey. 2010. Worksite environment intervention to prevent obesity among metropolitan transit workers. *Prev Med* 50(4): 180–5.

Friedmann, H. 2007. Scaling up: Bringing public institutions and food service corporations into the project for a local sustainable food system in Ontario. *Agr Hum Values* 24: 389–98.

Gittelsohn, J., H. J. Song, S. Suratkar et al. 2010a. An urban food store intervention positively affects food-related psychosocial variables and food behaviors. *Health Educ Behav* 37: 390–402.

Gittelsohn, J., M. Rowan, and P. Gadhoke. 2012a. Interventions in small food stores to change the food environment, improve diet, and reduce risk of chronic disease. *Prev Chronic Dis* 9: E59.

Gittelsohn, J., M. N. Laska, T. Andreyeva et al. 2012b. Small retailer perspectives of the 2009 Women, Infants and Children Program food package changes. *Am J Health Behav* 36: 655–65.

Gittelsohn, J., S. Suratkar, H. J. Song et al. 2010b. Process evaluation of Baltimore Healthy Stores: A pilot health intervention program with supermarkets and corner stores in Baltimore City. *Health Promot Pract* 11: 723–32.

Gittelsohn, J., V. Vijayadeva, N. Davison et al. 2010c. A food store intervention trial improves caregiver psychosocial factors and children's dietary intake in Hawaii. *Obesity* (Silver Spring) 18: S84–90.

Glanz, K. and A. L. Yaroch. 2004. Strategies for increasing fruit and vegetable intake in grocery stores and communities: Policy, pricing, and environmental change. *Prev Med* 39: S75–80.

Glanz, K., B. K. Rimer, and K. Viswanath. 2008. *Health Behavior and Health Education: Theory, Research, and Practice*. San Francisco, CA: Wiley.

Guptill, A. and J. Wilkins. 2002. Buying into the food system: Trends in food retailing in the U.S. and implications for local foods. *Agr Hum Values* 19: 39–51.

HFFI. 2011. CED Data Healthy Food Financing Initiative. Available at http://www.acf.hhs.gov /programs/ocs/resource/healthy-food-financing-initiative-0 (accessed June 25, 2013).

Hill, J. O. and J. C. Peters. 1998. Environmental contributions to the obesity epidemic. *Science* 280: 1371–4.

Ilbery, B. and D. Maye. 2006. Retailing local food in the Scottish-English borders: A supply chain perspective. *Geoforum* 37: 352–67.

Jeffery, R. W., S. A. French, C. Raether, and J. E. Baxter. 1994. An environmental intervention to increase fruit and salad purchases in a cafeteria. *Prev Med* 23: 788–92.

Jetter, K. M. and D. L. Cassady. 2010. Increasing fresh fruit and vegetable availability in a low-income neighborhood convenience store: A pilot study. *Health Promot Pract* 11: 694–702.

Kantor, L. S. 2001. Community food security programs improve food Access. *Food Rev* 24: 20–6.

Karpyn, A., M. Manon, S. Treuhaft, T. Giang, C. Harries, and K. McCoubrey. 2010. Policy solutions to the 'grocery gap'. *Health Affairs* (Millwood) 29: 473–80.

Kunkel, M. E., B. Luccia, and A. C. Moore. 2003. Evaluation of the South Carolina seniors farmers' market nutrition education program. *J Am Diet Assoc* 103: 880–3.

Larsen, K. and J. Gilliland. 2009. A farmers' market in a food desert: Evaluating impacts on the price and availability of healthy food. *Health Place* 15: 1158–62.

Leibowitz, J., J. T. Rosch, E. Ramirez, and J. Brill. 2012. A review of food marketing to children and adolescents: Follow-up report. Washington, DC: Federal Trade Commission. Available at http://www.ftc.gov/os/2012/12/121221foodmarketingreport.pdf (accessed November 9, 2013).

Lerman, T., G. Feenstra, and D. Visher. 2012. *A Practitioner's Guide to Resources and Publications on Food Hubs and Values-based Supply Chains: A Literature Review.* Davis, CA: Sustainable Agriculture Research and Education Program, Agricultural Sustainability Institute, University of California.

Lucan, S. C., A. R. Maroko, R. Shanker, and W. B. Jordan. 2011. Green carts in neighborhoods of high obesity—Are mobile produce vendors selling how and where they are most needed? *Obesity* 19: S145.

Maley, M. 2007. Learning the lay of the land: Needs assessment for a community environmental approach to obesity prevention. MS Thesis, Cornell University.

Marks, J. S. and R. Lavizzo-Mourey. 2012. Philadelphia freedom. *Prev Chronic Dis* 9: E144.

Martinez, S., M. Hand, M. Da Pra et al. 2010. Local food systems: Concepts, impacts, and issues. Economic Research Service Reports, USDA. Available at http://ers.usda.gov/media/122868/err97_1_.pdf (accessed November 9, 2013).

Morgan, K. 2009. Feeding the city: The challenge of urban food planning. *Int Plann Stud* 14: 341–8.

Morland, K. B. 2010. An evaluation of a neighborhood-level intervention to a local food environment. *Am J Prev Med* 39: e31–8.

NYC Economic Development Corporation. 2013. Food Retail Expansion to Support Health (FRESH). Available at http://www.nycedc.com/program/food-retail-expansion-support -health-fresh (accessed June 20, 2013).

NYS. 2013. WIC vegetables and fruits checks at farmers' markets. Available at http://www .agriculture.ny.gov/AP/agservices/fmnp-wic-vf.html (accessed June 26, 2013).

NYS Department of Agriculture and Markets. 2013. Pride of New York. Available at http://www.agriculture.ny.gov/AP/PrideOfNY/pride_index.html (accessed June 26, 2013).

People's Grocery. 2012. Available at http://www.peoplesgrocery.org/ (accessed June 26, 2013).

Perez, J., P. Allen, and M. Brown. 2003. Community supported agriculture on the Central Coast: The CSA member experience. Center Research Brief no. 1. Santa Cruz, CA: Center for Agroecology & Sustainable Food Systems, University of California.

Pothukuchi, K. 2004. Community food assessment—A first step in planning for community food security. *J Plann Educ Res* 23: 356–77.

Reger, B., M. G. Wootan, S. Booth-Butterfield, and H. Smith. 1998. 1% or less: A community-based nutrition campaign. *Public Health Rep* 113: 410–9.

Reinvestment Fund. 2006. Pennsylvania Fresh Food Financing Initiative. Available at http://www.trfund.com/pennsylvania-fresh-food-financing-initiative/ (accessed June 26, 2013).

REV Birmingham. 2013. The Urban Food Project. Available at http://www.revbirmingham .org/growing-business/the-urban-food-project/ (accessed June 26, 2013).

Robert Wood Johnson Foundation. 2011. Re/Storing Nashville. Available at http://www .rwjf.org/en/about-rwjf/newsroom/newsroom-content/2011/05/re-storing-nashville. html (accessed April 14, 2014).

Rose, D., J. N. Bodor, P. L. Hutchinson, and C. M. Swalm. 2010. The importance of a multi-dimensional approach for studying the links between food access and consumption. *J Nutr* 140: 1170–4.

Rose, D., J. N. Bodor, C. M. Swalm, J. C. Rice, T. A. Farley, and P. L. Hutchinson. 2009. Deserts in New Orleans? Illustrations of urban food access and implications for policy. Available at http://www.npc.umich.edu/news/events/food-access/rose_et_al.pdf (accessed November 9, 2013).

Ross, N. J., M. D. Andeson, J. P. Goldberg, R. Houser, and B. Rogers. 1999. Trying and buying local produce at the workplace: Results of a marketing intervention. *Am J Altern Agr* 14: 171–9.

RWJF. 2013. Robert Wood Johnson Foundation. Available at http://www.rwjf.org/en /about-rwjf.html (accessed June 26, 2013).

Sagan, C. 1980. *Cosmos*. New York: Random House.

Sallis, J. F., M. Story, and D. Lou. 2009. Study designs and analytic strategies for environmental and policy research on obesity, physical activity, and diet: Recommendations from a meeting of experts. *Am J Prev Med* 36: S72–7.

Sallis, J. F., N. Owen, and E. Fisher. 2008. Ecological models of health behavior. In *Health Behavior and Health Education: Theory, Research, and Practice*, pp. 465–86, edited by K. Glanz, B. K. Rimer, and K. Viswanath. San Francisco, CA: Wiley.

Schmidt, M., J. Kolodinsky, T. DeSisto, and F. Conte. 2011. Increasing farm income and local food access: A case study of a collaborative aggregation, marketing, and distribution strategy that links farmers to markets. *J Agr Food Syst Community Dev* 1: 157–75.

Sleator, R. D. and C. Hill. 2007. Food reformulations for improved health: A potential risk for microbial food safety? *Med Hypotheses* 69: 1323–4.

Smed, S. and A. Robertson. 2012. Are taxes on fatty foods having their desired effects on health? *BMJ* 345: e6885.

Sobal, J. and C. A. Bisogni. 2009. Constructing food choice decisions. *Ann Behav Med* 38: S37–46.

Song, H. J., J. Gittelsohn, M. Kim, S. Suratkar, S. Sharma, and J. Anliker. 2009. A corner store intervention in a low-income urban community is associated with increased availability and sales of some healthy foods. *Public Health Nutr* 12: 2060–7.

Story, M., K. M. Kaphingst, R. Robinson-O'Brien, and K. Glanz. 2008. Creating healthy food and eating environments: Policy and environmental approaches. *Annu Rev Public Health* 29: 253–72.

Strom, S. 2012. Walmart to label healthy foods. Available at http://www.nytimes. com/2012/02/08/business/walmart-to-add-great-for-you-label-to-healthy-foods.html? _r=0 (accessed June 20, 2013).

Suarez-Balcazar Y, Redmond L, Kouba J et al. 2007. Introducing systems change in the schools: The case of school luncheons and vending machines. *Am J Community Psychol* 39: 335–45.

Swinburn, B., G. Egger, and F. Raza. 1999. Dissecting obesogenic environments: The development and application of a framework for identifying and prioritizing environmental interventions for obesity. *Prev Med* 29: 563–70.

Thow, A. M., S. Jan, S. Leeder, and B. Swinburn. 2010. The effect of fiscal policy on diet, obesity and chronic disease: A systematic review. *Bull World Health Organ* 88: 609–14.

Truck Farm Chicago. 2013. Available at http://www.truckfarmchicago.org (accessed June 26, 2013).

Truck Farm Tampa. 2012. Truck Farm Tampa. Available at http://truckfarmtampa.com / (accessed June 26, 2013).

The Food Trust. 2012. Available at http://thefoodtrust.org/ (accessed June 25, 2013).

USDA. 2013. Know Your Farmer, Know Your Food. Available at http://www.usda.gov/wps /portal/usda/knowyourfarmer?navid=KNOWYOURFARMER (accessed June 26, 2013).

Ver Ploeg, M. V. Breneman, T. Farrigan et al. 2009. Access to affordable and nutritious food: measuring and understanding food deserts and their consequences. Economic Research Service, USDA. Available at http://ers.usda.gov/publications/ap-administra-tive -publication/ap-036.aspx (accessed November 9, 2013).

Waterlander, W. E., I. H. Steenhuis, M. R. de Boer, A. J. Schuit, and J. C. Seidell. 2012. Introducing taxes, subsidies or both: The effects of various food pricing strategies in a web-based supermarket randomized trial. *Prev Med* 54: 323–30.

Wekerle, G. R. 2004. Food justice movements—Policy, planning, and networks. *J Plann Educ Res* 23: 378–86.

Whitacre, P., P. Tsai, and J. Mulligan. 2009. *The Public Health Effects of Food Deserts: Workshop Summary*. Washington, DC: National Academies Press.

Wholesome Wave. 2013. Nourishing Neighborhoods across America. Available at http:// wholesomewave.org/ (accessed June 26, 2013).

Young, C., A. Karpyn, N. Uy, K. Wich, and J. Glyn. 2011. Farmers' markets in low income communities: Impact of community environment, food programs and public policy. *Community Dev* 42: 208–20.

Index